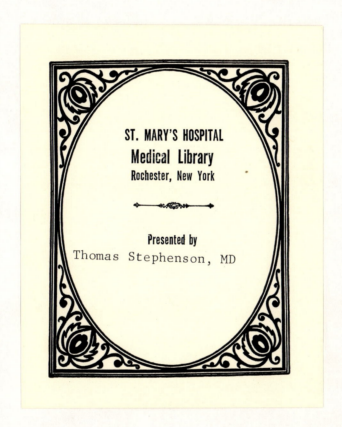

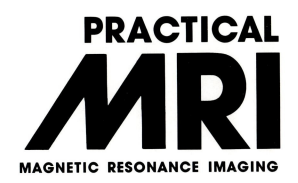

PRACTICAL MRI

MAGNETIC RESONANCE IMAGING

A CASE STUDY APPROACH

Wilson S. Wong, MD
Staff Radiologist
Huntington Memorial Hospital
Pasadena, California
Assistant Clinical Professor of Radiology
University of California, Los Angeles

Jay S. Tsuruda, MD
Magnetic Resonance Research Fellow
Huntington Medical Research Institutes
Pasadena, California and University of California, San Diego
Clinical Instructor
University of California, San Francisco

Keith E. Kortman, MD
Staff Radiologist
Huntington Memorial Hospital
Research Radiologist
Huntington Medical Research Institutes
Pasadena, California

William G. Bradley, Jr., MD, PhD
Staff Radiologist
Huntington Memorial Hospital
Director of MR Imaging Laboratory
Huntington Medical Research Institutes
Pasadena, California
Associate Clinical Professor of Radiology
University of California, San Francisco

AN ASPEN PUBLICATION®
Aspen Publishers, Inc.
Rockville, Maryland
Royal Tunbridge Wells
1987

Library of Congress Cataloging in Publication Data

Practical magnetic resonance imaging.

"An Aspen publication."
Includes bibliographies and index.
1. Magnetic resonance imaging — Case studies. 2. Magnetic resonance imaging —
Examinations, questions, etc. I. Wong, Wilson S. [DNLM: 1. Nuclear Magnetic
Resonance — diagnostic use. WN 445 P8955]
RC78.7.N83P73   1986   616.07′57   86–22337
ISBN: 0–87189–600–1

Editorial Services: Jane Coyle

Library of Congress Catalog Card Number: 86–22337
ISBN: 0–87189–600–1

Printed in the United States of America

1 2 3 4 5

*This book is dedicated
to our wives and children.*

WSW
JST
KEK
WGB

CONTENTS

PREFACE

Magnetic resonance (MR) imaging is a rapidly evolving technology that, in a relatively short period of time, has become a well-accepted modality, especially in the examination of the central nervous system (CNS), the head and neck, the spine, and the musculoskeletal system. Its distinct advantages include superb contrast resolution, multiplanar imaging capabilities, and the lack of ionizing radiation.

Unlike x-ray computed tomography (CT), the MR imaging parameters under the operator's control are greater in number and can be bewildering, especially to those who are unfamiliar with the technology's unique vocabulary. It is of extreme importance, however, that proper MR imaging techniques are used, since pathology can be masked or missed when improper pulsing sequences are employed.

We have been performing MR scans at the Huntington Medical Research Institutes since May 1983; during this time we have imaged more than 9,000 patients. A monthly visiting fellowship has been offered since August 1983, and an 8-week evening MRI course was held at the Huntington Memorial Hospital in January 1986. As an outgrowth of the visiting fellowship program, we started an "on-site" fellowship program in January 1985, whereby physicians essentially receive MR fellowship training at their own site on their own imager through a teleradiology link.

In the course of these teaching programs, we have often been asked questions related to imaging protocols. There were also frequent requests for MR teaching files demonstrating common pathology. In response to these requests, we undertook the writing of this workbook, which is composed of a series of review sections and a collection of interesting MR cases. These cases are chosen specifically to illustrate MR findings that exemplify the different disease categories that are frequently encountered in a clinical MR setting. We have presented these cases in a format that we hope will help others in learning MR imaging techniques and interpretation.

The first chapter provides the reader with a basic understanding of the principles of MR imaging. The second chapter provides an algorithmic approach to MR scanning techniques. Since pulsing sequences may be different on different MR imagers (depending on the field strength), a table (Appendix B) translating the techniques of one imager to another is provided to allow users to apply the protocols to their own machines.

An introductory section for each organ system is then presented prior to the case studies. These sections are designed to provide an overview of the current applications of MRI as well as to suggest imaging techniques pertaining to the specific organ system. A list of current references is provided for additional reading.

In each case study, the clinical history is presented. The readers are encouraged to design a pulsing sequence tailored to the specific clinical situation. The MR images are then displayed along with the actual pulsing technique that we used. Every attempt has been made to show as many images as possible so as to simulate the actual clinical setting. Explanations are then given as to why certain pulsing sequences were chosen. The findings on the images are described, and the differential diagnosis is discussed. A summary of the findings for the particular disease entity is then presented. This summary section is designed mainly as a quick reference. Companion cases are also added to illus-

trate additional points being discussed. Finally, current references are cited as a list for further reading on a given subject.

The main goal of this book is to provide a practical guide to MR imaging. Although we have presented the information as a series of case studies, we hope this book will also serve as a reference manual for physicians working with MRI in every-day practice.

Pasedena, CA
WSW
JST
KEK
WGB

ACKNOWLEDGMENTS

We wish to express our appreciation to our associates of the Hill Medical Corporation for their support of this project. We are especially indebted to Dr. Robert W. Henderson for writing the introductory section to the cardiothoracic system and to Dr. Richard A. Yadley for his review of and input to the neuroradiology material.

We extend a special thanks to Dr. Robert B. Lufkin, Assistant Professor at UCLA, for contributing his thoughts and materials to the head and neck section. Many physicians have loaned us materials and referred cases. These are acknowledged where they appear.

For their work that made this book possible, we are much indebted to our MR technologists at the Huntington Medical Research Institutes: Jay A. Mericle, Leslee M. Watson, Terry A. Andrues, and Jose Jiminez. We wish to thank Kaye R. Finley and Gail M. Thompson for their help in preparing this manuscript. We would also like to thank Valerie Gausche at UCLA and Jeanine J. Bohnsack and Gary Thomsen in Phoenix for printing images for us.

Finally, we want to acknowledge the excellent photographic work by Gordon Galloway and Salvatore Vallone.

1

FUNDAMENTALS
OF MR IMAGE INTERPRETATION

INTRODUCTION

Like its predecessor, x-ray computed tomography (CT), magnetic resonance (MR) is a computer-based imaging modality that displays the body in thin tomographic slices.[1] Unlike CT, which requires ionizing radiation, MR is based on an apparently safe interaction between radio waves and hydrogen nuclei in the body in the presence of a strong magnetic field. Physical characteristics of a volume element, or "voxel," of tissue are translated by the computer into a two-dimensional image comprised of picture elements, or "pixels." In CT, one must scan in the plane of the gantry—that is, axial or semicoronal. In MR, one is able to acquire images directly in any plane—that is, axial, sagittal, coronal, or oblique. It is useful to compare the determinants of pixel intensity in CT and MR to demonstrate differences in the imaging methods. The pixel intensity in CT reflects the electron density; in MR it reflects the density of mobile hydrogen nuclei modified by the chemical environment—that is, by the magnetic relaxation times, T1 and T2.[2]

In both CT and MR, certain parameters are fixed by the manufacturer and other parameters are under operator control. CT parameters under operator control include voltage, time, current, and number of views. In MR, the parameters of operation are less familiar and utilize a new vocabulary. Those that are generally determined by the manufacturer include field strength, acquisition technique (projection reconstruction or Fourier transform), and acquisition signal (spin echo or free induction decay). Factors under operator control include choice of pulsing sequence, sequence parameter times, matrix size (i.e., spatial resolution), slice thickness and gap between slices, field of view, number of repetitions, orientation of imaging plane, diameter and type of radio frequency (RF) coil, and use of cardiac gating.[3]

Improved spatial resolution in CT is generally associated with an increased radiation dose. Spatial resolution in MR can be calculated from matrix size and field of view and is determined by the strength of the gradient fields and the specific range of frequencies (bandwidth) that can be detected and discriminated. On a given MR imaging system, increased spatial resolution (at a given signal-to-noise ratio) requires longer acquisition times but does not increase risk to the patient.

Given these substantial differences between MR and CT, how is image interpretation affected? Certain elements of interpretation are unchanged. Although the transverse axial anatomy has a different appearance on MR, the normal morphologic relationships are the same. The pathophysiologic principles used in interpretation of CT scans still apply to MR, and alteration of normal anatomy should be apparent in both.

The MR image differs from the CT image in several respects. The effect of the magnetic relaxation times on MR pixel intensity has no parallel in CT. Magnetic relaxation effects depend on the choice of pulsing sequences and the sequence parameter times.[3,4] Flowing blood has a different appearance on MR than on CT.[5-7] On MR images, intraluminal blood can appear black, white, or gray—depending on the pulsing sequence, orientation of blood flow to the imaging plane, and velocity of flow. The intraluminal signal can yield information on velocity and characteristics of flow that is not available from CT.

The following discussion presumes a reasonable basic knowledge of the physical principles of MR.[8] The emphasis of this chapter is on the effect that magnetic relaxation times have on image appearance. For those interested in a more basic discussion of imaging physics, a bibliography is included at the end of the chapter.

MAGNETIZATION

The MR signal is proportional to a quantity called the magnetization.[8] The magnetization is a measurable property that results from placing the body in a magnetic field. The most abundant element in the body is hydrogen, and the nucleus of the hydrogen atom (a proton) possesses a property known as "spin." Spin gives the hydrogen nuclei "magnetic moments" and causes them to behave like small bar magnets. Like compass needles, they tend to align with a strong magnetic field. Immediately after the hydrogen-containing body is placed in a magnetic field, equal numbers of protons point north (parallel) and south (antiparallel); thus, the individual magnetic moments cancel, and there is zero net magnetization. Within a few seconds (in biologic substances), a redistribution occurs such that a slightly greater number of hydrogen nuclei align parallel to the field and the body is now said to be "magnetized" (Figure 1–1). Magnetization increases exponentially with a first-order exponential time constant known as the T1 relaxation time. The magnetization plateaus at an equilibrium value that is usually dependent only on the hydrogen density. In general, the ratio of the magnetic field temporarily induced in the substance to the applied magnetic field is called the "magnetic susceptibility." Certain substances with unpaired electrons (i.e., paramagnetic and ferromagnetic materials) have very high magnetic susceptibilities. The iron in hemosiderin is an example of such substances. A much stronger field may be induced in paramagnetic substances (e.g., tissues containing hemosiderin) than in normal tissues.

Although the *equilibrium* magnetization only points along the main z axis of the static magnetization field, the magnetization in general can point in any direction. The magnetiza-

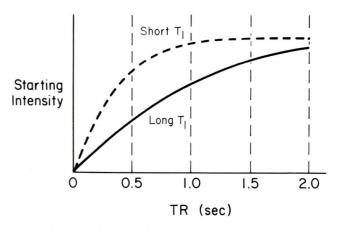

Figure 1–1. T1 relaxation following placement in a magnetic field or recovery from a 90° RF pulse. Magnetization recovers exponentially with a first-order time constant, T1, the spin-lattice relaxation time.

tion is a vector quantity that can be represented by a "longitudinal" component (along the z axis of the main magnetic field) and by a second component perpendicular to the first, called the "transverse" magnetization (in the xy plane).[8] Transverse magnetization results from application of short bursts of radio frequency (RF) energy (i.e., radiowaves) called "RF pulses." A 90° RF pulse produces transverse magnetization by causing the longitudinal magnetization to flip 90° from the z axis into the transverse xy plane. A 180° pulse causes 180° of rotation, so the longitudinal magnetization becomes directed along the -z axis. Unlike a 90° pulse, a 180° pulse cannot generate transverse magnetization. When transverse magnetization is present, however, application of a 180° pulse causes a 180° change in the phase of the magnetization in the xy plane. The maximum transverse magnetization results from a 90° flip angle. Flip angles smaller than 90° produce less transverse magnetization per flip but, because they can be repeated rapidly, may generate more signal per unit time.[9] This is the basis for some of the fast scanning techniques (e.g., FLASH: *Fast, Low Angle Shot . . .*) that have been developed.[10]

When transverse magnetization is present, it rotates about the z axis at a particular frequency determined by the magnitude of the magnetic field and the magnetic moment of the nuclei. This frequency, called the resonance or Larmor frequency, is that of the radio signal generated by the rotating transverse magnetization that is eventually processed into the MR image. Only transverse magnetization rotates and thereby yields a detectable MR signal.

Two types of MR signals can be produced by transverse magnetization. Immediately following a 90° pulse, a signal is produced by the freely rotating transverse magnetization. This signal is called a "free induction decay," or "FID" (Figure 1–2). Transverse magnetization decays rapidly due to nonuniformities in the main magnetic field that cause protons to resonate at slightly different frequencies at slightly different positions within the voxel. As these protons get out of phase, or "lose coherence," transverse magnetization (and induced signal) is lost at an exponential rate T2*. When a 90° pulse and a 180° pulse are applied sequentially, a "spin echo" signal is generated.[8] The purpose of the 180° pulse is to "refocus" the phase of the protons, causing them to regain coherence and thereby to recover transverse magnetization,[8] producing a spin echo. (Similar rephasing can be accomplished[9] rapidly by symmetrically reversing the gradient fields, producing a "gradient echo.") Following the spin echo, coherence is again lost as the protons continue to resonate at slightly different frequencies because of nonuniformities in the main magnetic field. If another 180° pulse is applied, coherence can again be established for a second spin echo. In fact, multiple spin echo signals can be produced if the original 90° pulse is followed by multiple 180° pulses (or gradient reversals). This "echo train" is illustrated in Figure 1–2.

Although the 180° pulses cause some rephasing to occur (because of fixed nonuniformities in the main field), complete rephasing is not possible due to randomly fluctuating magnetic fields within the substance itself. Thus, the maximum intensity of the spin echo signals in the echo train is limited by an exponentially decaying curve. The time constant of this decay curve is the second magnetic relaxation time, T2.[8]

To summarize—there are two types of decay: that which is reversible and that which is irreversible.[8] Immediately following the initial 90° pulse, transverse magnetization decays rapidly (at rate T2*) because of nonuniformities in the external magnetic field. As this transverse magnetization initially decays, a free induction decay is produced, although it is rarely acquired on MR imaging systems. Since the nonuniformities causing this initial rapid decay are fixed, transverse magnetization can be partially restored by a 180° RF pulse, producing a spin echo. Transverse magnetization

is also lost by magnetic nonuniformities within the substance that result from randomly fluctuating internal fields. Unlike the decay due to fixed nonuniformities in the main field, this decay is irreversible. It is represented by the T2 relaxation time of the substance. Like radioactive decay, this is a first-order exponential decay process with time constant T2.

In general, one must be careful to distinguish terms used to describe MR *signals* from those used to describe MR *pulsing sequences*. A "spin echo" signal and sequence results from a 90°–180° RF pulse pair. An FID signal results from a terminal 90° RF pulse. An inversion recovery (IR) sequence results from a 180°–90° pulse pair. Since the final pulse in the IR *sequence* is a 90° pulse, an FID *signal* is produced. By adding a terminal 180° pulse—that is, 180°–90°–180°—an IR *sequence* can be made to produce a spin echo *signal*.

PHYSICAL BASIS FOR T1 AND T2

T1 is variously called the "longitudinal," "thermal," or "spin-lattice" relaxation time. It indicates the time required for a substance to become magnetized after first being placed in a magnetic field or, alternatively, the time required to regain longitudinal magnetization following a 90° RF pulse. T1 is determined by thermal interactions between the resonating protons and other magnetic nuclei in the magnetic environment, or "lattice." These interactions allow the energy absorbed by certain protons during resonance to be dispersed to other nuclei in the lattice.

All molecules have natural motions due to vibration, rotation, and translation.[11] Smaller molecules, such as water, generally move more rapidly (i.e., they have higher natural frequencies), and larger molecules, such as proteins, move more slowly. When water is held in hydration layers around the protein by hydrophilic side groups, its rapid motion slows considerably.[12]

The T1 relaxation time reflects the relationship between the frequency of these molecular motions and the resonant Larmor frequency (which depends on the main magnetic field of the MR imager). When the two are similar, T1 relaxation is efficient and rapid; when they are different, T1 relaxation is prolonged.[12] Cholesterol, a medium-sized molecule, has natural frequencies close to those used for MR imaging[4] and has a short T1 (Figure 1–3). The water molecule is small and moves too rapidly; large proteins move too slowly. Both have natural frequencies significantly different from the Larmor frequency and thus have long T1 relaxation times.

Water in the bulk phase, like CSF, has a long T1 relaxation time because the frequency of its natural motions is much higher than the Larmor frequency.[12] When this same CSF is forced out into the periventricular white matter as interstitial edema due to ventricular obstruction, however, its T1 relaxation time is much shorter (Figure 1–4). The T1 shortening reflects the fact that water is now in hydration layers rather

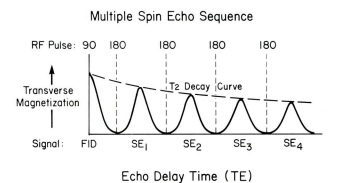

Multiple Spin Echo Sequence

RF Pulse: 90 180   180   180   180

Transverse Magnetization

T2 Decay Curve

Signal: FID   SE₁   SE₂   SE₃   SE₄

Echo Delay Time (TE)

Figure 1–2. Multiple spin echo sequence. Initial decay of transverse magnetization produces a signal known as an FID (free induction decay). Repeated 180° pulses produce multiple spin echoes that are limited in amplitude by the T2 decay curve.

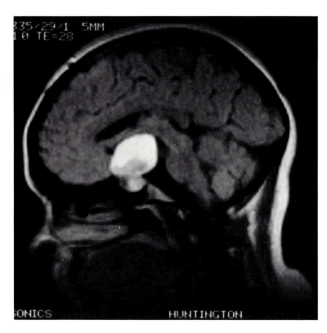

Figure 1-3. Craniopharyngioma. High intensity of tumor is due to short T1 from the presence of liquid cholesterol.

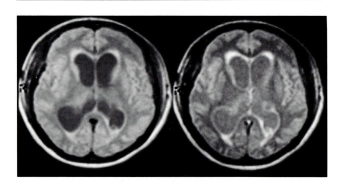

Figure 1-4. Interstitial edema. Water in the bulk phase as intraventricular CSF has a long T1 relaxation time and thus appears dark on T1-weighted images. When that same CSF is forced through the ependyma, it is partially bound by the myelin protein that shortens its T1 relaxation time, increasing its intensity. Thus water in the form of interstitial edema has a different appearance on MR images than water in the form of CSF.

than in the bulk phase (Figure 1-5). Proteinaceous solutions (such as abscesses and necrotic tumors) have a higher percentage of water in hydration layers and thus have a shorter T1 compared with that of "pure" aqueous solutions such as CSF.[12] A method for determining the percentage of bulk and hydration-layer water in a substance has been described.[12]

Subacute hemorrhage has a shorter T1 than the brain (Figure 1-6). This reflects the paramagnetic nature of the oxidized (ferric) iron in denatured methemoglobin.[13] T1 shortening is produced by dipole–dipole interaction between the paramagnetic iron and water protons in the solution. The short T1 allows hemorrhage to recover longitudinal magnetization very quickly relative to brain. Thus at short TR

Molecular Environment of Water

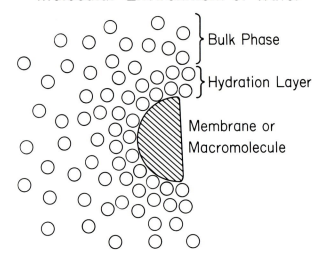

Figure 1-5. Molecular environment of water. Water in the bulk phase has natural motional frequencies much higher than the operating (Larmor) frequency of most MR imagers. Water in hydration layers around macromolecules (such as proteins) moves at frequencies much closer to the Larmor frequency. Water protons in this environment have shorter T1 times.

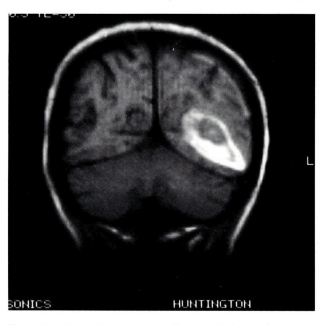

Figure 1-6 Subacute hemorrhage. One week following right occipital hemorrhage, hematoma has higher intensity than surrounding brain parenchyma. This is accentuated on a T1-weighted image that brings out the short T1 character of the paramagnetic methemoglobin.

times, subacute hemorrhage appears brighter than brain (with the longer T1) (Figure 1-6).

Paramagnetic contrast agents shorten the T1 of all mobile protons within several angstroms of the paramagnetic center,[14] increasing the signal. As the concentration of the

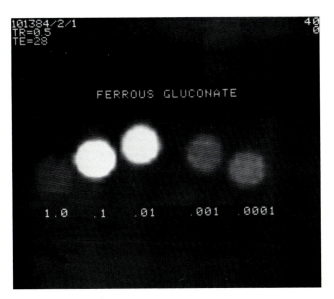

Figure 1–7. Effect of concentration on intensity of paramagnetic substance. Serial dilutions of ferrous gluconate first demonstrate increasing intensity due to T1 shortening and then decreasing intensity due to T2 shortening. This is a typical dipole–dipole interaction of paramagnetic centers in aqueous solution.

paramagnetic substance is increased, however, T2 is also shortened. Thus with increasing concentration, the intensity is initially increased due to accelerated T1 recovery and then decreased due to accelerated T2 decay (Figure 1–7). When both T1 and T2 are shortened, little signal may remain by the earliest time TE the signal can be received.

T2 is called the "transverse" or "spin-spin" relaxation time. It is a measure of how long transverse magnetization would last in a perfectly uniform external magnetic field. Alternatively, it is a measure of how long the resonating protons remain coherent or precess "in phase" following a 90° RF pulse. T2 decay is due to magnetic interactions that occur between spinning protons. Unlike T1 interactions, T2 interactions do not involve transfer of energy and only result in a change in phase that leads to loss of coherence.

T2 relaxation depends on the presence of static internal fields in the substance.[8] These are generally due to protons attached to larger molecules. These stationary or slowly fluctuating magnetic fields produce local regions of increased or decreased magnetic field, depending on whether the protons align with or against the main magnetic field. Local field nonuniformity causes the protons to precess at slightly different frequencies. Thus, following the 90° pulse, the protons lose coherence and transverse magnetization is lost; this results in T2 relaxation.

Stationary paramagnetic substances with high magnetic susceptibility lead to rapid loss of coherence and have a short T2. Paramagnetic deoxyhemoglobin within intact red blood cells (Figure 1–8) causes a local region of high magnetic field.[15] This results in rapid dephasing of water protons diffusing in the vicinity of an acute hematoma with second-

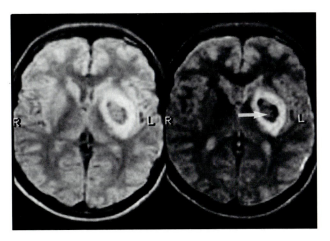

Figure 1–8. Acute hematoma. Paramagnetic, magnetically susceptible deoxyhemoglobin within intact red cells causes local magnetic nonuniformity leading to T2 shortening. Note decreased signal (arrow) on second echo (TE 56 msecond) image.

ary T2 shortening and loss of signal. A similar T2 shortening phenomenon is observed when magnetically susceptible ferritin is deposited in macrophages in hemochromatosis (Figure 1–9).

As the motional frequency of the proton increases, T2 relaxation becomes less and less efficient. Rapid fluctuating motions average out over the period of a precessional cycle, leading to a more uniform internal magnetic environment. This results in a long T2 relaxation time. It should be apparent that an environment that is efficient for one form of relaxation may not be efficient for another. Hydration-layer water (e.g., brain edema) has a much shorter T1 than bulk phase water such as CSF.[12] Yet the motion of the protons in brain edema is not so slow that T2 relaxation is efficient; so T2 remains long. (This accounts for the intense appearance of brain edema on T2-weighted MR images.)

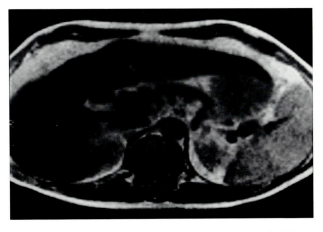

Figure 1–9. Hemochromatosis. Magnetically susceptible ferritin deposited in the liver causes T2 shortening and loss of signal.

A comment on the measurement of T1 and T2 relaxation times in current MR imagers: although they are useful in a qualitative sense, their absolute values have little meaning. With most MR imaging systems, there is significant RF nonuniformity throughout the imaging volume.[16] The double-saddle RF coil cannot produce an exact 90° pulse at each point in a large imaging volume. At some points, it overshoots; at others, the flip angle is less than 90°. The result is a nonuniform MR signal from otherwise comparable tissue throughout the volume. Because apparent T1 and T2 times can be calculated from these intensities, the calculated values are also position dependent. In addition, the particular TR and TE times chosen to calculate the T1 and T2 relaxation times affect the determined values since a single exponential model is often inaccurate.[17] Thus, even in the same imager, a substance may appear to have variable relaxation times depending on position and the TR and TE values used. There is an even greater difference in measured T1 and T2 relaxation times between different imaging systems operating at the same field because of differences in RF coil design and RF power input and gain settings. For imagers operating at different field strengths, T1 increases as the field strength increases while T2 remains essentially constant with increasing field.[11]

Measured values of T2 vary, not only because of RF nonuniformity but also because of differing strengths of the gradient fields. For bulk phase liquids in particular, self-diffusion during the time the slice-selecting gradient is on leads to additional dephasing and T2 shortening.[18] T2 measurements for such substances are different for different imagers and vary when different gradients are used in the same imager (e.g., to produce thinner slices).

SPIN ECHO

Since the intensity of the radio photon of MR is approximately 11 orders of magnitude weaker than the x-ray photon of CT, each MR pulsing sequence must be repeated to increase the signal-to-noise ratio. During the time between repetitions of the spin echo pulsing sequence, the longitudinal magnetization recovers along the z axis. Longitudinal recovery is identical to the process of initially becoming magnetized when the body was first placed in the magnet. "Relaxation," which indicates a return to equilibrium, is a better term than "recovery." While the body is in the magnet, the "equilibrium state" consists of being fully magnetized. Therefore, longitudinal "relaxation" represents the recovery of magnetization along the z axis that occurs between repetitions.[8]

In the first step of a spin echo pulsing sequence, a 90° RF pulse flips the existing longitudinal magnetization (which is traditionally oriented along the z axis) 90° into the transverse xy plane. Whenever transverse magnetization is present, it rotates at the Larmor frequency and produces an MR signal.

The magnitude of the transverse magnetization after the 90° pulse is approximately equal to the magnitude of the longitudinal magnetization that recovered during the interval allowed between repetitions. This interval is called the repetition time TR and is one of the programmable sequence parameters.

In the process of flipping the magnetization into the transverse orientation, the longitudinal component of magnetization is lost and must be allowed to recover before another signal can be generated. The amount of recovery that occurs in a given period of time depends on the particular pulsing sequence used, on the repetition time TR, and on the T1 relaxation time (Figure 1–1).

The magnitude of the signal detected depends not only on longitudinal recovery between repetitions but also on how well the signal persists or, alternatively, on how quickly the transverse magnetization decays from its initial maximum value (Figure 1–10). This decay depends on the T2 of the substance; the amount of time allowed for decay to occur— that is, the time between the initial 90° RF pulse and the detection of the spin echo—is called the echo delay time (TE) and is another programmable sequence parameter.

Mathematically, the intensity (I) of the spin echo signal can be approximated:[2]

$$I = N(H) f(v) (1 - e^{-TR/T1}) e^{-TE/T2}$$

where $N(H)$ is the NMR-visible, mobile proton density and $f(v)$ is an unspecified function of flow. This equation indicates that the intensity of the MR signal increases as hydrogen density and T2 increase and as T1 decreases. It should also be noted that T1 and T2 influences are both relative to TR and TE, the programmable sequence parameters. Thus the effect of the T1 and T2 times of the substance on signal intensity is subject to the specific values of TR and TE selected before the image is acquired.

When considered in the most simplistic terms, the magnitude of the measured MR signal depends on a two-step process. The first step (recovery between repetitions) determines the starting intensity for the second step (transverse decay). The starting intensity reflects the relationship between T1 and TR, modified by the proton density. The subsequent decay from this starting intensity reflects differences in T2 and TE. Consider the differentiation of brain and CSF (Figure 1–11). At TR = 0.5 seconds, the CSF signal starts to decay from a markedly decreased initial value. Despite the longer T2 of CSF, the intensity remains less than that of brain over the range of echo delay times used for routine imaging. If the repetition time TR is lengthened to 2.0 seconds, the CSF signal starts to decay from a greater initial intensity and still decays more slowly than the signal from brain. Thus the two signals will become isointense, and the CSF can even become relatively *more* intense than brain (Figure 1–12). The MR appearance of the CSF-filled ventricular and subarachnoid spaces can simulate a metrizamide CT study.

Signal Decay (T$_2$)

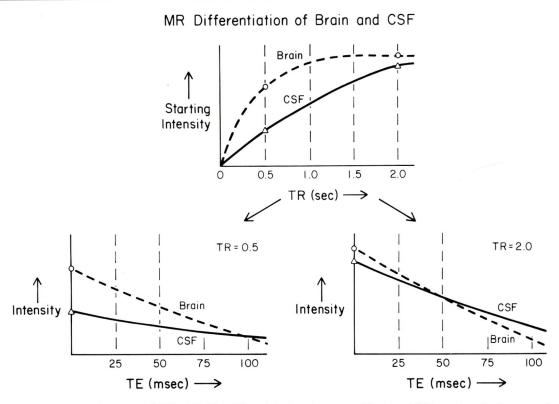

Long T$_2$

Signal

Short T$_2$

Long TR
(T$_1$ Irrelevant)

28   56

TE ⟶

Figure 1–10. T2 decay. Long repetition time TR. Individual T1 relaxation times become irrelevant, and full magnetization is achieved between repetitions. If it is assumed that two substances have comparable proton density, then they will begin to decay from the same complete magnetization. A substance with a long T2 will decay more slowly than one with a short T2. The decay curves are "sampled" by acquiring spin echo signals at variable echo delay times (TE). Two such echo delay times, 28 and 56 mseconds, are indicated for a standard dual echo sequence.

MR Differentiation of Brain and CSF

Brain

Starting
Intensity

CSF

0   0.5   1.0   1.5   2.0

TR (sec) ⟶

TR = 0.5

Intensity

Brain

CSF

25   50   75   100

TE (msec) ⟶

TR = 2.0

Intensity

CSF

Brain

25   50   75   100

TE (msec) ⟶

Figure 1–11. Differentiation of brain and CSF by MR. The differential rates of recovery of brain and CSF are given by the respective T1 relaxation times and illustrated in the top figure. The amount of time allowed for relaxation is the repetition time TR. Two cases (i.e., TR 0.5 second and TR 2.0 seconds) are illustrated in the lower two figures. In both cases, the small triangle and circle indicate the amount of recovery that had occurred by time TR. This then determines the starting point for the second (decay) step for CSF and brain, respectively. Brain recovers magnetization initially more rapidly but decays more rapidly because its T1 and T2 relaxation times are shorter than those of CSF. Notice that brain is more intense than CSF at TR 0.5 second and TE < 100 mseconds. When the TR is increased to 2.0 seconds, brain and CSF become isointense at 50 mseconds and then CSF becomes more intense than brain at longer TE.

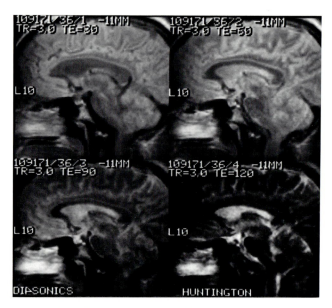

Figure 1–12. Effect of variable echo delay time on T2 contrast. Progressive prolongation of echo delay time (TE) from 30 mseconds to 60, 90, and 120 mseconds demonstrates progressive increase in intensity of long-T2 CSF compared with brain.

The difference in T1 values between brain parenchyma (shorter T1) and CSF (longer T1) can be used to enhance the contrast between the two. This is important when seeking abnormalities at the brain–CSF interface. As shown in Figure 1–1, a short TR time allows a short T1 substance (e.g., brain) to recover signal between repetitions to a much greater extent than a long T1 substance (e.g., CSF).

If the TR time is prolonged, all substances are allowed to recover between repetitions and the pixel intensity becomes independent of T1. At short echo delay times (TE), the effect of T2 is minimized, and one is left with an image that depends primarily on differences in proton density. The effect of variable T1 weighting is demonstrated in Figure 1–13. At TR = 2.0 seconds, the white matter in the corpus callosum is less intense than gray matter due to a lower proton density.[4] When the TR is shortened to 0.5 seconds, however, the relative signal from the corpus callosum increases because white matter has a shorter T1 than gray matter.

Substances with longer T2 times generate stronger signals than substances with shorter T2 times if both are acquired at the same TE and if proton density and T1 are comparable (Figure 1–10). When multiple spin echoes are acquired, the signal strength generally decreases as TE is lengthened because of T2 decay (Figure 1–2). As discussed later, an exception to this may occur in slow laminar blood flow where the intraluminal signal may be greater on the second echo image than on the first.[6]

Increasing the TE brings out the differences in the T2 relaxation times between substances, increasing the T2 weighting. Images obtained with a sufficiently long TR and TE in which the CSF is more intense than brain are regarded as ''heavily T2 weighted.'' Images in which brain and CSF are isointense are ''moderately T2 weighted'' (Figure 1–12).

A typical edematous lesion has prolongation of both T1 and T2 (Figure 1–14). On T1-weighted images, such a lesion appears dark; that is, it has negative contrast. On T2-

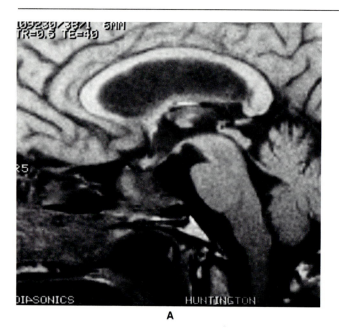

A

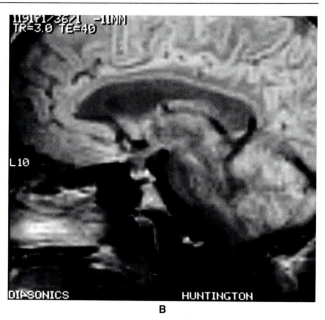

B

Figure 1–13. Effect of variable TR on T1 contrast. (A) At TR 0.5 second, CSF is dark relative to brain parenchyma because of T1 differences. Corpus callosum (arrow) is more intense than adjacent gray matter at shorter T1 values. (B) On TR 2.0 image, there is relatively less contrast between CSF and brain, the longer T1 CSF having "caught up" in signal intensity with the brain. Also, the white matter in the corpus callosum now appears dark relative to adjacent gray matter because of lower proton density.

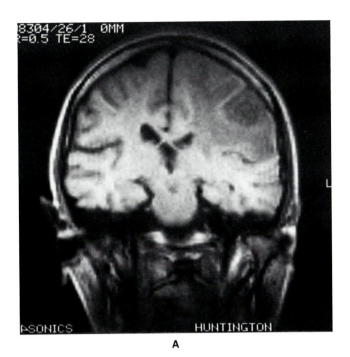

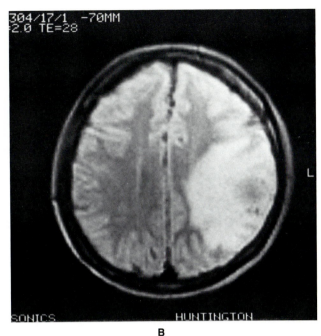

A   B

Figure 1–14. Edematous brain tumor. (A) T1-weighted image demonstrates low intensity edema (open arrow) surrounding lower intensity tumor (open arrow). (B) T2-weighted image demonstrates brain edema with high intensity (closed arrow) relative to surrounding brain and brain tumor (closed arrow).

weighted images, it appears bright; that is, it has positive contrast. If a short TR/long TE sequence is inadvertently chosen, the tendencies toward positive and negative lesion contrast cancel and the lesion may be undetectable (Figure 1–15).

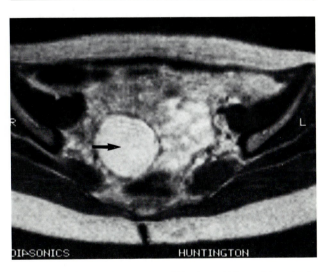

Figure 1–15. Hepatic cyst. On TR 1.0 second, TE 28-msecond image (top), hepatic cyst (arrow) has negative contrast relative to hepatic parenchyma. On second echo image (TR = 1.0 second, TE = 56 mseconds), cyst has become isointense with surrounding hepatic parenchyma, precluding visualization. Note also even echo rephasing in hepatic veins (arrowhead).

When proton densities are equal, the strongest signal is detected from those substances with the shortest T1 times (rapid recovery) and the longest T2 times (slowest decay). Such substances include fat (Figure 1–16), mucus (Figure 1–17), subacute hemorrhage (Figure 1–6), and gadolinium-enhanced brain tumors (Figure 1–18). The weakest MR signals come from areas of low proton density, tissues with long T1 values (slow recovery) or short T2 values (rapid decay), and rapidly flowing blood (Figure 1–19). Air (Figure 1–17), dense calcification (Fig-

Figure 1–16. Dermoid tumor. Fat within dermoid (arrow) has short T1 relaxation time and thus has high intensity.

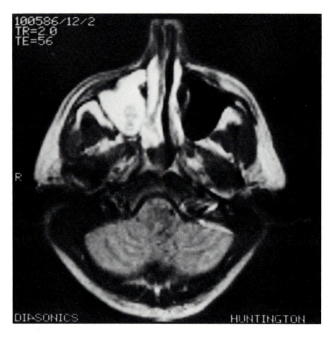

Figure 1–17. Sinusitis. Mucus in right maxillary sinus has high intensity because of the proteinaceous character of the fluid collection. This causes a relatively short T1 relaxation time (while maintaining a long T2 relaxation time) due to the hydration-layer environment of the water.

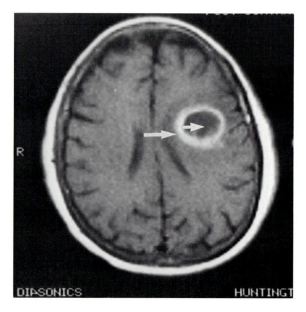

Figure 1–18. Gadolinium-DTPA-enhanced brain tumor. Enhancing portion of astrocytoma (arrow) is distinguished from necrotic central portion (arrowhead) and surrounding edema, which has been muted on this
T1-weighted image.

ure 1–20), and cortical bone (Figure 1–18) have low-mobile hydrogen density.

To summarize—the spin echo MR signal is increased if the T1 is short and the T2 value is long; it is decreased if the T1 is long and the T2 is short. The differentiation of lesions from normal tissues can be enhanced if one is aware of the differences in the magnetic relaxation times and selects the sequence times accordingly.

On images acquired with cardiac gating (e.g., by triggering off the R wave of the EKG), the TR is determined by the patient's heart rate (Figure 1–21). When images are gated to each heartbeat, a heart rate of 60 corresponds to a TR of 1.0 second; a heart rate of 120 corresponds to a TR of

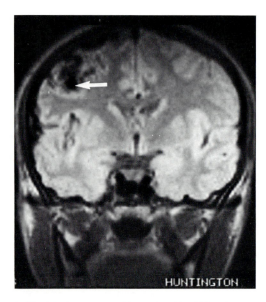

Figure 1–19. Arteriovenous malformation. Rapid flow in arteriovenous malformation produces signal loss (arrow) because of rapid motion and turbulence.

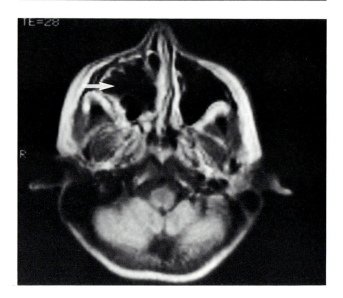

Figure 1–20. Calcified maxillary sinus rhabdomyosarcoma. Dense calcification in right maxillary sinus tumor produces marked signal loss (arrow) relatively indistinguishable from air in contralateral normal left maxillary sinus.

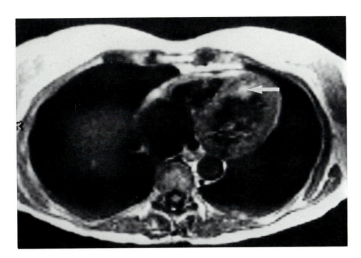

Figure 1–21. Viral myocarditis. High intensity (arrow) is noted in cardiac apex secondary to inflammation and edema from viral myocarditis. This area corresponded to focal wall motion abnormality on scintigraphic study (cardiac gated at TE of 28 mseconds).

0.5 second. To increase T2 weighting (i.e., to display myocardial edema with positive contrast similarly to brain edema), images can be acquired gating to *every other beat*. With this technique, a heart rate of 60 corresponds to a TR of 2.0 seconds.

FORMING AN MR IMAGE

Generating an MR image requires combining spatial and intensity information. Spatial information is encoded in the *frequencies* that comprise the spin echo signal.[8] As discussed earlier, the frequency of resonance depends on the local value of the magnetic field. Although the main magnetic field is designed to be quite uniform, additional magnetic fields can be temporarily superimposed on the main static field. This creates spatial variation in the *net* magnetic field, resulting in a magnetic field gradient. At each position along this gradient, there is a slightly different resonant frequency. By knowing the exact value of the magnetic field at each point, one can predict the resonant frequency. Thus the various frequencies in the RF signal detected indicate the position of the resonating protons that generated that signal. Since three coordinates (x, y, and z) must be specified to localize a point in space, MR images require three separate gradient fields. In practice these fields are generated by electromagnetic coils that can be turned on and off rapidly.

An MR image is the result of a complicated interplay between RF pulses and intermittently activated gradient fields, all of which are under computer control.[19] Depending on the programming, signal can be acquired from the whole volume simultaneously (3D acquisition) or from slices or planes within the volume (2D acquisition). A particularly efficient method of generating images from multiple slices within the volume of interest involves sequential acquisition from adjacent slices.[2] Thus while protons in one slice are recovering during the repetition time between pulses, other slices can be imaged by selective exposure to RF pulses containing very specific frequencies. Such selective pulses must be applied in the presence of a slice-selecting gradient so that only protons within the intended slice resonate.[8]

Two algorithms are generally used for image reconstruction. Projection reconstruction techniques (2DPR or 3DPR) are similar to the method used in CT and are thus prone to the same streak and motion artifacts present in CT. Spatial resolution is related to the number of different projections or angles used. Fourier transform techniques (2DFT or 3DFT) are less sensitive to motion artifact and are now the most commonly used for reconstruction. Spatial resolution in such techniques is determined by the number of phase-encoded projections and by the relationship between the strength of the gradient and the range of frequencies (i.e, the bandwidth) that are detected.

There are two axes in a 2DFT image: the "readout" axis and the "phase-encoded" axis. For a transaxial image in the traditional orientation (i.e., z axis along the main magnetic field), the z gradient is used to select the slice, the y gradient is used for "phase encoding," and the x gradient is used for "readout." If a constant range of frequencies is received (i.e., if the bandwidth is constant), increasing the gradient reduces the field of view, increasing the spatial resolution. Alternatively, if the gradient is held constant and the bandwidth is reduced, spatial resolution is improved (assuming the radio receiver can still divide the signal into the same number of frequency "bins" in both cases). Reduced-bandwidth techniques place greater demands on the RF electronics but benefit additionally by reducing noise (since noise is proportional to the square root of the bandwidth), increasing the signal-to-noise ratio.[19]

Spatial resolution along the readout axis is determined by the number of "frequency bins" into which the signal is divided. Increasing the number of bins requires better frequency discrimination characteristics in the radio receiver but takes no additional acquisition time. The only "penalty" for increasing spatial resolution along the readout axis is that there are fewer protons resonating in the smaller voxels, which decreases the signal-to-noise ratio.[20] Increasing spatial resolution along the phase-encoded axis requires increasing the number of phase-encoded projections N, each with a different strength of the phase-encoding gradient (i.e., the y gradient for our standard transaxial image). When the strength of the readout gradient and the strength of the strongest phase-encoded gradient are the same (and the bandwidths are the same), spatial resolution is comparable along the two axes.

Like the sequence parameter times (TR and TE), spatial resolution must be set prospectively during clinical operation of an MR imager. This is accomplished by specifying the size of the acquisition matrix and the field of view. Larger matrices (covering the same area or volume) result in better spatial resolution but not necessarily in greater lesion detectability. In addition, larger matrices (larger N) may require longer acquisition times since the acquisition time is equal to the product $TR \times n \times N$, where TR is the repetition time and n is the number of excitations. Spatial resolution can be increased along the readout axis without increasing the acquisition time. This may be useful when the aspect ratio of the image is other than 1:1, such that the readout direction corresponds to the longer side in the rectangular image. For example, a sagittal spine image might well be longer along the axis of the spine than from front to back in the patient. If the aspect ratio of the image were 1:2, then a 128×256 acquisition matrix could produce square pixels. Assigning the longer axis to the readout direction would result in greater spatial resolution (compared with dividing the same signal into 128 bins) without increasing the acquisition time. If such an asymmetric acquisition matrix is used for a square field of view, nonsquare pixels result.

Other considerations may influence the assignment of phase-encoding and readout gradients to particular axes in addition to the image aspect ratio. Most motion artifacts in a 2DFT image occur in the phase-encoded direction,[9] regardless of the axis of motion. Using a sagittal image of the spine as an example, one might assign the phase-encoded direction to the shorter anterior–posterior axis. This might result, however, in projection of motion artifact from the high-intensity subcutaneous fat onto the spinal cord itself. When such artifacts are unacceptable, they can be eliminated by phase encoding along the axis of the spine (although the longitudinal field of view would be reduced).

Other artifacts may arise when the object is larger than the field of view. These are known as wraparound, or "aliasing," artifacts. Increasing the field of view or changing the direction of the phased-encoded and readout axes may also modify these artifacts.

The "resolving power" as defined by Rose[22] is a useful measure of the machine-determined ability to discriminate a lesion from its background. Resolving power increases with increasing spatial resolution, signal-to-noise, and object contrast. The signal-to-noise (S/N) per pixel is determined by the voxel volume V, the number of excitations n, and the number of phase-encoded projections N:[22]

$$S/N \propto V \sqrt{n} \sqrt{N}$$

Using this equation, the effect of changing spatial resolution on S/N can be examined.[20] Spatial resolution is determined by the size of the acquisition matrix—that is, by the number of projections N along each axis in the image and by the field of view. (That one pixel is fully resolved from the next[22] is due to the sinc spread function used in 2DFT imaging.) If slice thickness is held constant and spatial resolution is doubled, the volume of an individual pixel will be reduced to 25% of its original value. This would tend to reduce S/N to one-quarter of the original value as well. (Since there are twice as many projections N, however, the S/N is only decreased to $\sqrt{2}/4$ or 35% of the original value.) If the number of repetitions is held constant, the acquisition time of the high-resolution image is twice that at normal resolution. Thus the S/N of each pixel in a "high-resolution" image has 35% of the S/N per pixel of its "normal resolution" counterpart. In addition, since the number of phase-encoded projections N in the high-resolution image is twice the value in the normal resolution mode, the image acquisition time is twice as great.

For small lesions where edge detection is important, it is appropriate to compare S/N per pixel. For diffuse lesions that are larger than the dimensions of an individual pixel, it is more appropriate to compare S/N per unit area.[20] (S/N increases as the square root of the number of pixels in the image.)

Since there are four times as many pixels per unit area in the high-resolution image (compared to normal resolution) the S/N is doubled. Thus the S/N per area of a high-resolution image will be 70% of the "normal resolution" image—but will still take twice as long to acquire. As should be apparent from the preceding discussion, the overall effect of increasing spatial resolution on resolving power may not be favorable.[20]

Like many imaging parameters, S/N is perceived logarithmically; that is, increasing the S/N is perceived as having a greater effect on image quality at low values than at high values. Thus for systems with high S/N, the loss of 30% to 65% may be barely perceptible, while the same drop for low-S/N systems may result in an unacceptable loss of image quality. Image quality is therefore quite machine-specific and depends not only on field strength and temporal stability but also on RF coil design (mainly filling factor) and electronics, gradient coils and their power supplies, and multiple software-related variables.

As an example of improved RF coil design, consider the surface coil. Although the imaging volume and field of view are reduced compared with a standard double-saddle coil, the filling factor of the coil is much improved, improving the S/N. Images obtained with surface coils can be expected to better tolerate S/N losses necessarily associated with improved spatial resolution than can larger whole-body or head coils using single-phase detection. When comparing single-phase detection surface coils to double-saddle coils using quadrature detection, the latter benefit by a $\sqrt{2}$ increase in S/N; thus the relative advantage of surface coils is reduced.

APPEARANCE OF FLOWING BLOOD

Flowing blood can appear bright or dark, depending on the selected parameter times and on the velocity, direction, and

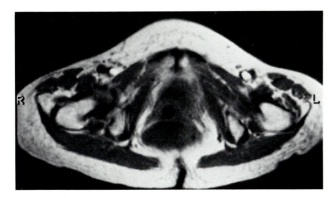

Figure 1–22. Variable appearance of flowing blood. High intensity is noted in the femoral veins (arrow) due to flow-related enhancement. Signal loss is noted in femoral arteries due to high-velocity signal loss and turbulence.

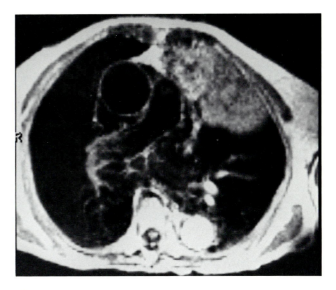

Figure 1–23. Lymphoma. On diastolic gated image of the mediastinum, high signal intensity (arrow) is noted in the descending aorta secondary to slow flow. Similar appearance can be seen when there is chance synchronization of cardiac and MR cycles due to diastolic pseudogating.

other characteristics of flow. Rapidly flowing blood can appear dark for two reasons: high velocity and turbulence.[7] At high velocity, the blood flows through the selected section too rapidly to acquire both a 90° and 180° pulse; thus it will not return a spin echo signal (Figure 1–19). This has been termed "high-velocity signal loss."[7] "Turbulence" is not synonymous with high velocity, although it does increase as the velocity increases. Turbulence is defined as random nonaxial motion of fluid elements.[7] Such random motion leads to loss of coherence and therefore to signal loss. Turbulence is increased with increasing velocity, increasing vessel diameter, endothelial roughening (due to atherosclerotic plaquing), vascular branching, and pulsatile flow. Thus arterial flow is generally turbulent. The motion of blood within the heart is generally turbulent and therefore has a low signal. When eddy currents (large-scale recirculation zones) are associated with turbulence—that is, downstream from a vascular stenosis—the nonaxial motion of fluid elements is not completely random and may demonstrate certain phenomena more characteristic of slow flow.

Slowly flowing blood can appear bright for at least three reasons: "flow-related enhancement" (FRE), "even-echo rephasing," and "diastolic pseudogating."[5] When fully magnetized, unsaturated blood enters the first few slices of a multislice imaging volume and is exposed to a spin echo sequence; it emits a strong signal commensurate with full magnetization (Figure 1–22). The adjacent stationary tissue exposed to the same pulsing sequence is still recovering from the previous excitation and thus emits a relatively weaker signal. FRE is maximal at low velocity such that the excited blood in the slice at the time of the previous 90° pulse is replaced by fresh blood in the time TR between repetitions. FRE is enhanced at short TR values that do not allow significant recovery of magnetization in the adjacent stationary tissues.[5] As the flow rate increases, the magnitude of FRE decreases, but the effect may penetrate several slices further into a multislice imaging volume. This reflects the influx of totally magnetized protons that occurs between application of successive 90° pulses.[7]

When multiple echoes are acquired by applying additional 180° pulses, the intensity of the even echoes can exceed that of the odd echoes.[6] The effect is due to a rephasing phenomenon that occurs after each full 360° of rotation (i.e., all even echoes) following the initial 90° pulse. The effect is particularly prominent in slow laminar flow and allows veins to be identified as bright structures on even-echo images (Figure 1–15). Rephasing can also occur in turbulent flow and in eddies associated with partial luminal obstructions.[7]

"Diastolic pseudogating" occurs when there is partial synchronization of the cardiac and MR cycles. For example, when the heart rate is 60 (i.e., one cardiac cycle per second) and the TR is 1.0 second, both the cardiac and MR cycles are 1 second in duration. Should the two cycles remain in phase for the 4- to 8-minute acquisition, several slices will be acquired by chance synchronization during cardiac systole and several during diastole. On sections acquired during mechanical systole, blood vessels will appear dark due to rapid, turbulent flow. On sections acquired during diastole, however, blood vessels will have increased intensity comparable to an image acquired during diastole with intentional cardiac gating (Figure 1–23).

When high intraluminal signal is found on an MR image and pathology (e.g., thrombus or tumor) is suspected, normal flow phenomena must first be excluded. FRE is generally found nearer the entry surface of the multislice imaging volume. Even-echo rephasing is found only on even-echo images. Even-echo rephasing, in fact, can only occur when there is flow. Thus its presence confirms the presence of flow and luminal patency. Diastolic pseudogating is difficult to exclude as a cause of increased signal. If thrombus is suspected, cardiac-gated images must be acquired during systole at the level of concern, although the delay from the R wave of the EKG should be adjusted so systole is not the first slice in the sequence (and would therefore be subject to FRE).

CHEMICAL SHIFT ARTIFACT

Although the majority of the NMR signal comes from the hydrogen nuclei of water molecules, lipid protons in fatty tissues can also contribute.[24] Fat and water protons do not resonate at exactly the same frequency. Fat protons resonate at a slightly higher frequency. The *difference* between these frequencies is usually described as a fraction of the resonant frequency. Since the difference in frequencies (or the "chemical shift") is very small, it is expressed as parts per million, or ppm. Fat protons resonate at a frequency that is 3 ppm higher than that of water protons. The absolute frequency difference depends on the strength of the main magnetic field (which determines the Larmor frequency). Thus at 0.35 tesla (15 MHz), a 3-ppm chemical shift will result in fat resonating at 45 Hz (15 MHz $\times$ 3 ppm) higher frequency than water. At 1.5 tesla (64 MHz), fat resonates at 192 Hz higher frequency than water.

Spatial information in the MR image is encoded in the specific frequencies comprising the spin echo. Such frequency discrimination is provided through the use of gradient fields. The minimum strength of the gradient field is determined by the degree of nonuniformity of the main magnetic field; that is, the net variation in field strength from point to point due to the gradient must be greater than that due to the random nonuniformity in the static field. Stronger static fields with comparable uniformity (e.g., 20 ppm) require stronger gradient fields. High-field magnets with spectroscopic capability are typically uniform to less than 1 ppm and thus require relatively weaker gradients.

If a 0.5 gauss (G) per centimeter gradient is applied across a 24-cm object, there will be a field difference of 12 G across the object and a frequency difference of 50 kHz (12 G $\times$ 42 MHz/Tesla $\times$ Tesla/10^4 G) from one end of the object to the other. (Since detection is usually sensitive to phase, the frequency across the object (relative to the center frequency) is $\pm$ 25 kHz. This is known as the "bandwidth.") If the object is divided into 256 pixels, there will be a frequency difference of 195 Hz (50,000/256) per pixel. If fat and water are both present in the pixel, they will resonate at frequencies

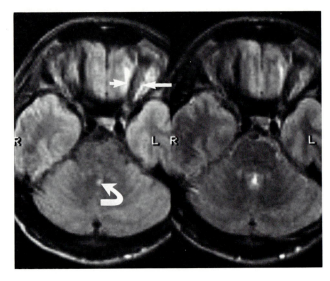

Figure 1–24. Chemical shift artifact. Note high intensity along medial border of superior rectus muscle (arrow) compared with dark border along lateral border (arrowhead). Notice also flow-related enhancement in fourth ventricle due to pulsatile motion of CSF (curved arrow).

that are separated by 45 Hz at 0.35 tesla and by 192 Hz at 1.5 tesla. Thus the frequency difference due to the chemical shift between fat and water is comparable to the frequency difference across a pixel at the high field. Therefore, at high field the fat image will be shifted two pixels along the readout (frequency-encoded) axis relative to the water image. This chemical shift artifact (Figure 1–24) is most noticeable at interfaces between tissues containing different amounts of fat and water.

Although chemical shift artifact may be more noticeable at high field, it is also increased when the strength of the gradient is reduced. As the intrinsic uniformity of lower field magnets has improved, weaker gradients can be used without sacrificing frequency discrimination. Weaker gradients narrow the bandwidth, which reduces the noise, increasing the signal-to-noise ratio. Thus an unwanted side effect of increasing signal-to-noise by weakening the gradients is increasing the clinical shift artifact.

While chemical shift artifact is a potential problem in most parts of the body, it is not so in the CNS. Fat in the brain is not NMR visible; thus there is no chemical shift artifact in the brain or cord, either at high-field or on intermediate-field systems using reduced-bandwidth techniques. When chemical shift artifact is present and bothersome, it can be eliminated by increasing the strength of the gradient fields (at a cost in the signal-to-noise ratio).

REFERENCES

1. Holland GN, Hawkes RC, Moore WS: Nuclear magnetic resonance (NMR) tomography of the brain: Coronal and sagittal sections. *J Comput Assist Tomogr* 1980;4:429–433.

2. Crooks LE, Arakawa M, Hoenninger JC, et al: NMR whole body imager operating at 3.5 kgauss. *Radiology* 1982;143:169.

3. Bradley WG: Effect of magnetic relaxation times on magnetic resonance image interpretation. *Noninvasive Medical Imaging* 1984;1: 193–204.

4. Wehrli FW, MacFall J, Newton TH: Parameters determining the appearance of NMR images, in Newton TH, Potts DG (eds): *Advanced Imaging Techniques*. San Francisco, Clavadel Press, 1983, vol 2, pp 81–118.

5. Bradley WG, Waluch V: Blood flow: Magnetic resonance imaging. *Radiology* 1985;154:443–450.

6. Waluch V, Bradley WG: NMR even echo rephasing in slow laminar flow. *J Comput Assist Tomogr* 1984;8:594–598.

7. Bradley WG, Waluch V, Fernandez E, et al: The appearance of rapidly flowing blood. *AJR* 1984;143:1167–1174.

8. Bradley WG, Crooks LE, Newton TH: Physical principles of NMR, in Newton TH, Potts DG (eds): *Advanced Imaging Techniques*. San Francisco, Clavadel Press, 1983, vol 2, chap 3, pp 15–62.

9. Nalcioglu O, Cho ZH, Lee SY, Kashmar G, Ahn CB: Fast hybrid 3D imaging by small tip angle excitation. *Mag Res Imaging* 1986;4:103.

10. Frahm J, Haase A, Matthaei D, Hänicke W, Merboldt KD: FLASH MR imaging. *Mag Res Imaging* 1986;4:104.

11. Farrar TC, Becker ED: *Pulse and Fourier Transform NMR: Introduction to Theory and Methods*. New York, Academic Press, 1971.

12. Fullerton GD, Cameron IL, Ord VA: Frequency dependence of magnetic resonance spin-lattice relaxation of protons in biological materials. *Radiology* 1984;151:135–138.

13. Bradley WG, Schmidt PS: The effect of methemoglobin formation on subarachnoid hemorrhage. *Radiology* 1984;153:166.

14. Brasch RC: Methods of contrast enhancement of NMR imaging and potential applications. *Radiology* 1983;147:781–788.

15. Gomori JM, Grossman RI, Goldberg HI, et al: Intracranial hematomas: Imaging by high-field MR. *Radiology* 1985;157:87–93.

16. Rosen BR, Pykett IL, Brady TJ: Spin-lattice relaxation time measurements in two-dimensional NMR imaging: Corrections for plane selection and pulse sequence. *J Comput Assist Tomogr* 1984;8:195–199.

17. Le Jeune JJ, Gallier J, Rivet P, et al: Is an interpretation model for proton relaxation times in biological tissue possible? abstracted. *Mag Res in Med* 1984;1:192.

18. Wesbey GE, Moseley ME, Ehman RL: Translational molecular self-diffusion in magnetic resonance imaging: Effects and applications, in James TL, Margulis AR (eds): *Biomedical Magnetic Resonance*. San Francisco, University of California Press, 1984, pp 63–78.

19. Feinberg DA, Crooks LE, Hoenninger JC, et al: Contiguous thin multisection MR imaging by two-dimensional Fourier transform techniques. *Radiology* 1986;158:811–817.

20. Bradley WG, Waluch V, Crues JV, et al: Central nervous system high-resolution magnetic resonance imaging: Effect of increasing spatial resolution on resolving power. *Radiology* 1985;156:93–98.

21. Wood M, Henkelman R: MR image artifacts from periodic motion. *Med Phys* 1985;12:143–151.

22. Rose AA: *Vision: Human and Electronic*. New York, Plenum Press, 1973, chap 1.

23. Crooks LE, Hoenninger J, Arakawa M, et al: High resolution magnetic resonance imaging. *Radiology* 1984;150:163–171.

24. Babcock EE, Brateman L, Weinreb JC, et al: Edge artifacts in MR images: Chemical shift effect. *J Comput Assist Tomogr* 1985;9: 252–257.

BIBLIOGRAPHY

Abraham A: *The Principles of Nuclear Magnetism*. International Series of Monographs on Physics, Oxford, Clarendon Press, 1961.

Andrew ER: *Nuclear Magnetic Resonance*. Cambridge, Cambridge University Press, 1969.

Bloembergen M: *Nuclear Magnetic Relaxation*. New York, WA Benjamin Inc, 1970.

Bradley WG, Adey WR, Hasso AN: *Magnetic Resonance Imaging of the Brain, Head and Neck: A Text Atlas*. Rockville, Md, Aspen Systems, 1985.

Carrington A, McLachlin AD: *Introduction to Magnetic Resonance*. New York, Harper & Row, 1967.

Farrar TC, Becker ED: *Pulse and Fourier Transform NMR: Introduction to Theory and Methods*. New York, Academic Press Inc, 1971.

Fukushima E, Roeder SBW: *Experimental Pulse NMR: A Nuts and Bolts Approach*. Reading, Mass, Addison-Wesley Publishing Co, Inc, 1981.

Gadian DG: *NMR and Its Applications to Living Systems*. Oxford, Clarendon Press, 1982.

James TL, Margulis AR (eds): *Biomedical Magnetic Resonance*. San Francisco, University of California Press, 1984.

Kaufman L, Crooks LE, Margulis AR (eds): *Nuclear Magnetic Resonance in Medicine*. Tokyo, Japan, Igaku-Shoin, 1981.

Newton TH, Potts DG (eds): *Modern Neuroradiology: Advanced Imaging Techniques*. San Francisco, Clavadel Press, vol 2, 1983.

Partain CL, Price RR, Patton JA, et al (eds): *Magnetic Resonance (MR) Imaging*. Philadelphia, WB Saunders Co, 1983.

Schumacher RT: *Introduction to Magnetic Resonance*. New York, WA Benjamin Inc, 1970.

Slichter CP: *Principles of Magnetic Resonance*. New York, Harper & Row, 1963.

2
OPTIMIZING THE MR IMAGE

Specifying the numerous parameters that constitute the MR imaging sequence is an exercise in assigning multiple interacting variables in a milieu of shifting clinical priorities and imager capabilities. A single parameter—for example, the repetition time (TR)—may have several effects on the pulsing sequence that are unrelated to image contrast. TR affects the acquisition time and determines the maximum number of slices that can be obtained in a single acquisition. Often as one variable is improved, another is worsened; for example, improving the spatial resolution by increasing the number of phase-encoded projections (N) increases the acquisition time and decreases the signal-to-noise (S/N) per pixel.[1] Furthermore, the net effect of such actions on the ability to detect disease is a continuously changing function of machine capability; that is, certain levels of improved spatial resolution can be tolerated only when S/N is at a certain high level.[1] In addition, it may be quite difficult to determine when a given system has sufficient S/N to tolerate such high spatial resolution without missing disease. The purpose of this section is to specify the variables that comprise the MR sequence, to consider interactions between these variables, and to evolve an algorithmic approach to setting up the MR pulsing sequence.

The parameters that comprise the MR pulsing sequence are listed in Table 2–1. "Primary" parameters are those that are specified directly; "secondary" parameters are indirectly determined by the primary parameters. Not all manufacturers allow the user the flexibility to specify all variables continuously over the complete range of values that may be considered necessary in clinical practice.[2] Additional software capabilities that may affect image quality are noted in Table 2–2.

Setting the variables that constitute the MR imaging sequence is a hierarchical process; that is, primary variables must be specified in a particular order, and the consequences on other (secondary) parameters must be considered. Choices may depend on clinical priorities. For example, there is a trade-off between image quality and acquisition time: the greater the acquisition time (to the point at which patient motion becomes excessive), the better the image quality. The total time that can be allotted is a clinical decision that depends on the particular patient's ability to remain motionless and on the desired level of patient throughput. While image quality may improve, this may or may not be correlated with improvement in the ability to detect disease or, more importantly, to affect the clinical

Table 2–1. Parameters That Characterize the MR Image

Primary Parameters	Secondary Parameters
Imaging plane	Spatial resolution
Field of view (FOV)	Signal-to-noise
Phase-coded projections (N)	Contrast
Slice thickness/gap	Coverage
Number of excitations (n)	Acquisition time
Repetition time (TR)	
Echo delay time (TE)	
Inversion time (TI)	

management of the patient.[3] Increasing the acquisition time decreases throughput and ultimately increases the cost of the examination. Improvements in S/N on a given imager may modify the trade-off between acquisition time and image quality. Thus, these choices are not static and must be considered in the context of the individual patient and the changing capabilities of the instrument with its continued upgrades.

Several primary variables can be selected first, since they have little effect on other parameters. The imaging plane and field of view can be selected without significantly affecting other software parameters, although the choice of certain hardware options—for example, the RF coil—may be affected. In general, the better the region of interest "fills" the coil, the better the S/N.[4] Whether this involves using a double-saddle coil with the smallest possible diameter or switching to a surface coil depends on the location of the area of interest and on the specific technology available to the user. If surface coils are used, the variable field of view (FOV) (which depends on the diameter of the coil) must be considered. Although larger coils have a larger FOV, the S/N is decreased for superficial structures compared with that achieved with smaller coils. As the surface coil diameter increases, the S/N advantage may be lost relative to double-saddle coils, particularly if the double-saddle coil is capable of quadrature detection (which increases the S/N by $\sqrt{2}$). If

Table 2–2. Specialized Imaging Capabilities

Multislice-multiecho acquisition

Variable slice thickness/gap ratio
   Contiguous slices
   Electronic offset from localizing scan
   Interchangeable frequency- and phase-encoded axes

Flow imaging

Chemical shift imaging

Fast scanning
   Echo planar
   Hybrid
   FLASH

Oblique planes of acquisition

Calculated images

the surface coil is used only to receive (and transmission is accomplished with a large "body" coil), the choice of plane may be affected, since the face of the flat surface coil must be perpendicular to the B1 field of the transmitting body coil.

Having specified the imaging plane and FOV, the user must select the primary parameters that may be interrelated in terms of their effect on the secondary parameters. These secondary parameters are also listed in Table 2–1 and include the variables that are often used to describe image quality: image contrast, in-plane spatial resolution, S/N, coverage (i.e., the volume spanned from the first to the last slice in the imaging sequence), and acquisition time. The combination of the often-interrelated primary and secondary parameters in Table 2–1 fully characterizes the MR image.

IMAGE CONTRAST

Image contrast is determined by the TR and TE if spin echo acquisition is performed and by these parameters plus the TI if inversion recovery (IR) is used.[5] Different clinical applications have different contrast requirements. T1 contrast is inversely related to the ratio TR/T1. Since T1 increases with increasing field strength, TR must increase a proportionate amount if TR/T1 is to remain constant. The field dependence of T1 depends on the particular tissue. The T1 of brain increases as the cube root of the field strength, while the T1 of skeletal muscle increases as the square root.[6] When comparing images at 0.35 T and 1.5 T, for example, the T1 of brain increases by 62%—$(1.5/0.35)^{1/3} = 1.62$. The T1 of skeletal muscle, on the other hand, increases by 107%—$(1.5/0.35)^{1/2} = 2.07$. Thus, to have comparable levels of T1 weighting, the TR of a brain study must be increased by 62% when going from 0.35 T to 1.5 T and the TR of muscle must be doubled. Leaving the TR fixed when going to a higher field increases the T1 weighting and decreases the S/N because of decreased longitudinal recovery.[7] While the increase in T1 weighting may be desirable for images that are intended to be T1 weighted, the effect is not desirable for images that are intended to be T2 weighted. Since most disease processes increase both T1 and T2, a lesion has negative contrast (i.e., appears black) on T1-weighted images and positive contrast (i.e., appears relatively bright) on T2-weighted images. Thus, increasing T1 weighting on a T2-weighted image (e.g., in the brain) tends to diminish lesion conspicuity. Where T1-weighted images are generally preferred—for example, in imaging of the body—the increased T1 weighting actually increases contrast and enhances lesion conspicuity.

The slice thickness profile results from the strength of the gradient and the particular blend of frequencies and amplitudes in the exciting RF pulses. The slice profile can affect T1 contrast as well.[8,9] Sloppy RF pulses may overlap the leading and lagging edges of adjacent slices and decrease the time of longitudinal recovery in the overlap region. Gaussian

Table 2–3. MR Contrast Jargon

| | 0.35 T | | 1.5 T | |
Contrast	TR	TE	TR	TE
Heavy T1	TR ≤ 300*	min	TR ≤ 400	min
Moderate T1	300 < TR ≤ 800	min	400 < TR ≤ 1200	min
Mild T1	800 < TR ≤ 1000	min	1200 < TR ≤ 1500	min
Proton density	TR > 2000	min	TR > 3000	min
Mild T2	1000 < TR ≤ 2000	30 < TE ≤ 50	1500 < TR ≤ 3000	30 < TE ≤ 50
Moderate T2	TR ≤ 2000	50 < TE ≤ 70	TR ≤ 3000	50 < TE ≤ 70
Heavy T2	TR ≥ 2000	TE ≥ 70	TR ≥ 3000	≥ 70

*All times in milliseconds.

pulses tend to be less sharp and have greater overlap than sinc pulses.[9] Thus, the effective TR is reduced and T1 weighting increases. As noted earlier, this has an adverse effect on S/N (decreased longitudinal recovery); it is helpful to T1-weighted images and detrimental to T2-weighted images.

Rather than specifying all combinations of TR and TE at every field strength, it is useful to describe contrast in terms of "degrees" of T1 and T2 weighting (Table 2–3). It should be apparent that these "degrees" are totally arbitrary, as the contrast changes are continuous rather than discrete. These terms serve in a qualitative sense to describe different levels of T1 or T2 weighting. "Proton density-weighted" images may be considered to be at the transition between the T1- and T2-weighted images in the following sense: if T1 weighting is produced by variation only in TR in combination with the shortest possible TE, and if T2 weighting is produced by variation in TE using the longest possible value of TR, then the proton density image is intermediate—having the longest possible TR and the shortest possible TE.

In general, T1-weighted images are obtained by keeping the TE as short as possible to minimize the complicating (and often competing) effects of T2 decay. The shortest possible TE (TE_{min}) currently available on many MR imaging systems is not very short (i.e., usually in the 20 to 40-mseconds range).[10] For tissues with T2 values of 50 mseconds (e.g., cerebral white matter), this represents up to 55% of T2 decay (i.e., $e^{-TE/T2} = e^{-40/50} = e^{-0.8} = 0.45$). Thus, there is significant T2 weighting on what should be a T1-weighted image. Unless the TE_{min} can be made significantly shorter than the T2 of the tissues of interest, the spin echo technique is relatively insensitive to T1 differences.[11] There are several reasons why the minimum TE is this long. During the interval TE, time is required for a 90° RF pulse (1 msecond), an FID (approximately 5 mseconds), a 180° RF pulse (approximately 5 mseconds), and half the time required to sample the spin echo signal (Figure 2–1A). Attempts to shorten the TE eventually involve starting the 180° pulse before the FID has fully decayed. Since the receiver frequency and Larmor frequency are rarely perfectly tuned, this off-resonance condition produces a low-frequency signal that persists into the spin echo. This results in an "FID artifact" in the image (Figure 2–1B).

The parameter T2* that specifies the decay envelope of the FID is a function of the main (Bo) field nonuniformity. More uniform and finely shimmed magnets have a longer T2* than do less uniform magnets. Thus, better, more uniform magnets have a more persistent FID and are more prone to FID artifacts as the TE is shortened; that is, artifacts may appear at longer values of TE than with less uniform magnets. One method of shortening the TE is to reverse the gradients (i.e., "gradient echo") rather than using a 180° RF pulse.[11] This is the basis for many fast scanning techniques.[12] Another way to shorten the TE is to decrease the time during which the echo is acquired (the "echo sampling time"); this has a beneficial effect on T1 weighting (because of the shorter TE) and on at least one aspect of S/N: shorter TE times allow less time for T2 decay and, therefore, allow for greater magnetization. Unfortunately, decreasing the echo sampling time also increases the bandwidth, which increases the noise and, thus, decreases the S/N.[9] The net effect on S/N depends on the T2 of the tissue and on the marginal change in overall bandwidth that results from the shorter echo sampling time.

T1-weighted images can be divided into three "degrees" of T1 weighting, as shown on Table 2–3. Since T1 increases with greater field strength, the TR values are given at 0.35 T and 1.5 T to "normalize" the T1 effect TR/T1. "Mildly" T1-weighted images are defined by their ability to demonstrate not only short T1 abnormalities but also long T2 lesions. This is accomplished by prolonging the TE to "intermediate values" (i.e., 50 to 70 mseconds). In practice, we have found the mildly T1-weighted images (e.g., TR = 1.0 second; TE = 30 and 60 mseconds) to be particularly useful in evaluation of the spinal cord. The first echo (TE_{min}) is sufficiently T1 weighted to produce very good contrast between cord and cerebrospinal fluid (CSF), yet the second echo (at intermediate TE) may still show cord or brain edema with positive contrast. On "moderately" T1-weighted images (TR approximately 0.5 second at 0.35 T), there is greater T1 contrast between cord and CSF at TE_{min} compared with the mildly T1-weighted images. There is, how-

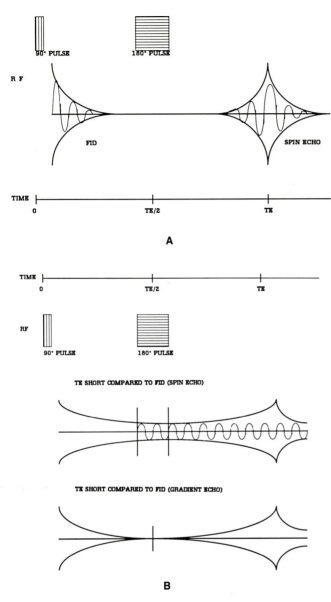

Figure 2–1. Spin echo NMR signal. Using traditional refocusing by 180° pulse centered at time TE/2, spin echo is produced centered at time TE (echo delay time). (A) TE is long compared to T2* such that FID has decayed at the time 180° pulse is initiated. (B) TE is short compared to T2* such that FID still has significant signal-to-noise at the time 180° pulse is initiated. Alternatively, focusing by means of gradient echo allows a longer period of time for FID to decay, minimizing FID artifact.

ever, little use for longer TE echoes because of the shorter TR and the marked degree of (competing) T1 weighting. In addition, longer TE echoes at a short TR have reduced S/N when only one or two excitations are used. On such sequences, therefore, we generally acquire only a single short TE echo. While S/N considerations may be more favorable on higher field systems or on intermediate field systems with reduced bandwidth technology, the competing effects of T1 and T2 weighting make such images less useful clinically.

"Heavily" T1-weighted images are defined as those with TR times shorter than 0.3 second at 0.35 T (or less than 0.4 second at 1.5 T). Such sequences may require more than two excitations on thin-slice, high-resolution images for an adequate S/N. The utility of one heavily T1-weighted technique (TR = 260 mseconds, TE = 15 mseconds) has recently been demonstrated in imaging of the upper abdomen.[13] In this clinical setting, the larger number of excitations (six to eight) required for good S/N is beneficial in that it tends to average out motion artifacts due to breathing.[13]

"Degrees" of T2 weighting may be defined by the relative intensity of brain and CSF; that is, on "heavily" T2-weighted images: CSF is more intense than brain; on "moderately" T2-weighted images: CSF is isointense with brain; and on "mildly" T2-weighted images: CSF is less intense than brain, but edematous lesions are still depicted with positive contrast.[5] Comparable levels of T2 weighting can be accomplished by varying either TR or TE. T2-weighted images obtained with a long TR have proportionally less T1 weighting and, therefore, greater proton density weighting. This has particular relevance in brain imaging, since the T1 and proton density differences that affect contrast between gray and white matter also affect contrast between edematous lesions and brain. Thus, while two sequences may have comparable T2 weighting in the terms of brain/ CSF contrast, the sequence with the longer TR will have better gray/white differentiation because of the greater mobile proton density of gray matter compared with that of white matter.[5] Similarly, edematous lesions have greater proton density than white matter; thus, long-TR, T2-weighted images benefit not only by differences in T2 but also by differences in proton density. While high-field images may have a S/N advantage as TE is increased to produce heavily T2-weighted images, they are at a relative disadvantage owing to the increasing "effective T1" at constant TR and the resultant loss of proton density weighting effects on otherwise similar T2-weighted images.

SPATIAL RESOLUTION CONSIDERATIONS

In-plane spatial resolution is determined by the FOV along a particular axis divided by the number of pixels in the same direction (Table 2–4). In 2DFT techniques, the two axes in the MR image are referred to as "phase encoded" and "frequency encoded."[7] For a given FOV, spatial resolution along the phase-encoded axis is determined by the number of phase-encoded projections (N).[14] Each projection is a separate spin echo acquisition obtained with a different value of the phase-encoding gradient. Each projection requires a time interval (TR) to complete; thus, the larger the N, the longer the acquisition time.[1] Simply stated, there is a time penalty for improved spatial resolution along the phase-encoded axis

Table 2–4. Spatial Resolution

Description	Resolution (mm)
Routine	>1.0
High	0.5–1.0
Very high	<0.5

(Figure 2–2). Spatial resolution along the frequency-encoded ("readout") axis is determined by the strength of the readout gradient and by the number of "frequency bins" into which the spin echo signal is divided.[12] (This is comparable to the number of points used to digitize the spin echo signal.) There is no time penalty for improving spatial resolution along the readout (frequency-encoded) axis. As shown later, however, improving spatial resolution along either the frequency- or phase-encoded axis carries an associated S/N penalty because of the smaller voxel volume (Figure 2–3).

On some systems, it is possible to exchange the axes used for phase encoding and readout. There are two circumstances

ACQUISITION TIME VS VOXEL VOLUME—HIGH S/N

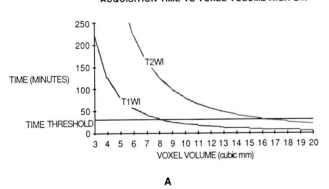

A

ACQUISITION TIME VS VOXEL VOLUME—LOW S/N

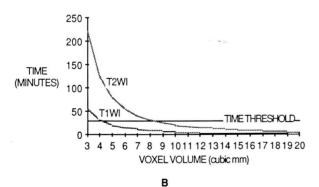

B

Figure 2–2. Acquisition time versus voxel volume for T1- and T2-weighted images. Arbitrary time threshold noted. (A) High signal-to-noise per pixel. (B) Low signal-to-noise per pixel.

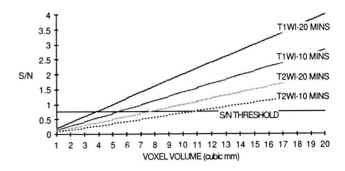

Figure 2–3. Signal-to-noise versus voxel volume for variable acquisition time and image contrast. Arbitrary signal-to-noise threshold noted.

under which this exchange may be desirable: if the image aspect ratio is not 1:1 (i.e., if the image is rectangular rather than square) or if there is motion artifact. Longitudinal images of the spine typically have a wider FOV along the axis of the spine than from front to back (in sagittal images) or from side to side (in coronal images). If the pixels remain square (i.e., when there is equal spatial resolution along the two axes in the image), then more pixels can be accommodated along the longitudinal axis. If there are more pixels along the frequency-encoded axis, there is no time penalty. Thus a 128 × 256 acquisition matrix could be used to double the coverage along the longitudinal, readout axis without incurring a time penalty. This would leave the anteroposterior direction to be described by the 128 phase-encoded projections in a sagittal image.

Motion along any axis results in artifacts in the phase-encoded direction.[15] Thus sagittal images of the thoracic spine may be hampered by cardiac or diaphragmatic motion anteriorly, projecting back on the spinal cord. If this artifact seriously degrades the image, one option that may be available to the user is to switch the frequency- and phase-encoded axes. This switching results in cardiac and respiratory motion artifacts being spread up and down along the anterior torso rather than from front to back. Unfortunately, it also decreases the longitudinal coverage for a given spatial resolution and the number of phase-encoded projections.

In-plane spatial resolution can generally be varied independent of slice thickness. Although spatial resolution certainly improves as larger (e.g., 256^2 or 512^2) matrices are used, the effect on overall image quality and lesion detectability is less certain.[1] As shown later, S/N (and therefore contrast-to-noise) decreases as spatial resolution improves. Depending on the absolute S/N of the imager, improvement in spatial resolution may decrease the resolving power—that is, the imager-determined ability to discriminate an object from its background.[1] Thicker slices are more prone to partial volume artifacts that will decrease contrast-to-noise and lesion detectability. We have thus found less utility for thick (e.g., 1-cm) slices in combination with submillimeter spatial resolution. "Screening" sequences are thus 128^2-1 cm thick, and "routine" sequences on our machine are 256^2-5 mm thick.

Coverage is defined here as the distance from the first to the last slice in a multislice imaging volume. Coverage is the product of the number of slices and the sum of the slice thickness plus the interslice gap (if any). The maximum number of slices that can be obtained in a single acquisition depends on the TR, on the longest TE (TE_n), and on the echo sampling time. In a 2DFT multislice acquisition, one or more echoes are acquired in one slice, and then (while the protons in that slice are relaxing during time interval $TR - TE_n$) the next slice is excited. The next slice may be adjacent or, within an interleaved data set, it may be subsequent and *next to* the adjacent slice (if the order of acquisition is even–odd: i.e., slices 1,3,5, . . . followed by slices 2,4,6, . . .). The amount of time spent at a particular slice position is determined by the TE of the last echo acquired (TE_n) and the length of echo sampling time. After this period, excitation of the next slice can begin. The maximum number of slices that can be obtained in the sequence is determined by dividing this time interval into the TR. As the time interval required at a particular slice level is prolonged (by prolonging TE_n or by using longer echo sampling times), the maximum number of slices is decreased, reducing the coverage.

In a particular clinical setting, the coverage may be critical. A screening sequence that covers three quarters of the brain is of limited utility; either the whole brain should be covered in a single sequence, or one half should be covered in each of two sequences. The coverage can be adjusted primarily by varying the TR, the slice thickness, the interslice gap, and the TE of the last echo. Often a range of TR and TE values is acceptable from a contrast standpoint. If a longer TR value allows the necessary anatomic area to be covered, then this value may be preferred over a shorter TR value that would require obtaining additional sequences, prolonging the examination time. Increasing coverage by thickening the slice or by increasing the size of the gap carries obvious penalties in terms of lesion detectability. Ideally, thin, contiguous slices should be used to detect small lesions optimally. If Gaussian or other "sloppy" RF pulses are found to have significant overlap or "cross talk" between slices, then two interleaved acquisitions may be necessary. In such sequences, the gap is equal to the slice thickness in two acquisitions, which are then software interleaved for display. The major disadvantage of such interleaved sequences is the time penalty incurred. When certain minimum coverage is necessary—for example, to span the distance between the neural foramina in the lumbar spine—electronic positioning may be important. Slice selection from an electronic localizing view in an orthogonal plane with variable electronic offset can be a most useful software feature when positioning is critical.

Table 2–5. Slice Thickness

Description	Thickness (mm)
Thick	>10
Routine	7–10
Thin	4–6
Very thin	3 or less

SIGNAL-TO-NOISE RATIO (S/N)

The signal-to-noise ratio (S/N) from a pixel is proportional to the product of the voxel volume (V) and square root of the number of excitations (n) and the number of phase-encoded projections (N):[1]

$$S/N \propto V\sqrt{nN}$$

Voxel volume V is determined by the in-plane spatial resolution and the slice thickness (Table 2–5). Spatial resolution is determined by the FOV divided by the number of pixels along a particular axis in the image. For purposes of discussion, the matrix is considered square with equal numbers of square pixels along both axes.

Thinner slices and higher spatial resolution carry a S/N penalty (Figure 2–4). When higher spatial resolution is achieved by increasing N (rather than decreasing the FOV), there is also a time penalty (Figure 2–5) since the acquisition time t is the product of TR, N, and n:

$$t = TR \times N \times n$$

S/N improves as the square root of the number of excitations. This is because as the two (or more) spin echoes of identical

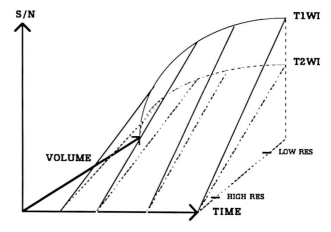

Figure 2–4. Signal-to-noise and acquisition time versus spatial resolution (voxel volume) and image contrast.

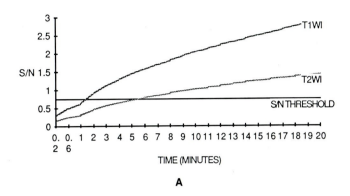

S/N VS ACQUISITION TIME-LARGE VOXEL: LOW RESOLUTION, THICK SLICE

A

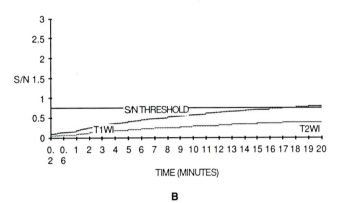

S/N VS ACQUISITION TIME-SMALL VOXEL:HIGH RESOLUTION, THIN SLICE

B

Figure 2–5. Signal-to-noise versus acquisition time, voxel volume, and image contrast. Arbitrary signal-to-noise threshold indicated. (A) Low-resolution thick-slice case. (B) High-resolution thin-slice case.

acquisitions are ''averaged'' together, the noise adds randomly and increases only as $\sqrt{n}$ while the signal adds linearly with n. The net result is thus $n/\sqrt{n} = \sqrt{n}$ increase in S/N. Similarly, if the number of phase-encoded projections N increases, the noise in the multiple spin echoes added together sums randomly (as $\sqrt{N}$) while the signal adds linearly for a similar net result: $N/\sqrt{N} = \sqrt{N}$ increase in S/N.[1]

For example, consider the net effect of S/N per pixel when the spatial resolution is improved by increasing from a 128^2 to 256^2 matrix at constant FOV, TR, TE, slice thickness, and number of excitations:

$$\frac{(S/N)_1}{(S/N)_2} = \frac{V_1}{V_2}\sqrt{\frac{n_1}{n_2}}\sqrt{\frac{N_1}{N_2}}$$

If subscript 1 refers to the high-resolution 256^2 image and subscript 2 to the 128^2, then:

$$\frac{(S/N)_1}{(S/N)_2} = \frac{1}{4}\sqrt{\frac{1}{1}}\sqrt{\frac{2}{1}} = 0.35$$

That is, the S/N per pixel of the high-resolution image is 35% of that of the low-resolution image. (Also, the acquisition time is twice as long, since $N_1 = 2N_2$ and the TR and number of excitations n is the same.) If the acquisition time is to be held constant, then the number of excitations must be halved in the high-resolution images. In this case, the S/N ratio is:

$$\frac{(S/N)_1}{(S/N)_2} = \frac{1}{4}\sqrt{\frac{1}{2}}\sqrt{\frac{2}{1}} = 0.25$$

That is, for equal acquisition times, the S/N of the high-resolution image is one fourth that of the low-resolution image.

Perception, like many other biologic processes, is a logarithmic process; that is, the eye does not respond linearly to stimuli but rather is more sensitive at low levels and less sensitive at higher levels of S/N. The perceived image quality is a logarithmic function of S/N. If there is a high ''baseline'' S/N (because of high fields or reduced bandwidth techniques), then reducing the S/N to 25% to 35% of its previous value may be tolerated without a significant perceptible loss in image quality. At lower S/N, however, such losses result not only in a ''grainy'' appearance in a normal image but also in loss of contrast-to-noise on abnormal images, so that small lesions may be missed.[1] Figures 2–6, 2–7, and 2–8 demonstrate progressive comparisons of image quality on 128^2 and 256^2 images on our unit from 1983 to 1986 as system upgrades improved S/N. Multiple sclerosis was chosen as the typical low-contrast lesion, and detectability was compared after each major upgrade. As is obvious, it was not until both reduced bandwidth technology and quadrature detection were implemented that a 256^2-5-mm thick, two-excitation image was considered diagnostically superior to the 128^2-5-mm, four-excitation image.

AN ALGORITHMIC APPROACH TO IMAGE OPTIMIZATION

The following algorithmic approach to setting up the MR pulsing sequence is suggested based on the preceding observations. The algorithm is iterative; that is, the parameters are adjusted during several cycles to achieve an ''optimal'' combination.

1. Set the plane and FOV, which may also involve specifying the direction of readout and phase encoding for rectangular images or images in which motion artifacts may be a problem. These selections have no consequences.

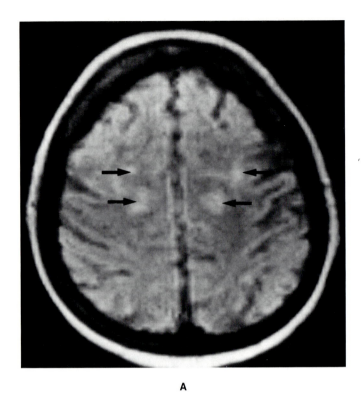

A

B   C

Figure 2–6. Signal-to-noise versus spatial resolution, 1983. Patient with MS plaques in centrum semiovale (arrows) scanned using TR = 2.0 seconds; TE = 28 mseconds and 7-mm-thick slice. (A) 128^2 image matrix using four excitations (17-minute acquisition). (B) 256^2 image matrix using two-excitation acquisition (17 minutes). (C) 256^2 four-excitation acquisition (34 minutes). Image quality is clearly better on 128^2 image than on 256^2 image because of intrinsically low signal-to-noise in 1983.

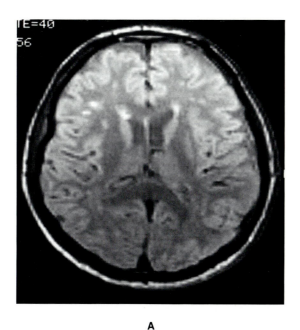
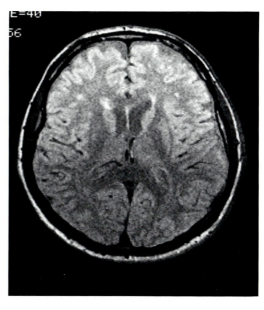

A   B

Figure 2–7. Signal-to-noise versus spatial resolution, early 1986 (with reduced bandwidth technique). Following installation of reduced bandwidth technology (Diasonics ASEP), an MS patient was scanned with a TR of 2.0 seconds and a TE of 40 mseconds using a 5-mm slice thickness. (A) 128^2, four-excitation acquisition (17 minutes). (B) 256^2, two-excitation acquisition (17 minutes). The 128^2 image still has greater "resolving power" because of the noise on the 256^2 acquisition image.

2. Set the value of TR and TE on the basis of anticipated contrast between suspected pathology and background. Set the slice thickness and gap (if any) on the basis of clinical applications—that is, anticipated lesion size and contrast—as well as the capabilities of the imager. The consequences of specifying particular values of TR, TE, slick thickness, and gap are to determine coverage. If this is adequate, go to step 3. If it is not adequate, adjust the primary parameters or, if coverage and contrast cannot be accommodated in a single acquisition, consider using more than one acquisition.

3. Set the number of phase-encoded projections (N) and the number of excitations (n). The FOV divided by N determines the spatial resolution. Spatial resolution and slice thickness determine voxel volume (V). Having determined V, N, and n, one can now measure (or visibly compare) S/N. The acquisition time can be determined from the specified values of TR, N, and n and the number of separate acquisitions. If S/N and acquisition time are acceptable, then the pulsing sequence is fully specified. If not acceptable, then one must adjust N and n.

For an example of the manner in which this algorithm may be implemented, consider the following: for a "screening" study (i.e., low probability of pathology, as in patients with headaches), one might use a 128^2, 1.0-cm-thick, T2-weighted (TR = 2.0 seconds, TE = 30 and 60 mseconds) sequence that takes 8.5 minutes. (While one can argue that small lesions may well be missed using such a technique, one should be aware that there is a threshold for the detection of disease on the higher resolution, thinner slice acquisition as well. Thus, detection of disease is a relative rather than an absolute function of image quality.) Our "routine" brain images utilize a similar T2-weighted technique (TR = 2.0 seconds, TE = 40 and 80 mseconds) with thinner 5-mm slices and better spatial resolution (0.95 mm: 256^2 matrix in a 24.3-cm FOV). While this acquisition takes 17 minutes (using two excitations), the sixteen 5-mm slices obtained (without a gap) cover only 8 cm. Since the craniocaudal extent of the brain is 12 to 14 cm, two such acquisitions are required or one may acquire a combination of 5-mm slices through the posterior fossa (17 minutes) and a "screening" 1-cm sequence through the entire brain (8.5 mm).

The cases that follow demonstrate uses of this algorithm in various clinical settings.

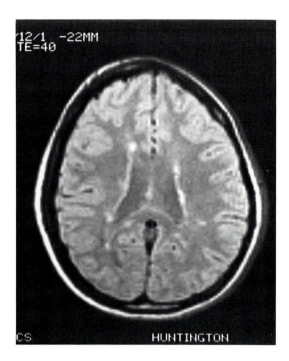

A

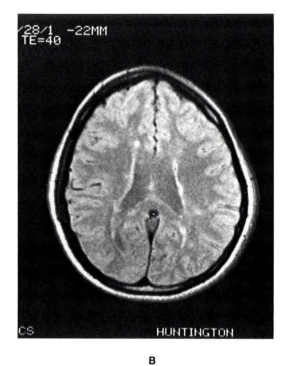

B

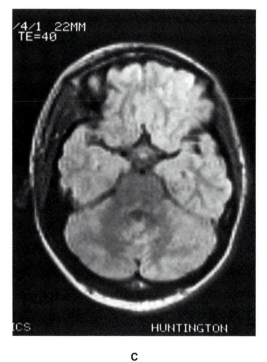

C

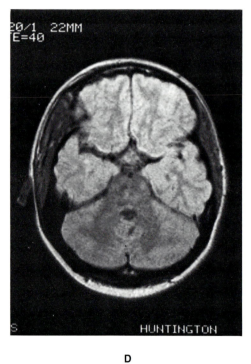

D

Figure 2–8. Signal-to-noise versus spatial resolution, mid 1986 (following installation of quadrature detection coil). MS patient scanned at level of lateral ventricles (A and B) and pons (C and D) using TR of 2.0 seconds and TE of 40 mseconds. (A) 128^2, four-excitation image (17-minute acquisition). (B) 256^2, two-excitation (17-minute acquisition). (C) 128^2, four-excitation image (17-minute acquisition). (D) 256^2, two-excitation image (17-minute acquisition). Signal-to-noise is now high enough that high-resolution images have greater resolving power than regular resolution images.

REFERENCES

1. Bradley WG, Kortman KE, Crues JV: Central nervous system high-resolution magnetic resonance imaging: Effect of increasing spatial resolution on resolving power. *Radiology* 1985; 156:93–98.

2. Bradley WG: Magnetic resonance imager survey, June 1985. *J Comput Assist Tomogr* 1985; 9:1155–1165.

3. Bradley WG: Comparing costs and ''efficacy'' of magnetic resonance imaging. *AJR* 1986; 146:1307–1310.

4. Edelman RR, McFarland E, Stark DD, et al: Surface coil MR imaging of abdominal viscera. *Radiology* 1985; 157:425–430.

5. Bradley WG: Fundamentals of MR image interpretation, in Bradley WG, Adey WR, Hasso AN: *Magnetic Resonance Imaging of the Brain, Head and Neck: A Text Atlas.* Aspen Systems, Rockville, Md, 1985, chap 1.

6. Chen C-N, Sank VJ, Hoult DI: Probing image frequency dependence. Presented at the Third Annual Meeting of Society of Magnetic Resonance in Medicine, New York, Aug 13–17, 1984.

7. Bradley WG, Crooks LE, Newton TH: Physical principles of NMR, in Newton TH, Potts DG (eds). *Modern Neuroradiology: Advanced Imaging Techniques.* San Francisco, Clavadel Press, 1983, vol 2, chap 3.

8. Kneeland JB, Shimakawa A, Wehrli FW: Effect of intersection spacing on MR image contrast and study time. *Radiology* 1986; 158:819–822.

9. Feinberg DA, Crooks LE, Hoenninger JC, et al: Contiguous thin multisection MR imaging by two-dimensional Fourier transform techniques. *Radiology* 1986; 158:811–817.

10. Hendrick RE, Newman FD, Hendee WR: MR imaging technology: Maximizing the signal-to-noise ratio from a single tissue. *Radiology* 1985; 156:749–752.

11. Mitchel MR, Tarr RW, Conturo TH, et al: Spin echo technique selection: Basic principles for choosing MRI pulse sequence timing intervals. *RadioGraphics* 1986; 2:245–260.

12. Haacke EM, Bearden FH, Clayton JR, et al: Reduction of MR imaging time by the hybrid fast-scan technique. *Radiology* 1986; 158:521–529.

13. Stark DD, Ferrucci JT: Technical and clinical progress in MRI of the abdomen. *Diagn Imaging* 1985; 7:118–131.

14. Crooks LE, Hoenninger J, Arakawa M, et al: High resolution magnetic resonance imaging. *Radiology* 1984; 150:163–171.

15. Wood ML, Henkelman R: MR image artifacts from periodic motion. *Med Phys* 1985; 12:143–151.

3

CNS IMAGING

Magnetic resonance (MR) imaging has proven highly effective in the evaluation of intracranial disease,[1-3] and in most cases its effectiveness surpasses that of conventional modalities, including CT. This is due largely to the superb contrast resolution of MR imaging—that is, its ability to define abnormal tissue by virtue of altered signal intensity. Contrast resolution is responsible for the modality's high sensitivity and, in part, for its tissue characterization capability. Compared with CT, MR imaging has additional advantages, including nonaxial scanning capability, absence of artifacts due to beam hardening, and lack of ionizing radiation or the need for contrast injection.

INDICATIONS FOR MR EXAMINATION

The choice of an imaging modality (MR vs. CT) should be influenced by a number of factors, including technical considerations, suspected pathology, patient/scanner "compatibility," logistics, and cost effectiveness. All factors should be considered carefully by the clinician and the imaging physician prior to the imaging workup.

Technical factors include relative sensitivity and specificity of the two modalities. Because of its high sensitivity to

neoplastic, inflammatory, and vaso-occlusive disease, MRI is ideally suited to be a screening examination of the central nervous system (CNS). With respect to suspected neoplasia, symptoms such as headaches, seizures, and altered mental status are traditionally "low-yield" indications for CT. The incidence of abnormalities demonstrated by MR imaging in these patients, although still low, may be significantly higher. For example, some investigators have reported a much greater incidence of pertinent positive MR findings in patients with temporal lobe seizures, as opposed to the relatively low incidence of positive CT findings.[4,5]

Similarly, noninfectious inflammatory conditions such as multiple sclerosis (MS) are difficult to diagnose by CT but are conspicuously demonstrated by MR.[6-8] In our experience, the sensitivity of MR imaging in evaluating MS is greater than 95% and is increasing with progressive implementation of improved software and coil design. Thus, patients with suspected MS should be studied with MR imaging rather than CT. MR imaging may also be used to supplant the need for other invasive and/or expensive tests, including electromyography, CSF analysis, and myelography.

Patients with suspected vaso-occlusive disease may be effectively evaluated with MR imaging,[9] particularly when confirmation of a suspected structural lesion is desired. Isolated infarcts can be localized precisely with respect to cortical association areas, white matter tracts, and central nuclei, permitting correlation with specific neurologic signs and symptoms. Demonstration of multifocal and/or extensive "deep infarction" by MR imaging may alter the management of patients with suspected presenile dementia (Alzheimer's disease) or normal pressure hydrocephalus (NPH).[10–12]

CT is relatively insensitive in the evaluation of posterior fossa pathology. This is largely due to the presence of beam-hardening artifacts from adjacent bone. MR imaging is not limited in this regard and therefore is the imaging modality of choice for suspected infratentorial disease,[13–15] including tumors, infarcts, and demyelinating disease.

Imaging specificity is largely, but not totally, influenced by the modality's tissue characterization capability. One can use MR imaging not only to distinguish pathology from normal tissue but also to indicate reliably the presence of fat, hematoma, and fibrous tissue. In addition, the protein content of cyst fluid can be estimated. Calcifications can be detected but are more conspicuously demonstrated with CT.

MR is generally more effective than CT in evaluating vascular abnormalities. Various flow phenomena discussed in Chapter 1 produce a natural contrast between vascular structures and adjacent brain parenchyma or CSF. The most useful of these phenomena is flow void, which permits an MR demonstration of intracranial aneurysms or vascular malformations, with a sensitivity at least as high as that of CT. When other flow-related phenomena can be excluded, the absence of flow void is indicative of vessel occlusion. This allows noninvasive evaluation of the patency of intracranial, large and medium-sized arterial and venous structures.

The resolution of direct sagittal, coronal, and oblique MR images surpasses that of reformatted CT sections. Thus, for pathology optimally demonstrated in a nonaxial plane, MR is the imaging modality of choice. This is particularly true in the evaluation of lesions at the cranial vertex or skull base, which may be obscured on CT by partial volume averaging and/or beam-hardening artifacts. Patients with obstructive hydrocephalus are also best evaluated with MR imaging, as sagittal sequences allow exact definition of the level of obstruction. Similarly, a number of congenital malformations primarily involve obliquely oriented midline structures and are thus best evaluated with direct sagittal MR sequences. Finally, coronal and/or sagittal scans best demonstrate the longitudinal extent of various pathologic processes and may be used to guide surgical planning or to determine radiation ports.

MR imaging may be less hazardous than CT in the evaluation of some patients, particularly those with allergies to iodinated contrast material. The lack of ionizing radiation is an advantage for those patients in whom radiation exposure should be minimized (e.g., children, pregnant patients, and individuals undergoing serial exams).

CONTRAINDICATIONS FOR MR IMAGING EXAMINATION

There are a number of contraindications for MR examination, both absolute and relative. Absolute contraindications are conditions under which MR imaging would be hazardous to the patient. Fortunately, these are few and familiar to all who work in the field. Patients with ferromagnetic aneurysm clips should not—under any circumstances—undergo MR examination. These devices torque in response to an externally applied magnetic field. Such a torque may dislodge the clip from the vascular structure to which it is applied. Local damage may also result from the shearing force produced by the clip handles. Conventional dural and vascular clips are composed of stainless steel and are nonferromagnetic, posing no hazard to the patient undergoing MR examination.[16]

Metal workers may harbor iron-containing foreign bodies and are at risk for injury when exposed to an externally applied magnetic field. There has been at least one documented report of a significant ocular injury in a patient with an unsuspected/undetected intraorbital metallic fragment. Such patients must be stringently screened during the interview process. If necessary, radiographs of the patient's skull should be obtained prior to MR examination.

The U.S. Food and Drug Administration (FDA) does not permit MR imaging examination of patients with cardiac pacemakers, because exposure to rapidly changing gradient magnetic fields may induce currents within the pacemaker leads, with resulting deleterious effects on the patient's heart rate.[17] Patients with sternotomy sutures, bypass graft clips, and artificial heart valves are not at risk, although examination of such patients may require approval by the imager manufacturer and/or the local investigative review board (IRB).

In certain situations, logistics may influence the choice of imaging modality. In inpatient facilities without an in-house MR imager, the relative advantages of MR imaging may be offset by the cost, effort, and delay involved in transporting patients to another facility. In addition, acutely ill patients may require continuous monitoring and/or mechanical support during an imaging exam, and this is more readily accomplished in the CT suite.

MR imaging requires greater patient cooperation than does CT, as patient motion leads to a much greater degree of MR imaging degradation. Potential causes of patient motion include pain, spasticity, anxiety, and altered mental status. Thus, CT may be the more effective modality in traumatized or acutely ill patients, children, those with dementia, and those with claustrophobia.

Less commonly, the sensitivity and/or specificity of MR imaging may be less than that of CT, rendering the latter examination more effective. The most commonly cited example of this is acute hemorrhage. While fresh hemorrhage can occasionally be recognized by virtue of T2 shortening in addition to edema and mass effect,[18] the specificity of MR imaging in this circumstance is relatively low compared with that of CT. In the setting of acute stroke, CT's greater specificity allows a more confident application of anticoagulant therapy for nonhemorrhagic lesions. In the setting of acute subarachnoid hemorrhage, earlier detection by CT allows more timely angiographic evaluation and surgical treatment of underlying aneurysms or other vascular etiologies. In the setting of head trauma, while CT may be less sensitive in the detection of contusions,[19] it is at least as sensitive in the evaluation of surgically amenable intracranial pathology, and it allows concurrent evaluation of associated injuries to the skull, face, spine, and torso.

Small calcified or fibrous lesions may be more conspicuously demonstrated with CT than with MR imaging.[20] Examples include small meningiomas and the calcified lesions associated with tuberous sclerosis and cysticercosis. At other times, a CT pattern of tumoral calcification may strongly suggest a specific diagnosis (e.g., craniopharyngioma or oligodendroglioma). Even the most pathognomonic CT pattern, however, does not preclude the need for biopsy to determine tumor type, prognosis, and appropriate therapy.

Contrast-enhanced CT may depict focal breakdown of the blood–brain barrier. Although a nonspecific indicator of pathology, in the proper clinical setting, CT with contrast may be used to separate tumor from edema or to detect residual/recurrent tumor in postoperative patients. This capability yields an advantage of CT over MR, as paramagnetic contrast materials are not yet available for noninvestigational use in the United States. Blood–brain barrier breakdown, however, can often be inferred from an MR examination by the presence and pattern of associated edema.

EXAMINATION PLANNING: GENERAL PRINCIPLES

Relative to CT, MR requires a greater amount of pre-examination planning. Programmable imaging parameters include the type of pulsing sequence, repetition time(s) (TR), echo delay time(s) (TE), imaging plane, slice thickness, interslice gap, and matrix size. Another consideration is the type of radio frequency coil (volume vs. surface) to be used. As discussed in Chapter 2, these decisions not only affect the type of information conveyed but also determine the duration of the exam and the volume of tissue (field of view, coverage) examined.

Each examination should be tailored in light of suspected pathology. Imaging goals are threefold. First, lesion conspicuity (and by definition, imaging sensitivity) should be maximized. Second, the exact location of any pathologic process should be determined. Finally, tissue characterization should be optimized, so that a primary diagnosis or a limited differential diagnosis may be offered. The indi-

vidualization of an MR imaging examination requires a proportionate increase in physician time and effort. The imaging physician should have a working knowledge of the basic physical principles of MR imaging, not only to determine imaging parameters properly but also to interpret information resulting from changes in those parameters. A thorough knowledge of the patient's history and results of prior imaging examinations is needed to optimize the information conveyed by the MR exam. In many instances, the initial MR sequence(s) should be reviewed at the time of the examination, so that other sequences may be added or altered in light of the information obtained.

EXAMINATION PLANNING: SPECIFIC EXAMPLES

Screening examinations for low-yield indications (e.g., headaches, lethargy, and memory loss) should be designed to maximize sensitivity while preserving efficiency and cost effectiveness. We use a moderate, T2-weighted spin echo sequence performed in the axial plane. Thick slices (7 to 10 mm) with or without a small interslice gap are sufficient, and such an examination can be performed with 8 to 15 minutes of imaging time. In screening for small lesions, such as MS plaques, acoustic neuromas, and aneurysms, thin and continuous slices are used. If an abnormality is demonstrated on the screening sequence, a second sequence can be added to yield additional information.

When evaluating an intracranial neoplasm, either suspected or previously demonstrated, a combination of T2- and T1-weighted pulsing sequences should be utilized to demonstrate and characterize the lesion. We typically obtain these sequences in two different orthogonal planes in order to determine lesion location and extent optimally. Thus, a tumor located within a cerebral or cerebellar hemisphere can be effectively demonstrated with T2-weighted axial and T1-weighted coronal sections, requiring 20 to 30 minutes of actual imaging time. Masses at the cranial vertex or skull base are imaged with a combination of T2-weighted coronal and T1-weighted axial sections.

The contour and mass effect of midline lesions are best appreciated on T1-weighted sagittal sections. Additional T2-weighted axial sections are used for lesions involving the corpus callosum, the pineal region, the brainstem, and/or the cerebellar vermis, while coronal sections are more effective in evaluating pituitary and/or hypothalamic neoplasms.

Infarcts and inflammatory lesions, such as abscess or focal cerebritis, are most conspicuous on T2-weighted images, which are usually obtained in the axial plane. T1-weighted sagittal and/or coronal scans can be added when appropriate. In the evaluation of hydrocephalus or congenital anomalies involving midline structures, we use a combination of T2-weighted axial and T1-weighted, thin-slice sagittal sections.

These and other protocols are outlined in Appendix C.

IMAGE INTERPRETATION

As with other imaging modalities, MRI can occasionally be evaluated with a gestalt approach. Accurate image interpretation can be optimized, however, by consistent application of an algorithm that addresses both lesion *recognition* and *characterization*.

Lesion recognition relies on the careful scrutiny of all images obtained. Unlike CT, there are few "blind spots" with MRI; thus the imaging physician is responsible for evaluating all structures included within the imaging volume. Axial and coronal sections allow evaluation of left-to-right symmetry, the loss of which is usually the first indication of intracranial pathology. Paired and unpaired midline structure should be carefully assessed for alterations in their normal course and contour.

A lesion, once recognized, should be characterized in as detailed a manner as possible. The characterization should address the MR depiction of a lesion's gross pathologic appearance and its histologic composition. A gross pathologic description entails the use of principles established by other imaging modalities, primarily CT. Determination of histologic composition relies largely on information unique to MR imaging.

The first issue to be addressed is the number of lesions present. In the setting of intracranial neoplasia, multiplicity can be regarded as the hallmark of metastatic disease. Multiple abscesses may mimic metastases in MRI as in CT, and biopsy may be needed to distinguish these processes. Occasionally, primary brain neoplasms may be multifocal. Tumors that appear multicentric by CT, however, may actually represent contiguous lesions connected by "CT-occult" foci of tumor. This continuity of lesions is usually apparent on T2-weighted MR imaging sequences.

Multiple sclerosis is, by definition, a multifocal process. The MR scans of affected patients typically demonstrate multiple plaques in the periventricular white matter and/or brainstem. The presence of an isolated lesion militates against MS. In middle-aged or older patients, such a finding can be more accurately attributed to lacunar-type infarction.

Appropriate MR imaging sequences allow accurate localization of intracranial pathology. Obvious considerations include lesion laterality (left vs. right) and location relative to the tentorial incisura (supratentorial vs. infratentorial). Proximity to adjacent internal and external landmarks should be addressed. Whenever possible, a lesion should be characterized as being intra-axial or extra-axial. This can usually be determined by using an appropriate imaging plane. Extra-axial lesions typically result in displacement of adjacent white matter and cortical vessels, structures that are readily apparent on moderately T2-weighted images.

The size of a lesion should be expressed in standardized units, such as centimeters. The presence of mass effect or atrophy may indicate the chronicity and etiology of a pathologic process. Both mass effect and atrophy are readily demonstrated on T1-weighted images and are manifested by distortion, displacement, or enlargement of adjacent CSF-containing structures.

The margins of moderate-sized and large lesions may be characterized as sharp or ill defined, and as smooth or irregular. Malignant lesions often have ill-defined and irregular margins, while benign processes tend to be characterized by smooth, sharp margins. The presence of a capsule or pseudocapsule is more indicative of a benign process.

Application of heavy T1- and/or T2-weighted images may allow differentiation between an inciting pathologic process and surrounding reactive edema. The T1 relaxation time of edema may be less than that of the inciting process, while the T2 relaxation time of edema is often greater than that of the inciting process. Thus, a tumor appears less intense than surrounding edema on both T1- and T2-weighted images. Such a distinction may be helpful in biopsy planning.

Tissue characterization is largely based on signal intensity patterns. The use of multiecho sequences with different TR values allows one to determine the T1 and T2 values of a lesion relative to normal brain parenchyma and CSF. Differences in the T1 and T2 relaxation times largely reflect pathologic but nonspecific increases in relative water content. Conversely, fibrous tissue and calcification result in relative decreases in the T1 and T2 relaxation times, reflecting a relative paucity of water content.

The presence of hemorrhage is manifested by characteristic alterations of signal intensity, the nature of which depends on the chronicity and chemical state of the blood products.[18,21] These changes are discussed in detail in Chapter 1 and in Cases 19 to 21.

The presence of fat (adipose) results in T1 shortening and thus can readily be demonstrated with MR imaging. Cholesterol may also result in T1 shortening, but this effect appears to depend on the degree to which the cholesterol is hydrolyzed.

SUMMARY

MR imaging is highly effective in the evaluation of a number of intracranial pathologic processes and appears to be the imaging modality of choice in most instances. The efficacy and accuracy of MR imaging can be optimized by careful examination planning and meticulous scan interpretation. The MR findings in a number of specific CNS disease entities are described in the case studies that follow.

REFERENCES

1. Bydder GM, Steiner RE, Young IR, et al: Clinical NMR imaging of the brain: 140 cases. *AJNR* 1982;3:455–480.

2. Brant-Zawadzki M, Davis PL, Crooles LE, et al: NMR demonstration of cerebral abnormalities: Comparison with CT. *AJR* 1983; 140:847–854.

3. Bradley WG, Waluch V, Yadley RA, et al: Comparison of CT and MR in 400 patients with suspected disease of the brain and cervical spinal cord. *Radiology* 1984;152:695–702.

4. Latack JT, Abou-Khalil BU, Siegel GU, et al: Patients with partial seizures: Evaluation by MR, CT, and PET imaging. *Radiology* 1986; 159:139–163.

5. Blom RJ, Vinuela F, Fox AJ, et al: Computed tomography in temporal lobe epilepsy. *J Comput Assist Tomogr* 1984;8:401–405.

6. Lukes SA, Crooks LE, Aminoff MJ, et al: Nuclear magnetic resonance imaging in multiple sclerosis. *Ann Neurol* 1983;13:592–601.

7. Runje VM, Price AC, Kirshner HS, et al: Magnetic resonance imaging of multiple sclerosis: A study of pulse-technique efficacy. *AJNR* 1984;5:691–702.

8. Sheldon JJ, Siddhanthan R, Tobias J, et al: MR imaging of multiple sclerosis: Comparison with clinical and CT examinations in 74 patients. *AJNR* 1985;6:683–690.

9. Bryan RN, Willcott MR, Schneiders NJ, et al: Nuclear magnetic resonance evaluation of stroke. *Radiology* 1983;149:189–192.

10. Bradley WG, Waluch V, Brant-Zawadzki M, et al: Patchy periventricular white matter lesions in the elderly: A common observation during MR imaging. *Noninvasive Medical Imaging* 1984;1:35–41.

11. Brant-Zawadzki M, Fein G, Van Dyke C: Magnetic resonance imaging (MRI) of the aging brain: Patchy white matter lesions and dementia. *AJNR* 1985;6:675–682.

12. Zimmerman RO, Fleming CA, Lee BCP, et al: Periventricular hyperintensity as seen by magnetic resonance: Prevalence and significance. *AJNR* 1986;7:13–20.

13. McGinnis BD, Brady TJ, New PJF, et al: Nuclear magnetic resonance (NMR) imaging of tumors in the posterior fossa. *J Comput Assist Tomogr* 1983;7:575–589.

14. Bydder GM, Steiner RE, Thomas DJ, et al: Nuclear magnetic resonance imaging of the posterior fossa: 50 cases. *Clin Radiol* 1984; 34:173–188.

15. Lee BCP, Kneeland JB, Deck MDF, et al: Posterior fossa lesions: Magnetic resonance imaging. *Radiology* 1984;153:137–143.

16. New PJF, Rosen BR, Brady TJ, et al: Potential hazards and artifacts of ferromagnetic and nonferromagnetic surgical and dental materials and devices in nuclear magnetic resonance imaging. *Radiology* 1983; 147:139–148.

17. Paulicek W, Geisenger M, Castle L, et al: Effects of nuclear magnetic resonance on patients with cardiac pacemakers. *Radiology* 1983; 147:149–153.

18. Gomori JM, Grossman RI, Goldberg HI, et al: Intracranial hematomas: Imaging by high-field MR. *Radiology* 1985;157:87–93.

19. Han JS, Kaufman B, Alfidi RJ, et al: Head trauma evaluated by magnetic resonance and computed tomography: A comparison. *Radiology* 1984;150:71–77.

20. Holland BA, Kucharcyzk W, Brant-Zawadzki M, et al: MR imaging of calcified intercranial lesions. *Radiology* 1985;157:353–356.

21. Bradley WG, Schmidt PC: Effect of methemoglobin formation on the MR appearance of subarachnoid hemorrhage. *Radiology* 1985; 156:99–103.

CASE 1

HISTORY

A 60-year-old woman with a longstanding history of "muscle tension" headaches. The neurologic examination was unremarkable. A screening examination of the brain was requested.

QUESTIONS

1. What are your differential considerations?

   _____

   _____

2. What MR techniques would you use?

	1	2	3
a. Coil	____	____	____
b. Centering point	____	____	____
c. Imaging plane(s)	____	____	____
d. Contrast	____	____	____
e. Slice thickness	____	____	____

3. What do you expect to find?

   _____

   _____

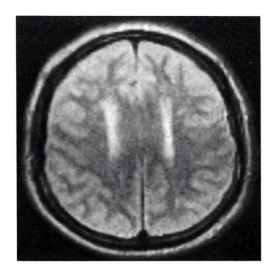

Figure 1.1 (SE 2000/56). Axial scans through the supraventricular level.

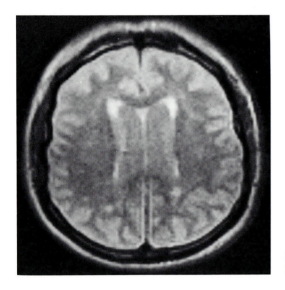

Figure 1.2 (SE 2000/56). Axial scans through the bodies of the lateral ventricles.

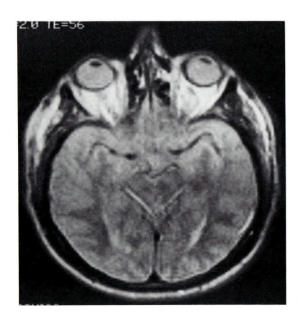

Figure 1.3 (SE 2000/56). Axial scan through the level of the occipital horns.

MR TECHNIQUES

a. Coil — Head
b. Centering point — CML (canthomeatal line)
c. Imaging plane — Axial
d. Contrast — Mild–moderate T2W
e. Slice thickness — Routine

This is the standard screening sequence of the brain. The use of spin echo sequences with mild-to-moderate T2 weighting provides the best contrast to screen for most intracranial abnormalities.[1] The axial plane is preferred since it depicts anatomic relationships in a familiar fashion and allows the assessment of right–left symmetry readily.

MR FINDINGS

Figure 1.1. Areas of confluent increased signal are seen along the lateral margin of the ventricular bodies.

Figure 1.2. There are small symmetric foci of increased signal intensity in the white matter adjacent to the frontal horns.

Figure 1.3. Small, high-intensity foci are also seen adjacent to the occipital horns.

DIFFERENTIAL DIAGNOSIS

In the absence of mass effect or surrounding edema, these high intensity foci are unlikely to be neoplastic or infectious in nature. The differential diagnosis includes demyelinating diseases and deep white matter infarcts. Although the patient's age is atypical for multiple sclerosis (MS), up to 10% of affected individuals may present after the age of 50. The symmetry of the lesions and the lack of other lesions in the periventricular white matter or brainstem (not shown) speak strongly against MS.[2]

Final Diagnosis

Minimal (age-related) deep white matter infarction.

SUMMARY OF MR FINDINGS FOR AGE-RELATED, DEEP WHITE MATTER INFARCTION[2,3]

1. Symmetric punctate foci about the frontal and occipital horns.
2. Symmetric, confluent, high intensity foci along the lateral ventricular bodies.
3. Increasingly prevalent after age 50.

COMMENTS

Small, high intensity foci are seen about the frontal horns in the majority of adult patients and thus should be considered a normal variant. Histologically, the white matter in this area differs from that found elsewhere, being slightly decreased in myelin content. Focal disruption of the ventricular ependyma is frequently seen at the frontal horn tips, and this may also play a role in alteration of signal intensity. High intensity foci near the occipital horns are seen less frequently in young adults but are increasingly common with people in advancing age, as are the bandlike areas about the superolateral margin of the ventricular bodies (which also include the bodies of the caudate nuclei). These should be considered normal involutional findings and are no more significant than the slight but progressive age-related increase in ventricular and sulcal size.

REFERENCES

1. Brant-Zawadzki M, Norman D, Newton TH, et al: Magnetic resonance of the brain: The optimal screening technique. *Radiology* 1984; 152:71–77.
2. Kortman KE, Bradley WG, Rauch RA, et al: Multiple sclerosis versus cerebral vascular disease: Differentiation by MRI. *AJR*, publication pending.
3. Bradley WG, Waluch V, Brant-Zawadzki M, et al: Patchy, periventricular white matter lesions in the elderly: A common observation during NMR imaging. *Noninvasive Medical Imaging* 1984; 1:35–41.
4. Brant-Zawadzki M, Fein G, Van Dyke C, et al: MR imaging of the aging brain: Patchy white-matter lesions and dementia. *AJNR* 1985; 6:675–682.

CASE 2

HISTORY

A 35-year-old man presenting with a 3-month history of seizures. An enhanced CT scan is shown in Figure 2.1. MR was requested for further evaluation.

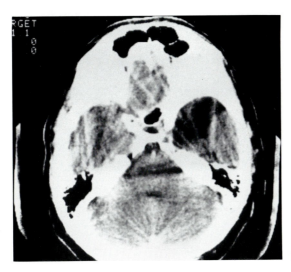

Figure 2.1. Enhanced CT scan through the temporal lobes.

QUESTIONS

1. What are your differential considerations?

2. What MR techniques would you use?

	1	2	3
a. Coil			
b. Centering point			
c. Imaging plane(s)			
d. Contrast			
e. Slice thickness			

3. What do you expect to find?

Look at Figures 2.2A and 2.2B first. Why was a second sequence performed?

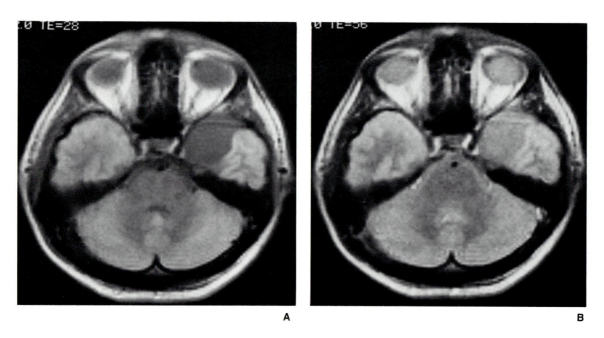

Figures 2.2A (SE 2000/28) and **2.2B** (SE 2000/56). Axial scans through the posterior fossa.

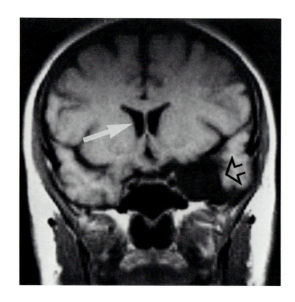

Figure 2.3 (SE 500/28). Coronal scan through the area of interest.

MR TECHNIQUES

	1	2
a. Coil	Head	Head
b. Centering point	CML	Vertex
c. Imaging planes	Axial	Coronal
d. Contrast	Mild–moderate T2W	Moderate T1W
e. Slice thickness	Routine	Routine

The first sequence is the routine CNS screening study, as described in Case 1. The second sequence was used for tissue characterization and for additional localizing information.

MR FINDINGS

Figure 2.1. The CT study demonstrates a nonenhancing focal area of low density within the left middle cranial fossa. Detailed examination of the lesion is limited by the streak artifacts from the adjacent bone.

Figure 2.2. Both images are from the initial pulsing sequence and show an extra-axial lesion within the anterior aspect of the left middle cranial fossa. The intensity of this lesion is similar to CSF fluid on both the first and second echos. There is relatively little mass effect relative to the size of the lesion.

Figure 2.3. This T1-weighted coronal image verifies the extra-axial location of the lesion (open arrow). Note the similarity of intensity of this lesion and the low intensity CSF within the lateral ventricles (closed arrow). Fluid with low protein content will have low intensity signal characteristics because of prolonged T1 relaxation times.

DIFFERENTIAL DIAGNOSIS

An extra-axial location, relatively little mass effect, and an intensity pattern like that of CSF are findings charac-teristic of an *arachnoid cyst*. Other extra-axial diagnostic considerations include *meningioma, epidermoid tumor, neuroma, metastasis,* and *subdural hematoma*. All these lesions have MR relaxation times that are quite different from those of CSF. (See individual case studies for additional discussion of these lesions.)

In this example, the advantages of MR compared to CT are an artifact-free image, depiction in more than one orthogonal plane (for better anatomic localization), and improved tissue characterization.

Final Diagnosis

Arachnoid cyst of the left middle cranial fossa.

SUMMARY OF MR FINDINGS FOR ARACHNOID CYST[1]

1. A well-defined, homogeneous, extra-axial lesion that has signal intensity similar to that of CSF (unless complicated by hemorrhage or infection).
2. A complicated arachnoid cyst—that is, a cyst with hemorrhage or infection—will have a signal intensity greater than CSF on T1-weighted or mildly to moderately T2-weighted images because of elevation in protein content and/or the presence of blood.
3. Mass effect is usually minimal, although there are exceptions (see Figures 2.4 and 2.5).

REFERENCE

1. Kjos BO, Brant-Zawadzki M, Kucharzyk W, et al: Cystic intracranial lesions: Magnetic resonance imaging. *Radiology* 1985;155:363–369.

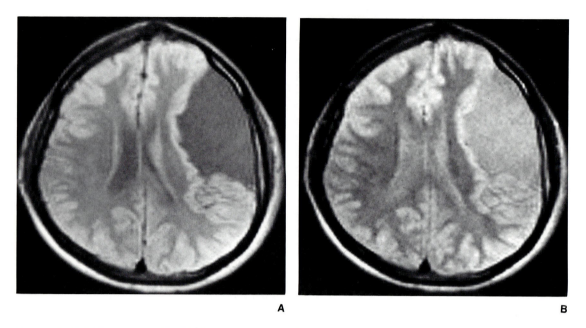

A   B

Figures 2.4A (SE 2000/28) and **2.4B** (SE 2000/56). Axial section through a large arachnoid cyst.

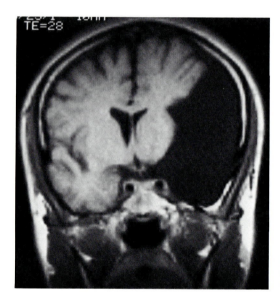

Figure 2.5 (SE 500/28). Coronal section through the same cyst as in Figure 2.4. Note the mass effect on the ipsilateral lateral ventricle.

CASE 3

HISTORY

A 25-year-old woman presented with right-sided numbness of 6 months' duration. MR was requested to rule out multiple sclerosis (MS).

QUESTIONS

1. What are your differential considerations?

_____

_____

2. What MR techniques would you use?

	1	2	3
a. Coil	_____	_____	_____
b. Centering point	_____	_____	_____
c. Imaging plane(s)	_____	_____	_____
d. Contrast	_____	_____	_____
e. Slice thickness	_____	_____	_____

3. What do you expect to find?

_____

_____

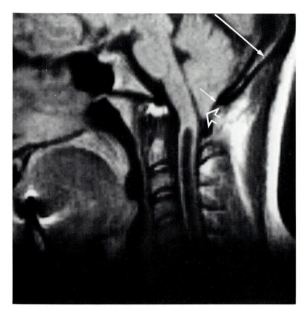

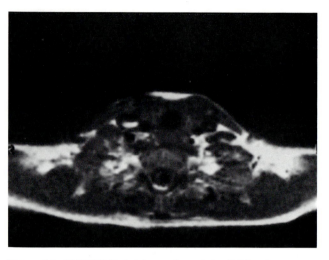

Figure 3.2 (SE 500/28). Axial scan through the C-7 level.

Figure 3.1 (SE 1000/28). Midline sagittal section through the head and neck.

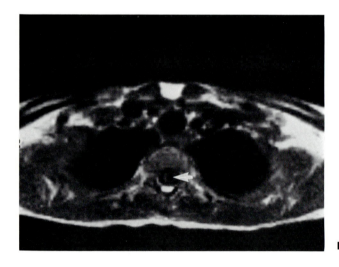

Figure 3.3 (SE 500/28). Axial scan through the T-2 level.

MR TECHNIQUES

	1	2	3
a. Coil	Head	Head	Head
b. Centering point	CML	Midline	Midneck
c. Imaging planes	Axial	Sagittal	Axial
d. Contrast	Mild to moderate T2W	Mild T1W	Moderate T1W
e. Slice thickness	Thin	Thin	Routine

The first pulsing sequence (not shown) is the routine screening head sequence for MS (see Case 19). Because of the clinical findings of paresthesias referable to spinal cord disease, the second and third sequences were performed to examine the spine and cord. Although MS involvement of the cord may dominate the clinical presentation, the brain should always be examined because of MR's greater sensitivity to intracranial disease, particularly MS.

The second sequence was performed with the head coil centered as low as possible. (Note the drop-off of signal peripherally at the limit of the RF field.) A mildly T1-weighted sequence was chosen to provide contrast between low intensity CSF and higher intensity cord or disc. On a second echo image (e.g., in the range of 50 to 70 mseconds), the CSF has a higher intensity but can still be distinguished from cord parenchyma. Additionally, there is sufficient T2 weighting to enable recognition of focal long T2 intramedullary lesions. We have found this additional sequence helpful in detecting cord abnormalities (see Cases 20 and 52).

Heavy T1- or T2-weighted images are less useful as a screening examination of the spine. With heavy T1 weighting, the cortical bone (e.g., osteophytes), CSF, and degenerated discs all have low signal, hence, low contrast discrimination. With heavy T2 weighting, the signal from CSF and cord are both intense, making discrimination between these two structures difficult. In addition, sequences with T2 weighting require longer scanning times and are more susceptible to patient motion and CSF flow artifacts.[1] In light of this, we use mild T1 weighting and mild T2 weighting for the screening sagittal sequence. Mild T1 weighting yields sufficient contrast between cord and CSF to define cord contours accurately. The use of mildly T2-weighted images gives enough T2 weighting to identify alterations of water content within the cord; it also produces contrast between light gray CSF and darker extradural structures.

Axial images (sequence 3) are helpful for further evaluation, and the TR can be adjusted according to pathology. A moderately T1-weighted sequence was used in this case to emphasize the differences between the dark CSF surrounding and within the cord and the brighter spinal cord parenchyma (Figures 3.2 and 3.3). If a lesion such as a cord tumor had been suspected from the first sagittal series, however, a moderately T2-weighted sequence would have been used to emphasize the longer T2 of the tumor and edema.

MR FINDINGS

Figure 3.1. There is caudal extension of the cerebellar tonsil (open white arrow) below the foramen magnum. The posterior margin of the foramen magnum (small white arrow) is easily identified because of the lack of signal from the cortical bone. High intensity marrow signal (long white arrow) is noted within the cortical bone. Note that the fourth ventricle is normally located.

A large, central, low intensity abnormality is seen within the cervical cord extending rostrally. Its intensity is similar to that of CSF; compare it with the CSF intensity anterior to the brainstem.

Figures 3.2 and 3.3. The intramedullary low intensity cyst (white arrow) is again demonstrated within the spinal cord at these levels. The signal intensity is similar to CSF.

DIFFERENTIAL DIAGNOSIS

Cerebellar ectopia with abnormal tonsil morphology and position is characteristic of a Chiari malformation. In the case of *Chiari I malformation*, the fourth ventricle is normal in location, in contrast to the inferior displacement of the fourth ventricle seen with *Chiari II malformation*. Other findings associated with Chiari I malformations include craniovertebral junction anomalies, Klippel-Feil syndrome, hydromyelia, and hydrocephalus.

The differential diagnosis for cystic lesions in the spinal cord includes the following:

1. *Hydromyelia* or *syringomyelia*. If uncomplicated (i.e., without hemorrhage or infection), these lesions have signal intensities similar to that of CSF on all pulsing sequences.
2. *Cystic cord tumor.* These lesions are inhomogeneous with increased intensity due to higher protein content. A component of solid tumor, often present, will produce cord expansion and a focal increase in cord parenchymal intensity on T2-weighted images. The findings associated with spinal cord tumors may not be entirely specific, since posttraumatic cystic myelomalacia may have a similar appearance.[2]

Final Diagnosis

Chiari I malformation with upper cervical cord hydromyelia.

SUMMARY OF MR FINDINGS FOR CHIARI I MALFORMATION[3,4]

1. Abnormal cerebellar tonsil morphology and position can be identified on sagittal images.
2. The fourth ventricle is nondisplaced.
3. Hydromyelia, seen as a CSF-intensity cyst within the cord, can be an associated finding.

REFERENCES

1. Bradley WG, Kortman KE, Burgoyne B: Flowing CSF in normal and hydrocephalic states: Appearance on MR images. *Radiology* 1986; 159:611–616.
2. Pojunas K, Williams AL, Daniels DL, et al: Syringomyelia and hydromyelia: Magnetic resonance evaluation. *Radiology* 1984;153:679–683.
3. Lee BCP, Zimmerman RD, Manning JJ, et al: MR imaging of syringomyelia and hydromyelia. *AJR* 1985;144:1149–1156.
4. Spinos E, Laster DW, Moody DM, et al: MR evaluation of Chiari I malformations at 0.15 T. *AJR* 1985;144:1143–1148.

CASE 4

HISTORY

This 37-year-old woman had a long history of seizures and subnormal intelligence.

QUESTIONS

1. What are your differential considerations?

_____

_____

2. What MR techniques would you use?

	1	2	3
a. Coil	___	___	___
b. Centering point	___	___	___
c. Imaging plane(s)	___	___	___
d. Contrast	___	___	___
e. Slice thickness	___	___	___

3. What do you expect to find?

_____

_____

Source: Courtesy of Irwin Grossman MD, Beverly Hills, CA.

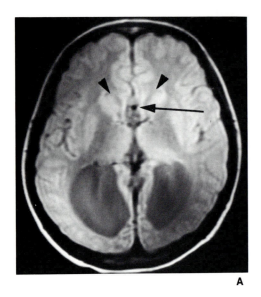

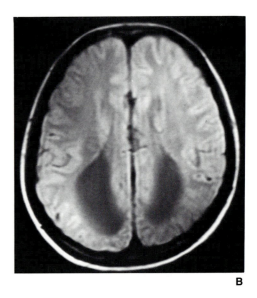

Figure 4.1A (SE 2000/30). Axial scan through the atrial and occipital horns.

Figure 4.1B (SE 2000/30). Axial scan 1 cm superior to Figure 4.1A.

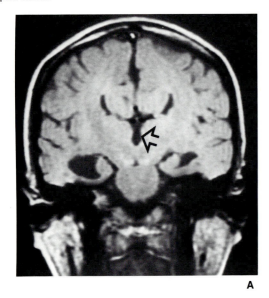

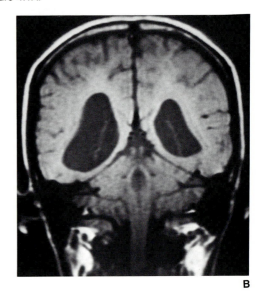

Figure 4.2A (SE 1000/25). Coronal section at the level of the third ventricle.

Figure 4.2B (SE 1000/25). Coronal section at the level of the atria.

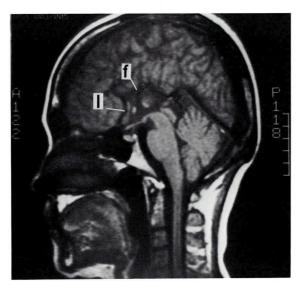

Figure 4.3 (SE 400/25). T1-weighted midsagittal image.

MR TECHNIQUES

	1	2	3
a. Coil	Head	Head	Head
b. Imaging planes	Axial	Coronal	Sagittal
c. Centering point	CML	Coronal midline	Sagittal midline
d. Contrast	Mild T2W	Mild T1W	Moderate T1W
e. Slice thickness	Thin	Thin	Thin

The first sequence is a routine screening study. T1-weighted coronal and sagittal sequences were used to define abnormal ventricular morphology more accurately.

MR FINDINGS

Figure 4.1A. The atria and occipital horns are moderately and symmetrically dilated. The frontal horns (arrowheads) are slitlike in configuration and widely separated. Between the frontal horns and posterior to the interhemispheric fissure as an unpaired midline structure with flow void (arrow). This represents a single (azygous) anterior cerebral artery trunk. No corpus callosum can be seen anterior to the foramen of Monro or posterior to the third ventricle.

Figure 4.1B. One centimeter more superior, at the expected level of the corpus callosum, the interhemispheric fissure is continuous from front to back.

Figure 4.2A. The frontal horns are widely spread and have a "beaked" appearance laterally. The third ventricle (open arrow) extends superiorly between the frontal horns and is continuous with the interhemispheric fissure.

Figure 4.2B. More posteriorly, the atria are moderately dilated bilaterally. The interhemispheric fissure is continuous inferiorly with the supravermian cistern.

Figure 4.3. The midsagittal section demonstrates complete absence of the corpus callosum. The lamina terminalis (1) is normal, but the fornix (f) is hypoplastic.

DIFFERENTIAL DIAGNOSIS

These findings are pathognomonic for agenesis of the corpus callosum.[1,2] No other diagnoses need be considered.

Comment

Arrested development of the commissural plate between the 12th and 20th weeks of gestation results in a spectrum of midline cerebral anomalies, including agenesis of the corpus callosum. This may occur as an isolated finding or in conjunction with other anomalies, such as holoprosencephaly, Dandy-Walker cysts, or gray matter heterotopia. None of these are present in the reference case. Callosal agenesis may be partial or complete. In complete agenesis, no callosal tissue can be identified. The lack of a midline commissure results in superior extension of the third ventricle and splaying of the lateral ventricular bodies. The third ventricle is continuous superiorly with the interhemispheric fissure or, occasionally, a midline interhemispheric cyst. The cortical axons that would otherwise form the corpus callosum are arranged in thick longitudinal bundles running from front to back along the medial surface of the lateral ventricles. (This can readily be appreciated in Figure 4.2A.) The fornices may be absent or hypoplastic, as in this case.

Callosal agenesis may be noted as an incidental finding in otherwise normal patients. More frequently, affected patients are retarded and/or have seizures.

Final Diagnosis

Agenesis of the corpus callosum.

SUMMARY OF MR FINDINGS FOR AGENESIS OF THE CORPUS CALLOSUM[1,2]

1. Absent corpus callosum.
2. Splayed frontal horns.
3. Dilated and splayed posterior horns.
4. Abnormal superior extension of the third ventricle.
5. Interhemispheric cyst (occasional).
6. Midline lipoma (occasional).
7. Azygous anterior cerebral artery (occasional).

REFERENCES

1. Kendall BE: Dysgenesis of the corpus callosum. *Neuroradiology* 1983;25:239–256.
2. Davidson HH, Abraham R, Steiner RF: Agenesis of the corpus callosum: Magnetic resonance imaging. *Radiology* 1983;155:371–373.

CASE 5

HISTORY

This 57-year-old man presented with severe headaches. An enhanced CT scan is shown in Figure 5.1.

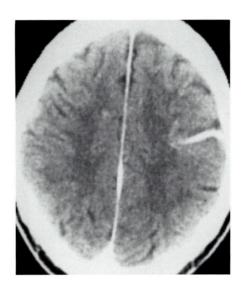

Figure 5.1. Enhanced CT scan through the parietal lobes. (Courtesy of Kenneth Kidd, MD, Santa Barbara, CA.)

QUESTIONS

1. What are your differential considerations?

   _____

   _____

2. What MR techniques would you use?

	1	2	3
a. Coil	___	___	___
b. Centering point	___	___	___
c. Imaging plane(s)	___	___	___
d. Contrast	___	___	___
e. Slice thickness	___	___	___

3. What do you expect to find?

   _____

   _____

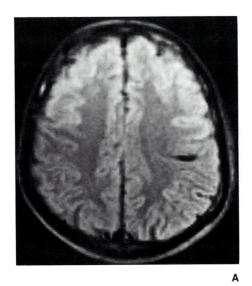
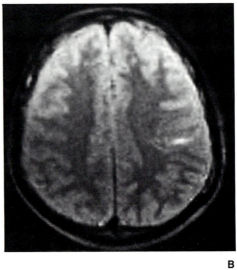

Figures 5.2A (SE 2000/28) and
5.2B (SE 2000/56). Axial scan at the
same level as Figure 5.1.

A   B

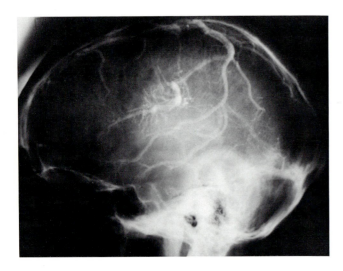

Figure 5.3. Venous phase of a cerebral angiogram performed in
the lateral projection. (Courtesy of Kenneth Kidd, MD, Santa
Barbara, CA.)

MR TECHNIQUES

a. Coil   Head
b. Centering point   CML
c. Imaging plane   Axial
d. Contrast   Mild to moderate T2W
e. Slice thickness   Thin

This pulsing sequence is the routine screening sequence for CNS abnormalities. A thin-slice thickness was utilized to ensure detection of the linear abnormality seen on the CT study.

MR FINDINGS

Figure 5.1. There is a linear, contrast-enhancing lesion located in the left parietal cortex.

Figure 5.2. The same lesion is seen on a comparable MR section. Note that the lesion has low signal intensity on the first echo image but high signal intensity on the second echo image. This is due to even-echo rephasing, indicating that the lesion is a vascular structure with slow, laminar flow.[1]

Figure 5.3. The venous phase of the cerebral angiogram demonstrates the typical appearance of a venous angioma with a central transcerebral draining vein surrounded by dilated medullary veins in a spoke–wheel pattern.

DIFFERENTIAL DIAGNOSIS

With this combination of studies, there is little doubt that this is a venous angioma. The CT and angiographic findings have been well described.[2] Venous angiomas are relatively common intracranial vascular abnormalities and are usually detected in an incidental fashion. The clinical presentation may be variable; the vast majority of these lesions do not produce symptoms. Rarely, an angioma may bleed.

Final Diagnosis

Venous angioma of the left parietal cortex.

SUMMARY OF MR FINDINGS FOR VENOUS ANGIOMA

1. Tubular structure demonstrating characteristic slow MR flow phenomenon.
2. No mass effect.
3. *Even-echo rephasing*[1] may be helpful in detecting the venous nature. (Multiple echo imaging is necessary to demonstrate this phenomenon.)
4. Occasionally, associated prior hemorrhage may produce changes in the adjacent parenchyma, including encephalomalacia or calcifications.[2]
5. MRI is very sensitive in detecting venous angiomas.[3,4]

REFERENCES

1. Waluch V, Bradley WG: NMR even echo rephasing in slow laminar flow. *J Comput Assist Tomogr* 1984;8:594–598.
2. Olson E, Gilmor RL, Richmond B: Cerebral venous angiomas. *Radiology* 1984;151:97–104.
3. Augustyn GT, Scott JA, Olson E, et al: Cerebral venous angiomas: MR imaging. *Radiology* 1985;156:391–395.
4. Cammarata C, Han JS, Haaga JR, et al: Cerebral venous angiomas imaged by MR. *Radiology* 1985;155:639–643.

CASE 6

HISTORY

A middle-aged woman was noted to have a left middle cerebral artery aneurysm. This was first diagnosed on an enhanced CT scan (Figure 6.1) and later confirmed on a left internal carotid angiogram (Figure 6.2). Because of other medical problems, she was considered a poor operative candidate and therefore was referred for MR scanning as a noninvasive method to follow this lesion.

QUESTIONS

1. What MR techniques would you use?

	1	2	3
a. Coil	_____	_____	_____
b. Centering point	_____	_____	_____
c. Imaging plane(s)	_____	_____	_____
d. Contrast	_____	_____	_____
e. Slice thickness	_____	_____	_____

2. What do you expect to find?

_____

_____

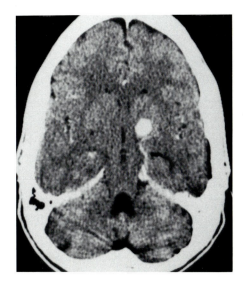

Figure 6.1. Enhanced axial CT through the inferior temporal fossa.

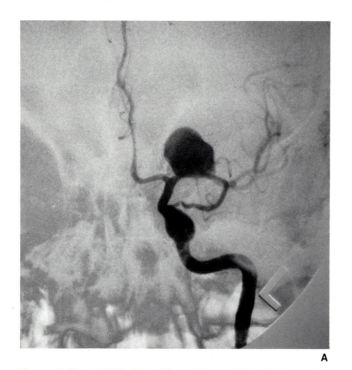
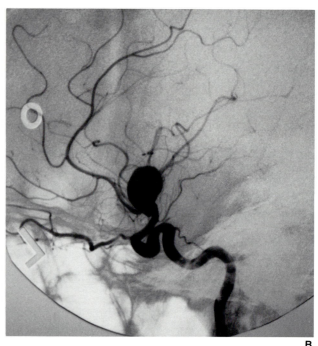

A

B

Figures 6.2A and **6.2B.** AP and lateral views obtained during a left internal carotid angiogram.

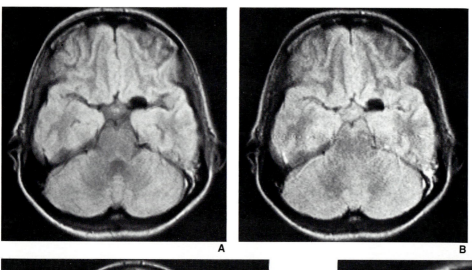

A

B

Figure 6.3A (SE 2000/30) and **6.3B** (SE 2000/60). Axial section through the circle of Willis.

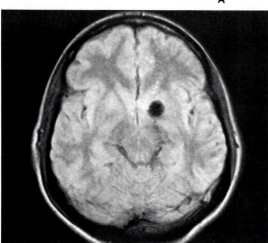

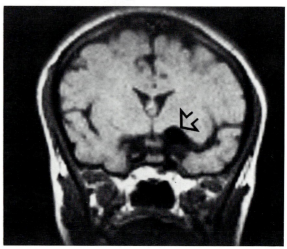

Figure 6.4 (SE 2000/30). Axial section 10 mm superior to Fig. 6.1.

Figure 6.5 (SE 500/40). Coronal section through the region of interest.

MR TECHNIQUES

		1	2
a.	Coil	Head	Head
b.	Centering point	CML	Midvertex
c.	Imaging planes	Axial	Coronal
d.	Contrast	Mild to moderate T2W	Moderate T1W
e.	Slice thickness	Thin	Thin

The initial study with mild to moderate T2 weighting is part of our routine study of the brain. Although we were primarily interested in the aneurysm, we make it a policy to screen the remainder of the brain for any additional findings. Thin sections were used to examine the major intracranial vessels. The second sequence provides an additional view of the aneurysm. The moderate T1 weighting is helpful in detecting the presence of methemoglobin if subacute hemorrhage is suspected.

MR FINDINGS

Figures 6.1 and 6.2. Both the CT and angiogram demonstrate a large aneurysm projecting superiorly from the proximal segment of the left middle cerebral artery.

Figures 6.3 to 6.5. A focal area of low signal intensity (arrow in Figure 6.5) is noted on both sequences and correlates well with the CT and angiographic findings. The adjacent brain parenchyma appears normal, and there is no evidence of subacute hemorrhage, which would appear as increased signal intensity on the moderately T1-weighted image.

DIFFERENTIAL DIAGNOSIS

Focal areas of very low signal intensity on MR usually can be attributed to one of the following: (1) tissue with *low proton density*, such as air or calcium; (2) *rapidly flowing or turbulent blood*; or (3) focal changes in *magnetic susceptibility*, such as produced by hemosiderin deposition in chronic hemorrhage (see Case 11). In this example, low intensity can be attributed to flow within an aneurysm.

Final Diagnosis

Aneurysm of the left middle cerebral artery.

SUMMARY OF MR FINDINGS FOR ANEURYSMS[1,2]

1. Aneurysms commonly involve the internal carotid artery, the anterior communicating artery, and the trifurcation of the middle cerebral artery.
2. The signal intensity changes may serve to characterize the aneurysm and include the following:

    a. low signal intensity on all pulsing sequences due to either rapidly flowing blood or turbulence.
    b. increased second echo signal intensity due to even-echo rephasing in areas of slow flow. (This was not seen on the second echo image, Figure 6.3B, in this demonstration case.)
    c. intermediate or increased heterogeneous signal due to thrombosis (see Figure 6.6).
    d. Peripheral foci of low signal intensity due to hemosiderin deposition (on T2WI) and/or mural calcium.

3. Giant aneurysms may have a ''laminar'' appearance, reflecting complex flow patterns and thrombus formation.

REFERENCES

1. Bradley WG, Waluch V: Blood flow: Magnetic resonance imaging. *Radiology* 1985;154:443–450.
2. Lee BCP, Deck MDF: Sellar and juxtasellar lesion detection with MR. *Radiology* 1985;157:143–147.

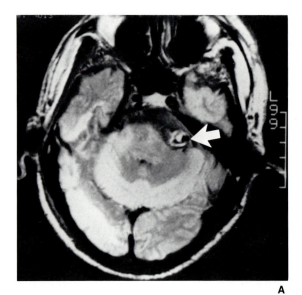

A

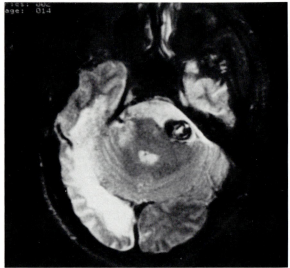

B

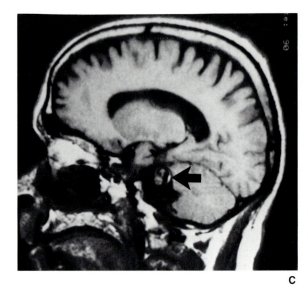

C

Figures 6.6A (SE 2500/20), 6.6B (SE 2500/70), and 6.6C (SE 600/250). Axial (A and B) and left parasagittal (C) views of a basilar artery aneurysm (arrow). Note the heterogeneous signal intensity in this region due to partial thrombosis, calcification, and possible hemosiderin deposition. (Courtesy of Washington MR Center, Whittier, CA.)

CASE 7

HISTORY

A 45-year-old man with a history of recurrent seizures. Papilledema and a right systolic carotid bruit were noted on physical exam.

QUESTIONS

1. What are your differential considerations?

   _____

   _____

2. What MR techniques would you use?

	1	2	3
a. Coil	_____	_____	_____
b. Centering point	_____	_____	_____
c. Imaging plane(s)	_____	_____	_____
d. Contrast	_____	_____	_____
e. Slice thickness	_____	_____	_____

3. What do you expect to find?

   _____

   _____

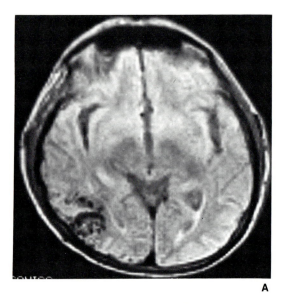 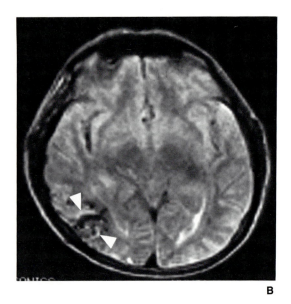

Figures 7.1A (SE 2000/28) and **7.1B** (SE 2000/56). Axial scans through the occipital horns.

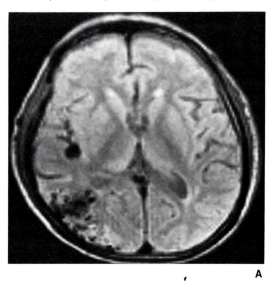 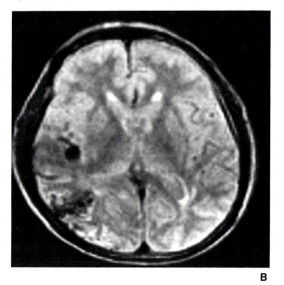

Figures 7.2A (SE 2000/28) and **7.2B** (SE 2000/56). Axial scans 1 cm superior to Figure 7.1.

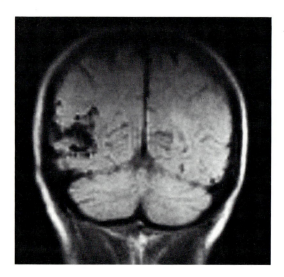

Figure 7.3 (SE 1000/28). Coronal scan through the region of the occipital horns.

MR TECHNIQUES

	1	2
a. Coil	Head	Head
b. Centering point	CML	Vertex
c. Imaging planes	Axial	Coronal
d. Contrast	Mild to moderate T2W	Moderate T1W
e. Slice thickness	Routine	Routine

The first pulsing sequence is the standard screening sequence. The second sequence with moderate T1 weighting provides additional localizing information and tissue characterization.

MR FINDINGS

Figure 7.1. There are multiple serpiginous and punctate low intensity structures in the right posterior temporal and anterior occipital regions. On the second echo images, several of these demonstrate even-echo rephasing with increased intensity (arrowheads).[1,2]

Figure 7.2. The lesion is seen extending into the posterior temporal area. In addition, there is a 1-cm round signal-void lesion in the right Sylvian fissure representing a large draining vein.

Figure 7.3. The large vessel seen in Figure 7.2 is shown to be tubular in configuration and to extend peripherally. Additional serpiginous vessels are evident.

DIFFERENTIAL DIAGNOSIS

This is the typical appearance of an arteriovenous malformation (AVM). Other differential considerations are:

1. *Vascular neoplasm.* Enlarged tumor vessels may resemble those of a malformation, but the absence of soft tissue intensity or mass effect excludes vascular neoplasm.

2. *Parenchymal calcifications.* Although the punctate loss of signal on the first echo image may be similar to rapidly flowing blood, it would be very unusual for calcified lesions to have this morphology or to appear this distinct.

Extensive calcifications are usually associated with gliosis (which is not seen in this case). The even-echo rephasing (increased signal) noted on the second echo image is seen only in slow laminar flow and would not be seen with calcification alone. On the other hand, an AVM may also have calcifications that may be difficult to distinguish from abnormal veins.

Final Diagnosis

Arteriovenous malformation.

SUMMARY OF MR FINDINGS FOR ARTERIOVENOUS MALFORMATION[3,4]

1. Serpiginous and punctate areas of signal void due to rapid blood flow and turbulence in abnormal vessels.
2. Characteristically, there is minimal mass effect unless there is associated hemorrhage (see Case 8).
3. Even-echo rephasing may be observed in vessels with slow flow.[2]
4. Associated calcification, although demonstrated readily by CT, may be difficult to detect by MR imaging.

REFERENCES

1. Bradley WG, Waluch V: Blood flow: Magnetic resonance imaging. *Radiology* 1985;154:443–450.
2. Waluch V, Bradley WG: NMR even echo rephasing in slow laminar flow. *J Comput Assist Tomogr* 1984;8:594–598.
3. Kucharczyk W, Lemme-Pleghos L, Uske A, et al: Intracranial vascular malformation: MR and CT imaging. *Radiology* 1985;156:383–389.
4. Lee BCP, Herzberg L, Zimmerman RD, et al: MR imaging of cerebral vascular malformations. *AJNR* 1985;6:863–870.

CASE 8

HISTORY

A 53-year-old epileptic man presented with a several-day history of progressive headaches and minimal left-sided hemiparesis.

QUESTIONS

1. What are your differential considerations?

   _____

   _____

2. What MR techniques would you use?

	1	2	3
a. Coil	___	___	___
b. Centering point	___	___	___
c. Imaging plane(s)	___	___	___
d. Contrast	___	___	___
e. Slice thickness	___	___	___

3. What do you expect to find?

   _____

   _____

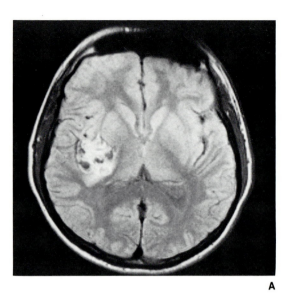
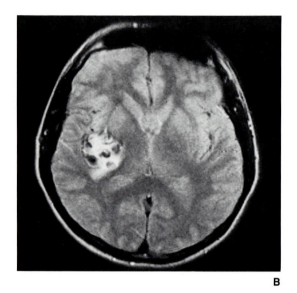

A   B

Figures 8.1A (SE 2000/30) and **8.1B** (SE 2000/60). Axial scans through the basal ganglia.

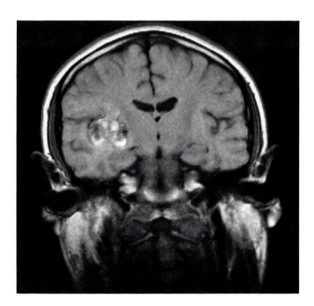

Figure 8.2 (SE 500/30). Coronal section through the region of interest.

MR TECHNIQUES

	1	2
a. Coil	Head	Head
b. Centering point	CML	Midvertex
c. Imaging planes	Axial	Coronal
d. Contrast	Mild to moderate T2W	Moderate T1W
e. Slice thickness	Routine	Routine

The first pulsing sequence was used for a standard screening examination. The second sequence gives additional T1 weighting in the coronal plane. In retrospect, an argument for the use of thin slices could be made, as these would increase the anatomic detail in the region of interest.

MR FINDINGS

Figure 8.1. There is a large, well-defined, slightly heterogeneous, high intensity mass involving the right insular cortex, the adjacent basal ganglia, and portions of the internal capsule. In addition, there are irregular and curvilinear foci of decreased signal intensity on both the first and second echo images. These are surrounded by areas of high signal intensity, possibly representing edema. Since central high signal intensity is noted on the first echo image, the presence of T1 shortening due to methemoglobin is suspected. A more heavily T1-weighted sequence is needed to confirm this (see Case 10).

Figure 8.2. On this coronal T1-weighted image, both the low intensity and high intensity foci are again seen. Mass effect with compression of the Sylvian cistern is better appreciated in this plane. Since the foci of signal void are noted on all pulsing sequences, this finding is consistent with either rapidly flowing blood[1] or calcification, although even large calcifications are seldom so distinct or hypointense. Within and surrounding the mass, there is T1 shortening indicating the presence of methemoglobin, compatible with subacute hemorrhage.[2]

DIFFERENTIAL DIAGNOSIS

As discussed in Case 7, an uncomplicated vascular malformation usually does not present a diagnostic problem. In this case, there is mass effect and evidence of hemorrhage, which makes the differentiation between *vascular malformation associated with a hematoma* and a *hemorrhagic neoplasm* more difficult. The low signal intensity areas are suspicious for abnormal vascular structures. Subsequently, an angiogram confirmed the presence of an arteriovenous malformation.

Final Diagnosis

Arteriovenous malformation associated with a subacute hematoma.

SUMMARY OF MR FINDINGS FOR VASCULAR MALFORMATION WITH HEMATOMA

1. Serpiginous and punctate areas of signal void due to rapid blood flow and turbulence in abnormal vessels.[3,4]
2. Even-echo rephasing may be observed in vessels with slow flow.[1]
3. Hematoma may result in varying signal intensities, depending on the pulsing sequences used and the chronicity of the hemorrhage.[5] See summary in Case 11.
4. Significant mass effect may be identified.
5. Associated calcification may be difficult to detect with MR imaging, unlike CT.

REFERENCES

1. Bradley WG, Waluch V: Blood flow: Magnetic resonance imaging. *Radiology* 1985;154:443–450.
2. Bradley WG, Schmidt PG: Effect of methemoglobin formation on the MR appearance of subarachnoid hemorrhage. *Radiology* 1985;156:99–103.
3. Lee BCP, Herzberg L, Zimmerman RD, et al: MR imaging of cerebral vascular malformations. *AJNR* 1985;6:863–870.
4. Kucharczyk W, Lemme-Pleghos L, Uske A, et al: Intracranial vascular malformation: MR and CT imaging. *Radiology* 1985;156:383–389.
5. Gomori JM, Grossman RI, Goldberg HI, et al: Intracranial hematomas: Imaging by high-field MR. *Radiology* 1985;157:87–93.

CASE 9

HISTORY

A 65-year-old hypertensive man presenting with a 1-day history of headaches and weakness on the right side. A CT examination without contrast is shown in Figure 9.1.

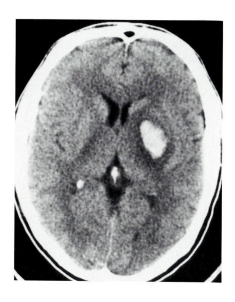

Figure 9.1. Nonenhanced axial CT through the basal ganglia.

QUESTIONS

1. What are your differential considerations?

_____

_____

2. What MR techniques would you use?

	1	2	3
a. Coil	___	___	___
b. Centering point	___	___	___
c. Imaging plane(s)	___	___	___
d. Contrast	___	___	___
e. Slice thickness	___	___	___

3. What do you expect to find?

_____

_____

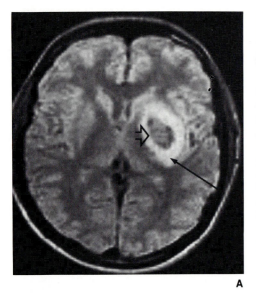 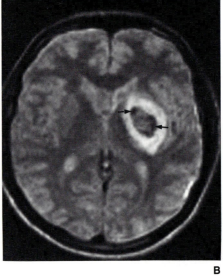

A   B

Figures 9.2A (SE 2000/28) and **9.2B** (SE 2000/56). Axial scans through the same level as Figure 9.1.

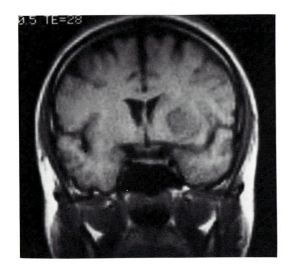

Figure 9.3 (SE 500/28). Coronal scan through the basal ganglia.

MR TECHNIQUES

		1	2
a.	Coil	Head	Head
b.	Centering point	CML	Midvertex
c.	Imaging planes	Axial	Coronal
d.	Contrast	Mild to Moderate T2W	Mild T1W
e.	Slice thickness	Routine	Routine

The first sequence is the standard CNS screening sequence with mild to moderate T2 weighting. The second sequence was performed to provide additional localizing information and tissue characterization.

MR FINDINGS

Figure 9.1. The nonenhanced CT study demonstrates a focal area of increased density within the left basal ganglia compatible with an acute intraparenchymal hemorrhage. Note the surrounding rim of low density consistent with edema.

Figures 9.2A and 9.2B. Within the left basal ganglia, there is a well-circumscribed, low intensity elliptical mass (open black arrow) surrounded by a thick, high intensity rim (long black arrow). There are foci (small black arrows, Figure 9.2B) within this central mass with very low intensity, reflecting focal T2 shortening. These become more conspicuous as the TE is increased on the second echo image.

When the MR study is compared with the CT study, one notes a reversal in lesion "brightness"; that is, the high density of acute blood on CT is now low intensity on MR, and the low-density edamatous rim on CT is now high intensity on MR. As discussed later, these findings can be readily explained from some basic principles of MR.

Figure 9.3. Both the acute central hemorrhage and peripheral edema have similar T1 values and are less distinguishable on this T1-weighted image. A pertinent negative finding is the absence of T1 shortening attributable to paramagnetic methemoglobin, as would be seen in *subacute* hemorrhage.[1] (See Case 10.)

DIFFERENTIAL DIAGNOSIS

The differential diagnosis includes any cause of acute parenchymal hemorrhage, such as *hypertensive bleed, vascular malformation,* or *tumor.* As with CT, it may be difficult to differentiate between these entities. The absence of enlarged vessels or mass separate from the hemorrhage militates against AVM and hemorrhagic tumor, respectively. In this case, this lesion was felt to be a hypertensive hemorrhage.

Final Diagnosis

Acute hypertensive hemorrhage of the left basal ganglia.

SUMMARY OF MR FINDINGS FOR ACUTE HEMORRHAGE

1. Acute hematomas are characterized by central low intensity on T2-weighted images.[2] The T2 shortening is attributed to the presence of hypoxic red blood cells containing "magnetically susceptible" deoxyhemoglobin. This creates regions of high local magnetic field strength. When water protons diffuse near the region of high field they dephase, losing signal.[1] This causes shortening of T2 (without affecting T1).

2. These findings are usually present in the first few days after hemorrhage, prior to the formation of methemoglobin. The T2 shortening is accentuated with higher magnetic field strengths[2] and produces an area of low signal intensity on images with T2 weighting.

3. Typically, there is edema surrounding the acute hematoma. The edema is better differentiated from the hematoma on a T2-weighted image because of the marked difference between their respective T2s. On T1 weighting, however, there is little difference between the T1 values of edema and acute hematomas, accounting for the findings in Figure 9.3.[1]

4. These findings should be distinguished from those of *subacute* hemorrhage (see Case 10) and *chronic* hematoma (see Case 11).

REFERENCES

1. Bradley WG: MRI of intracranial hemorrhage, in Partain CL, Price RR, Patton JA, et al (eds): *Magnetic Resonance Imaging,* ed 2. Philadelphia, Saunders, in press.

2. Gomori JM, Grossman RI, Goldberg HI, et al: Intracranial hematomas: Imaging by high-field MR. *Radiology* 1985;157:87–93.

CASE 10

HISTORY

A 55-year-old man with hemorrhagic foci in the left frontal lobe and cerebellar vermis demonstrated on a CT scan 6 weeks earlier. A four-vessel cerebral angiogram was performed and was interpreted as normal. MR was requested as a follow-up study.

QUESTIONS

1. What are your differential considerations?

_____

_____

2. What MR techniques would you use?

	1	2	3
a. Coil	_____	_____	_____
b. Centering point	_____	_____	_____
c. Imaging plane(s)	_____	_____	_____
d. Contrast	_____	_____	_____
e. Slice thickness	_____	_____	_____

3. What do you expect to find?

_____

_____

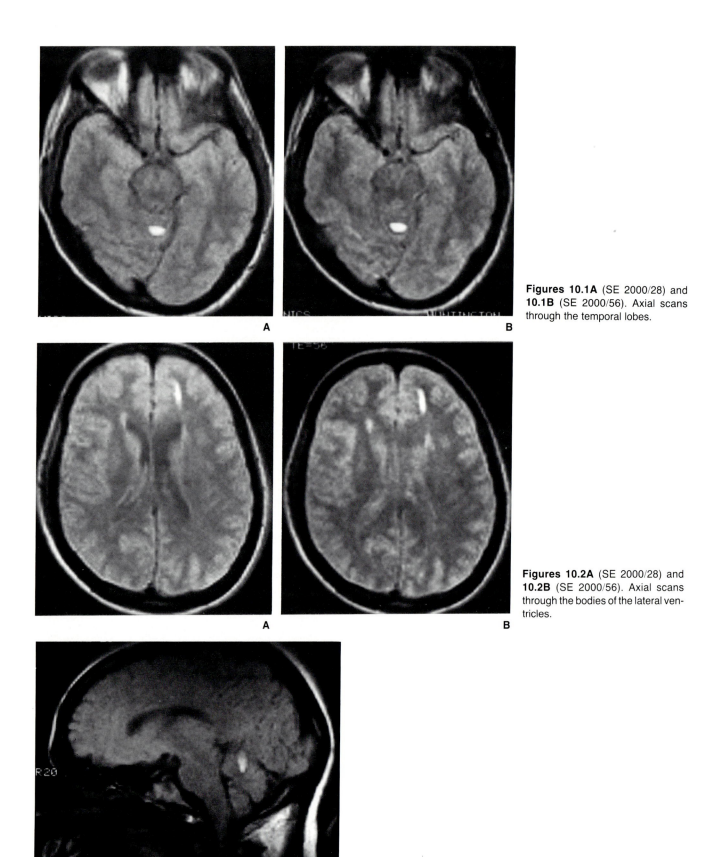

Figures 10.1A (SE 2000/28) and **10.1B** (SE 2000/56). Axial scans through the temporal lobes.

Figures 10.2A (SE 2000/28) and **10.2B** (SE 2000/56). Axial scans through the bodies of the lateral ventricles.

Figure 10.3 (SE 1000/28). Sagittal scan through the midline.

MR TECHNIQUES

	1	2
a. Coil	Head	Head
b. Centering point	CML	Midline
c. Imaging planes	Axial	Sagittal
d. Contrast	Mild to moderate T2W	Mild T1W
e. Slice thickness	Routine	Routine

The first sequence is the standard CNS screening sequence. The second pulsing sequence is to provide additional localizing information and tissue characterization.

MR FINDINGS

Figure 10.1. There is a 1.3-cm, well-circumscribed superior vermian lesion with a high intensity signal on both first and second echo images. Because of the abnormally high signal intensity on the first echo image (Fig. 10.1A), T1 shortening is suspected.

Figure 10.2. There is a left frontal and well-defined linear lesion with similar signal intensity. Also note the foci of increased intensity involving the deep white matter adjacent to the frontal horns (Fig. 10.2B). The latter are normal, age-related changes (see Case 1, normal aging brain).

Figure 10.3. On this relatively T1-weighted image, the vermian lesion shows some T1 shortening manifested by increased signal intensity relative to that of adjacent brain parenchyma.

DIFFERENTIAL DIAGNOSIS

The preceding findings are consistent with multiple parenchymal subacute hemorrhagic foci. T1 shortening is due to the presence of methemoglobin.[1] There is no associated mass effect. The differential diagnosis is extensive and includes:

1. *Embolic disease.* This is unlikely given the distribution of the lesions.
2. *Vasculopathy and/or coagulopathy.*
3. *Metastases.* The lack of surrounding edema or mass effect makes this unlikely.
4. *Occult vascular malformations.*
5. *Trauma.* Again, unlikely by virtue of lesion distribution.

Clinical evaluation revealed no embolic source or coagulopathy, and there was no history of primary tumor or trauma. *Occult* cerebrovascular malformations, though unusual, may be multiple and should be considered.

Final Diagnosis

Left frontal and vermian subacute hemorrhagic foci, of uncertain etiology.

SUMMARY OF MR FINDINGS FOR SUBACUTE HEMORRHAGE[1,2]

1. Subacute hemorrhage characteristically contains methemoglobin.[1]
2. The formation of methemoglobin from hemoglobin generally takes about 3 to 4 days in an environment of low oxygen tension. Methemoglobin generally forms first in the periphery of the hematoma and extends inward with time.[2] (See Figure 10.4.)
3. Since methemoglobin is paramagnetic, T1 is shortened and results in high intensity on T1-weighted images.
4. On a T2-weighted image, the lesion also has a high intensity signal. This is secondary to lengthening of the T2 as a result of hydration-layer water bound to protein.

REFERENCES

1. Bradley WG, Schmidt PG: Effect of methemoglobin formation on the MR appearance of subarachnoid hemorrhage. *Radiology* 1985;156: 99–103.
2. Gomori JM, Grossman RI, Goldberg HI, et al: Intracranial hematomas. Imaging by high-field MR. *Radiology* 1985;157:87–93.

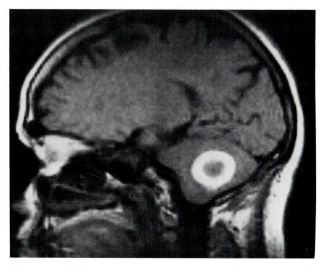

Figure 10.4 (SE 500/28). Moderately T1-weighted image showing a parasagittal section through the cerebellum 5 days after resection of a hemangioblastoma. Note the high intensity peripheral rim of methemoglobin surrounding a relatively lower intensity center.

CASE 11

HISTORY

Four months prior to the MR study, this 71-year-old man presented with headaches and a right homonomous hemianopsia. A CT obtained at the onset of symptoms demonstrated an intraparenchymal hematoma within the left occipital lobe. The current CT study is shown on Figure 11.1. An MR scan was also requested.

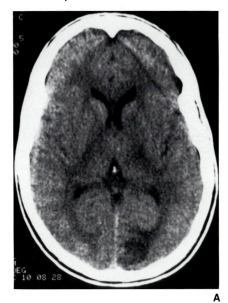 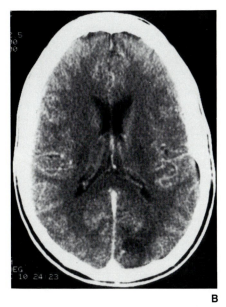

A   **B**

Figures 11.1A and **11.1B.** Nonenhanced (A) and enhanced (B) CT sections through the occipital lobes.

QUESTIONS

1. What are your differential considerations?

_____

_____

2. What MR techniques would you use?

	1	2	3
a. Coil	____	____	____
b. Centering point	____	____	____
c. Imaging plane(s)	____	____	____
d. Contrast	____	____	____
e. Slice thickness	____	____	____

3. What do you expect to find?

_____

_____

Source: Courtesy of Irwin Grossman MD, Beverly Hills, CA.

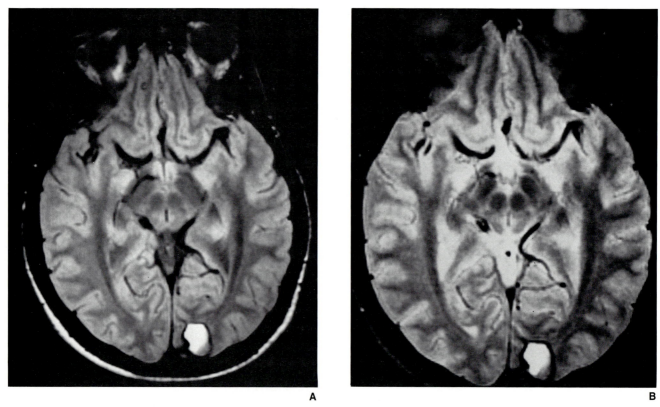

Figures 11.2A (SE 2500/25) and **11.2B** (SE 2500/50). Axial MR scans through the occipital poles.

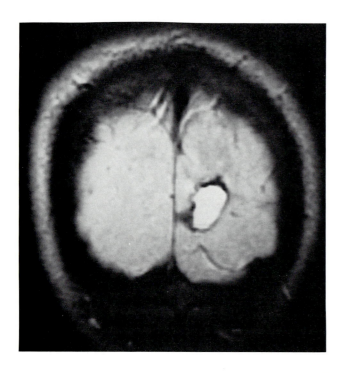

Figure 11.3 (SE 600/25). Coronal view through the area of interest.

MR TECHNIQUES

	1	2
a. Coil	Head	Head
b. Imaging planes	Axial	Coronal
c. Centering point	CML	Posterior cranium
d. Contrast	Mild to moderate T2W	Moderate T1W
e. Slice thickness	Routine	Routine

A routine screening sequence with mild to moderate T2 weighting was performed. In this case, since a higher field unit was used for imaging, the TR is slightly longer than that used for screening in other reference cases (see Chapter 2). The moderately T1-weighted coronal images provided additional localizing information and tissue characterization.

MR FINDINGS

Figure 11.1. A focal low-density and nonenhancing area is noted in the left occipital lobe. This corresponded to the area of acute hemorrhage 4 months earlier. The findings are compatible with a resolving hematoma.

Figures 11.2. In the same region shown by CT, the MR study demonstrates a focal area of increased signal intensity on both the first and second echos. This appearance is similar to the findings in Case 9—that is, hemorrhage with T1 shortening due to the presence of methemoglobin. This lesion has a low intensity rim, however, which becomes even lower in intensity on the second echo image (moderate T2 weighting). This finding indicates hemosiderin deposition around what can now be considered a chronic hematoma.[1]

Figure 11.3. The moderately T1-weighted coronal scan confirms the presence of central T1 shortening, which yields increased signal intensity.

DIFFERENTIAL DIAGNOSIS

The differential diagnostic considerations should be the various causes of parenchymal hemorrhage, including vascular malformation, aneurysm, tumor, hypertension, trauma, and bleeding disorders. In elderly patients, an additional cause of lobar hemorrhage is amyloid angiopathy. There is no MR evidence of a vascular malformation. A tumor was not demonstrated on the initial CT or on the MR; however, it is conceivable that a small tumor could be hidden within this hematoma. There is no history of hypertension, trauma, or coagulopathy. At the time of the MR scan, the etiology for the intracerebral hemorrhage was not known, and the patient was treated conservatively.

Final Diagnosis

Chronic intracerebral hematoma.

SUMMARY OF MR FINDINGS FOR INTRACEREBRAL HEMORRHAGE

The evolution of an intracranial hemorrhage (Table 11–1) may be divided into three phases:[2]

1. Acute
   a. Less than 3 days.
   b. Characterized by the presence of magnetically susceptible deoxyhemoglobin within intact RBCs, which causes preferential T2 shortening because of increased dephasing of diffusing water protons.
   c. Surrounding edema in the white matter.
2. Subacute
   a. Greater than 3 days but less than 1 month.
   b. Primarily characterized by the formation of paramagnetic methemoglobin[3] within the hematoma, which causes T1 shortening due to dipole–dipole interaction, enhancing proton relaxation.
   c. As methemoglobin is further oxidized[3] to nonparamagnetic substances (hemichromes), less pronounced T1 shortening can be attributed to hydration-layer water bound to protein.

Table 11–1. Intensities of Hematoma

	Hematoma		RIM	White Matter Edema
	Inner Core	Outer Core		
1. Acute				
a. T1WI	Iso	Iso	NP	Hypo
b. T2WI	Marked hypo	Marked hypo	NP	Hyper
2. Subacute				
a. T1WI	Iso	Marked hyper	NP	Hypo
b. T2WI	Variable	Hyper	NP/hypo	Hyper
3. Chronic				
a. T1WI	Hyper	Marked hyper	NP/hypo	Iso
b. T2WI	Hyper	Hyper	Marked hypo	Iso

Marked hypo = markedly hypointense compared with normal brain parenchyma.
Hypo = hypointense compared with normal brain parenchyma.
Iso = isointense compared with normal brain parenchyma.
Hyper = hyperintense compared with normal brain parenchyma.
Marked hyper = markedly hyperintense with normal brain parenchyma.
NP = not present.
T1WI = T1-weighted image.
T2WI = T2-weighted image.

Sources: Radiology (1985;157:87–93), Copyright © 1985, Radiological Society of North America, Inc; and *Magnetic Resonance Imaging* by CL Partain et al, WB Saunders Company, in press.

d. There is usually some residual edema in the surrounding white matter.
3. Chronic
   a. Greater than 1 month.
   b. The hematoma is increased in intensity on all pulsing sequences because of the presence of residual methemoglobin and proteinaceous material.
   c. The deposition of magnetically susceptible hemosiderin in macrophages surrounding the hematoma gives rise to the low intensity rim, which is most pronounced on T2-weighted images. This effect is best seen on higher field units; however, we have noted similar findings at 0.35 tesla (see Figure 11.4).
   d. Surrounding white matter edema resolves.

REFERENCES

1. Gomori JM, Grossman RI, Goldberg HI, et al: Intracranial hematomas: Imaging by high-field MR. *Radiology* 1985;157:87–93.

2. Bradley WG: MRI of intracranial hemorrhage, in Partain CL, Price RR, Patton JA, et al (eds): *Magnetic Resonance Imaging*. Philadelphia, Saunders, in press.

3. Bradley WG, Schmidt PG: Effect of methemoglobin formation on the MR appearance of subarachnoid hemorrhage. *Radiology* 1985; 156:99–103.

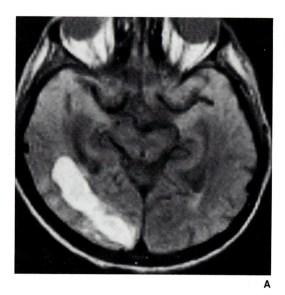

A

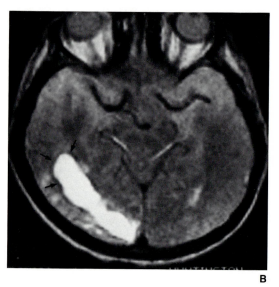

B

Figures 11.4A (SE 2000/28) and **11.4B** (SE 2000/56). Large, chronic right temporal–occipital hematoma. Note the low-intensity rim of hemosiderin, which is more pronounced on the second echo image (arrows).

CASE 12

HISTORY

A 70-year-old man presenting with a 1-month history of declining mental status. A CT study is shown in Figure 12.1.

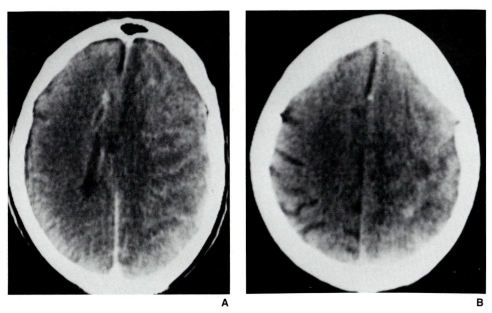

Figures 12.1A and **12.1B.** Enhanced CT examination at the level of the lateral ventricles (A) and the upper convexity (B). (Courtesy of Hans-Udo Juttner, MD, San Marino, CA.)

QUESTIONS

1. What are your differential considerations?

_____

_____

2. What MR techniques would you use?

	1	2	3
a. Coil	___	___	___
b. Centering point	___	___	___
c. Imaging plane(s)	___	___	___
d. Contrast	___	___	___
e. Slice thickness	___	___	___

3. What do you expect to find?

_____

_____

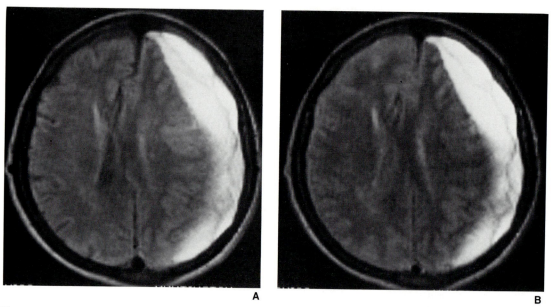

Figures 12.2A (SE 2000/28) and **12.2B** (SE 2000/56). Axial scans through the lateral ventricles.

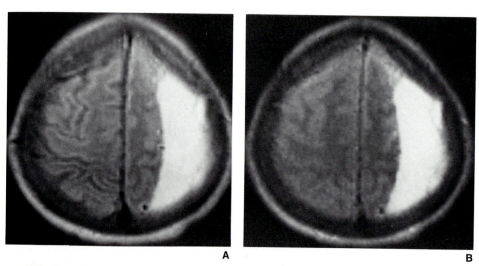

Figures 12.3A (SE 2000/28) and **12.3B** (SE 2000/56). Axial scans through the upper convexity.

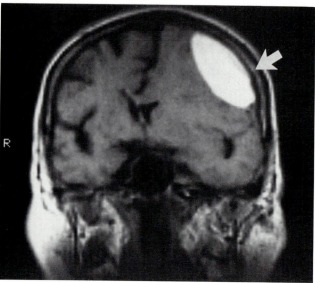

Figure 12.4 (SE 500/28). Coronal scan through the area of interest.

MR TECHNIQUES

	1	2
a. Coil	Head	Head
b. Centering point	CML	Midvertex
c. Imaging planes	Axial	Coronal
d. Contrast	Mild to moderate T2W	Moderate T1W
e. Slice thickness	Routine	Routine

The first sequence is a routine screening study using mild to moderate T2 weighting. This not only characterizes the CT abnormality but also provides sensitivity to the presence of associated parenchymal lesions. Moderate T1 weighting in the coronal sequence was used to define the longitudinal extent of the lesion and to detect the presence of paramagnetic methemoglobin.[1]

MR FINDINGS

Figure 12.1. There is obvious left-sided mass effect, manifested by ventricular deformity and a rightward midline shift. The left cerebral sulci are compressed and displaced from the inner table. An isodense, subacute subdural hematoma can be suspected but is poorly characterized in terms of size and extent. An irregular margin of contrast enhancement is due to an enhancing membrane.

Figures 12.2 and 12.3. A large, crescentic, extra-axial lesion between the dark calvarial inner table and brain parenchyma can readily be identified. The signal intensity of the lesion is increased on both the mildly (Figure 12.2A) and moderately (Figure 12.2B) T2-weighted images. This pattern is indicative of a proteinaceous fluid collection with T1 shortening due to the presence of methemoglobin.

Figure 12.4. The subdural collection is separated from the high signal of the diploic marrow (white arrow) by the low signal intensity of the inner table of the calvarium.

DIFFERENTIAL DIAGNOSIS

Differential diagnostic considerations include extra-axial fluid collections and masses. Epidural hematomas have a characteristic biconvex shape, and the displaced dura can readily be identified by MR. Subarachnoid hemorrhages appear less localized and extend into the surrounding sulci. Thus, the morphology and intensity of the lesion are most compatible with a subacute subdural hematoma.

Recognition of T1 shortening virtually excludes neoplasms and nonhemorrhagic fluid collections (i.e., effusions or empyemas).

Final Diagnosis

Subacute subdural hematoma.

SUMMARY OF MR FINDINGS FOR SUBDURAL HEMATOMA[1-4]

1. As with CT, extra-axial mass effect and crescentic shape are important distinguishing features.
2. The MR signal intensity pattern may help in characterizing the fluid content (also see discussion in Case 11 on the MR appearance of hematomas).
   a. Acute hemorrhage may have T2 shortening due to the presence of ferrous deoxyhemoglobin, resulting in decreased intensity on T2-weighted images.[2,3]
   b. Subacute blood contains paramagnetic methemoglobin,[1] which has a short T1 and appears bright on T1-weighted images. T1 shortening can be seen within two to five days of the onset of hemorrhage and will persist for weeks to months. Thus, hyperintensity due to T1 shortening is not necessarily an indication of "subacute" hemorrhage. Rather, it relates to a longer period of time during which the CT appearance of a hematoma may be of low, intermediate, or high density.
   c. After a period of weeks to months, the blood products within a "chronic" hematoma will be broken down to nonparamagnetic hemichromes.[1] Such hematomas have intermediate intensity because of the high protein content and hydration-layer water.[2]
   d. The T1-shortening effect of methemoglobin may be used to help distinguish a subdural hematoma from a subdural effusion. This distinction may have important therapeutic implications.
   e. CT is generally more effective in detecting acute hemorrhage and should be used during the first postictus week.

REFERENCES

1. Bradley WG, Schmidt PG: Effect of methemoglobin formation on the MR appearance of subarachnoid hemorrhage. *Radiology* 1985; 156:99–103.
2. Fullerton GD, Cameron IL, Ord VA: Frequency dependency of magnetic resonance spin-lattice relaxation of protons in biological materials. *Radiology* 1984;151:135–138.
3. Bradley WG: MRI of intracranial hemorrhage, in Partain CL, Price RR, Patton JA, et al (eds): *Magnetic Resonance Imaging*, ed 2. Philadelphia, WB Saunders Co, in press.
4. Gomori JM, Grossman RI, Goldberg HI, et al: Intracranial hematomas: Imaging by high-field MR. *Radiology* 1985;157:87–93.

CASE 13

HISTORY

While undergoing cardiac catheterization, this 41-year-old man suffered the acute onset of right hemiparesis, areflexia, and hemianesthesia. On the same day, an MR study was requested.

QUESTIONS

1. What are your differential considerations?

_____

_____

2. What MR techniques would you use?

	1	2	3
a. Coil	_____	_____	_____
b. Centering point	_____	_____	_____
c. Imaging plane(s)	_____	_____	_____
d. Contrast	_____	_____	_____
e. Slice thickness	_____	_____	_____

3. What do you expect to find?

_____

_____

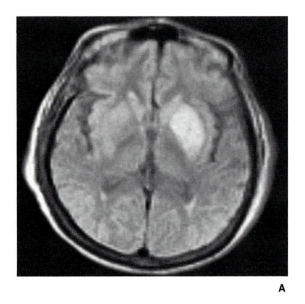 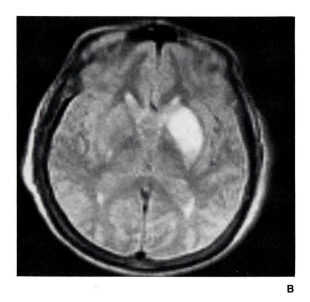

A

B

Figures 13.1A (SE 2000/30) and **13.1B** (SE 2000/60). Axial scans through the level of the basal ganglia.

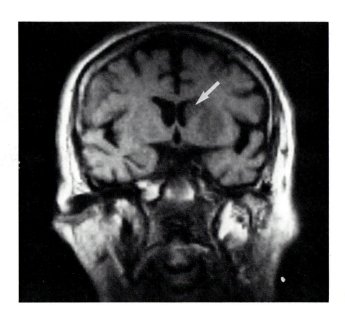

Figure 13.2 (SE 500/30). Coronal scan through the region of interest.

MR TECHNIQUES

		1	2
a.	Coil	Head	Head
b.	Centering point	CML	Midvertex
c.	Imaging planes	Axial	Coronal
d.	Contrast	Mild to moderate T2W	Moderate T1W
e.	Slice thickness	Routine	Routine

The first sequence is used for routine screening of CNS abnormalities. An additional moderately T1-weighted sequence in the coronal plane was used to provide more localizing information and tissue characterization.

MR FINDINGS

Figure 13.1. There is a well-defined, high intensity lesion involving the left anterior limb of the internal capsule and basal ganglia. There is mild mass effect. The lesion becomes more intense on the second echo image, indicating a prolonged T2. The remainder of the study was normal, except for a small hyperintense focus in the posterior limb of the right internal capsule. Is subacute hemorrhage (methemoglobin) present? Probably not. Since the T1 relaxation times would be shortened, the mildly T2-weighted image (first echo) would qualitatively have a higher signal intensity (compare with Case 10). Acute hemorrhage (less than 72 hours) would likely have been manifested as an area of T2 shortening. This effect is less apparent, however, on "low field" images.

Figure 13.2. This image demonstrates a focal area of low signal intensity within the affected region, as well as the head of the caudate nucleus (arrow). This is compatible with edema, which generally has prolonged T1 relaxation times compared with brain parenchyma. The absence of increased signal intensity argues against subacute hemorrhage. This confirmed our impression from the first sequence.

DIFFERENTIAL DIAGNOSIS

Since the intensity pattern is nonspecific, the differential diagnosis in the absence of clinical history would include vaso-occlusive, neoplastic, and inflammatory disease processes. In general, neoplasms and active inflammatory processes would produce a greater amount of surrounding vasogenic edema.

Given the history and the location of this lesion, a diagnosis of acute basal ganglia infarction can be made with confidence. The small right internal capsule lesion is probably a lacunar infarct of indeterminate chronicity.

Final Diagnosis

Acute cerebral infarct.

SUMMARY OF MR FINDINGS FOR ACUTE INFARCT[1,2]

1. Hyperacute infarcts produce cytotoxic edema. This causes intracellular swelling and decreased extracellular space. At the periphery of the infarct, the decreased extracellular space may limit the diffusion of vasogenic edema related to blood–brain barrier breakdown. As a result, sharply circumscribed borders are generally seen with acute infarcts. Prolongation of T2 is apparent within a few hours after onset of symptoms. Thus, within the first 24 hours, MRI is more sensitive than CT in the detection of infarcts.

2. As time progresses, vasogenic edema will predominate and the border of the lesion may become less well defined.

3. All forms of edema have prolonged T2 and are thus more intense on the second echo images. (Compare the intensity differences of the lesion in Figures 13.1A and 13.1B.)

4. Larger infarcts follow a vascular distribution and are often associated with mass effect.

REFERENCES

1. Bradley WG: Review: Magnetic resonance imaging of the central nervous system. *Neurol Res* 1984;6:91–106.

2. Flannigan BD, Bradley WG, Kortman KE, et al: MRI in cerebral infarction, in Rossi DR, Gerard G (eds): *Seminars in Neurology.* New York, Woodbury, in press.

CASE 14

HISTORY

A 53-year-old man with a 3-year history of left hemiparesis, slurred speech, and loss of memory.

QUESTIONS

1. What are your differential considerations?

   _____

   _____

2. What MR techniques would you use?

	1	2	3
a. Coil	____	____	____
b. Centering point	____	____	____
c. Imaging plane(s)	____	____	____
d. Contrast	____	____	____
e. Slice thickness	____	____	____

3. What do you expect to find?

   _____

   _____

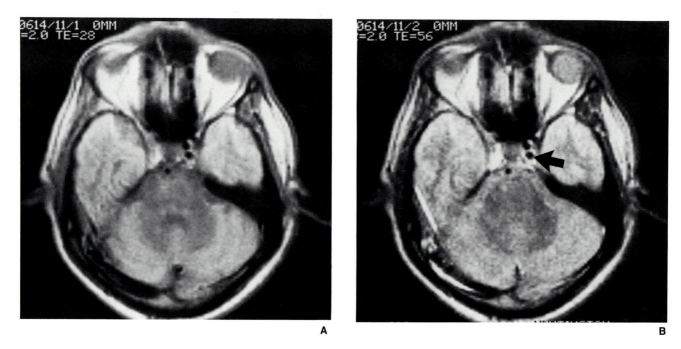

A

B

Figures 14.1A (SE 2000/28) and **14.1B** (SE 2000/56). Axial scans through the level of the cavernous sinuses. (Reprinted from Magnetic Resonance Annual 1986 (p 106) with permission of Raven Press, © 1986.)

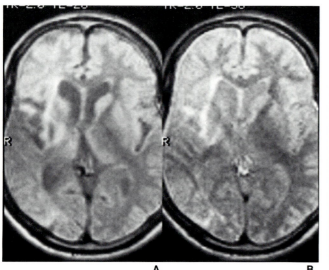

A   B

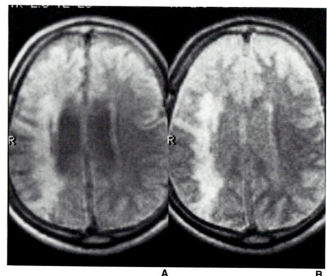

A   B

Figures 14.2A (SE 2000/28) and **14.2B** (SE 2000/56). Axial scans at the level of the basal ganglia.

Figures 14.3A (SE 2000/28) and **14.3B** (SE 2000/56). Axial scans through the superior margins of the lateral ventricular bodies.

MR TECHNIQUES

a. Coil   Head
b. Centering point   CML
c. Imaging plane   Axial
d. Contrast   Mild to moderate T2W
e. Slice thickness   Routine

This sequence is used for a general screening examination of the brain.

MR FINDINGS

Figure 14.1. The right internal carotid artery is completely thrombosed as indicated by the presence of a high signal within the lumen of the vessel. Patent arteries are characterized by the absence of signal produced by rapidly flowing blood (flow void phenomenon), as seen in the normal left internal carotid artery (black arrow).[1]

Figure 14.2 and 14.3. There are irregular high intensity areas within the right hemisphere, including the parietal and frontal lobes, the insular cortex, and the basal ganglia. Contiguous areas of focal atrophy (CSF intensity), best noted on the first echo images, are evident.

DIFFERENTIAL DIAGNOSIS

The MR findings are characteristic of a chronic cerebrovascular accident, and no other diagnoses need be considered.

Final Diagnosis

Chronic cerebrovascular accident (CVA) involving the right middle cerebral artery territory.

SUMMARY OF MR FINDINGS FOR CHRONIC CVA

1. Large chronic infarcts often have two different components:
   a. *Microcystic encephalomalacia* is characterized by hydration-layer water in small cysts within a zone of gliosis. A short T1 (relative to CSF) and long T2 (relative to normal brain parenchyma) result in high signal intensity on moderately T2-weighted images. This is well demonstrated in this case[2] and in Figure 14.4 from another patient.
   b. *Macrocystic encephalomalacia* is characterized by bulk phase water in large cystic regions and has an intensity similar to that of CSF. This is better demonstrated in Figures 14.4 and 14.5.
2. This two-zone appearance may not be seen in all chronic infarcts. Occasionally, only areas of CSF-like intensity may be seen with associated atrophy. Also

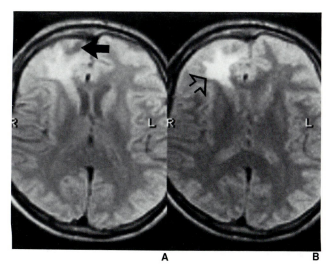

Figures 14.4A (SE 2000/28) and **14.4B** (SE 2000/56). Axial scans through the level of the basal ganglia from another patient with a chronic stroke. Note the zone of high intensity microcystic encephalomalacia (open arrow) and the more peripheral zone of CSF-intensity macrocystic encephalomalacia (solid arrow).

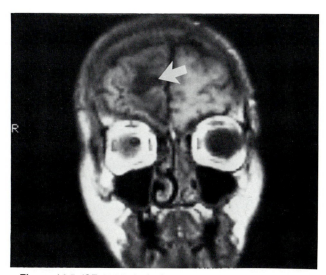

Figure 14.5 (SE 500/28). Corresponding T1-weighted coronal scan through the frontal lobes. Note the low signal focus (arrow) of CSF intensity corresponding to macrocystic encephalomalacia.

this two-zone appearance may not be readily apparent on heavily T2-weighted images, since both areas would have an increased signal intensity.

3. Rarely, alterations in signal intensity within major arterial structures may be seen, indicating slow flow or thrombosis.

REFERENCES

1. Bradley WG, Waluch V: Blood flow: Magnetic resonance imaging. *Radiology* 1985;154:443–450.
2. Flannigan BD, Bradley WG, Kortman KE, et al: MRI in cerebral infarction, in Rossi DR, Gerard G (eds): *Seminars in Neurology.* New York, Woodbury, in press.

CASE 15

HISTORY

A 74-year-old hypertensive woman presenting with a 6-month history of left hemiparesis and dizziness.

QUESTIONS

1. What are your differential considerations?

   _____

   _____

2. What MR techniques would you use?

	1	2	3
a. Coil	___	___	___
b. Centering point	___	___	___
c. Imaging plane(s)	___	___	___
d. Contrast	___	___	___
e. Slice thickness	___	___	___

3. What do you expect to find?

   _____

   _____

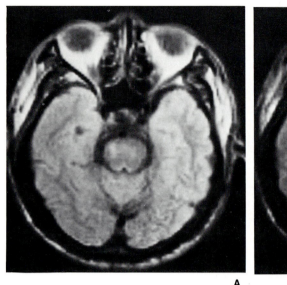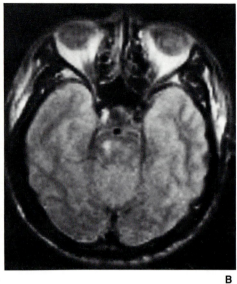

Figures 15.1A (SE 2000/28) and **15.1B** (SE 2000/56). Axial scans through the temporal lobes and brainstem.

A   B

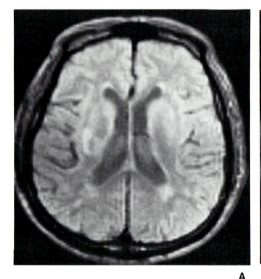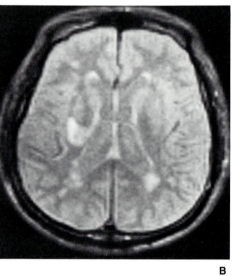

Figures 15.2A (SE 2000/28) and **15.2B** (SE 2000/56). Axial scans through the bodies of the lateral ventricles.

A   B

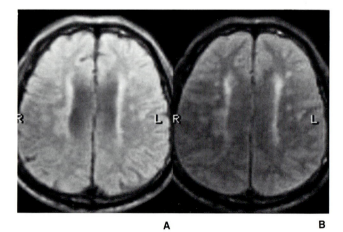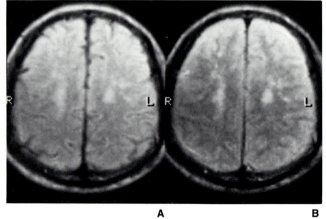

A   B   A   B

Figures 15.3A (SE 2000/28) and **15.3B** (SE 2000/56). Axial scans 1 cm superior to Figure 15.2.

Figures 15.4A (SE 2000/28) and **15.4B** (SE 2000/56). Axial scans at the supraventricular level.

MR TECHNIQUES

a. Coil   Head
b. Centering point   CML
c. Imaging plane   Axial
d. Contrast   Mild to moderate T2W
e. Slice thickness   Routine

This sequence is a standard routine screening examination of the brain.

MR FINDINGS

Figure 15.1. Multiple upper-pontine high intensity foci (more prominent on the right) are shown.

Figure 15.2. Similar foci are found in the posterior limb of the right internal capsule and the adjacent basal ganglia.

Figures 15.3 and 15.4. There are extensive, predominately confluent, periventricular, high intensity foci that extend into the centrum semiovale superiorly (Figure 15.4).

DIFFERENTIAL DIAGNOSIS

In view of the patient's clinical history and the MR findings, the most likely diagnosis is chronic deep infarcts. The differential diagnosis in this case is limited. The most important diagnosis to exclude is *multiple sclerosis (MS)*. It would be unusual for MS to present in this age group, and the history is not compatible with that diagnosis. The pattern of white matter involvement has some features of MS,[1] especially the focal lesions in the periventricular white matter and within the brainstem. On the other hand, the symmetric, predominately confluent, increased signal intensity along the bodies of the lateral ventricles (Figure 15.3: compare with Case 1) is more consistent with an ischemic etiology. These rules are not foolproof, and the MR findings should not be interpreted without the clinical history.

Final Diagnosis

1. Deep white matter infarcts.
2. Lacunar infarcts of the right basal ganglia and internal capsule.
3. Vertebrobasilar infarcts.

SUMMARY OF MR FINDINGS

1. Deep White Matter Infarcts

a. Multiple high intensity foci, predominately confluent and symmetrically distributed within the periventricular white matter, are seen on T2-weighted images. These findings become more marked with increasing age, and the process is accelerated in patients with risk factors for cerebrovascular disease.[1] The term *infarcts* is used advisedly, as abnormalities in this distribution are seldom associated with acute clinical events. Further, to some degree these findings can be regarded as "normal" involutional changes of advancing age.

b. Extensive periventricular infarction may produce progressive dementia, or so-called subcortical arteriosclerotic encephalopathy (SAE).[2,3]

2. Vertebrobasilar and Basal Ganglia Infarcts

Lesions of the basal ganglia are more likely to be lacunar infarcts and are less characteristic of MS. The vertebrobasilar infarcts cannot be differentiated from MS plaques. Therefore, the history should take precedence.

REFERENCES

1. Kortman KE, Bradley WG, Rauch RA, et al: Multiple sclerosis versus cerebral vascular disease: Differentiation by MRI. *AJR,* publication pending.

2. Brant-Zawadzki M, Gein G, Van Dyke C, et al: MR imaging of the aging brain: Patchy white-matter lesions and dementia. *AJNR* 1985; 6:675–682.

3. Bradley WG, Waluch V, Brant-Zawadzki M, et al: Patchy, periventricular white matter lesions in the elderly: A common observation during NMR imaging. *Noninvasive Medical Imaging* 1984;1:35–41.

CASE 16

HISTORY

A 73-year-old man who suffered perioperative hypotension 3 years ago presenting now with memory loss and visual problems.

QUESTIONS

1. What are your differential considerations?

_____

_____

2. What MR techniques would you use?

	1	2	3
a. Coil	___	___	___
b. Centering point	___	___	___
c. Imaging plane(s)	___	___	___
d. Contrast	___	___	___
e. Slice thickness	___	___	___

3. What do you expect to find?

_____

_____

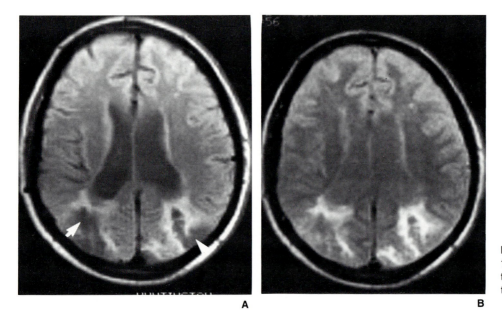

Figures 16.1A (SE 2000/28) and 16.1B (SE 2000/56). Axial scans through the bodies of the lateral ventricles.

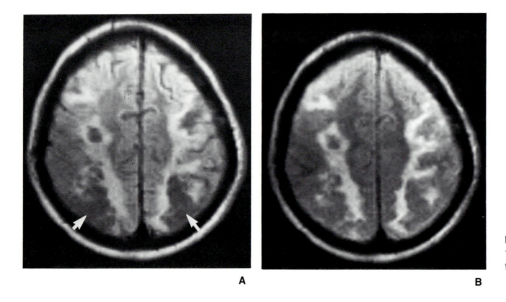

Figures 16.2A (SE 2000/28) and 16.2B (SE 2000/56). Axial scans through the supraventricular region.

MR TECHNIQUES

a. Coil — Head
b. Centering point — CML
c. Imaging plane — Axial
d. Contrast — Mild to moderate T2W
e. Slice thickness — Routine

This sequence is the routine screening sequence for CNS abnormalities.

MR FINDINGS

Figure 16.1 and 16.2. There are coarse, symmetric, and confluent high intensity lesions primarily involving the white matter of the occipital and parietal lobes, between the distribution of the anterior, middle, and posterior cerebral arteries. These lesions have higher intensity on the second echo images, indicating a long T2 compared with brain parenchyma, and are consistent with *microcystic encephalomalacia*. The high intensity areas border more peripheral regions of CSF intensity (white arrows), the latter compatible with *macrocystic encephalomalacia* (see Case 14).

DIFFERENTIAL DIAGNOSIS

The clinical history of hypotension and the MR findings of mixed intensity lesions located between vascular distributions are characteristic of watershed infarcts. The symmetry of the lesions and associated atrophy argue against a multifocal neoplastic process. Chronic inflammatory disease ("burned-out" encephalitis) could result in similar findings, but the clinical history is not compatible with that diagnosis.

Final Diagnosis

Watershed infarcts secondary to hypotension.

SUMMARY OF MR FINDINGS FOR WATERSHED INFARCT

1. Symmetric areas of abnormal signal intensity located in the expected watershed areas between the anterior, middle, and posterior cerebral artery distributions.
2. Chronic infarcts of sufficient size often result in microcystic and macrocystic encephalomalacia, as demonstrated in this case.[1] (See also Case 14.)
3. There is often a history of hypotension and/or hypoperfusion. Common etiologies include cardiac arrest and complications related to cardiopulmonary bypass.

REFERENCES

1. Flannigan BD, Bradley WG, Kortman KE, et al: MRI in cerebral infarction, in Rossi DR, Gerald G (eds): *Seminars in Neurology*. New York, Woodbury, in press.

CASE 17

HISTORY

A 28-year-old woman with fever, nuchal rigidity, and altered mental status.

QUESTIONS

1. What are your differential considerations?

_____

_____

2. What MR techniques would you use?

	1	2	3
a. Coil	_____	_____	_____
b. Centering point	_____	_____	_____
c. Imaging plane(s)	_____	_____	_____
d. Contrast	_____	_____	_____
e. Slice thickness	_____	_____	_____

3. What do you expect to find?

_____

_____

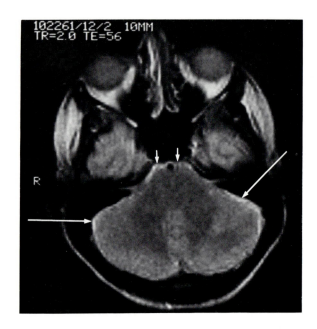 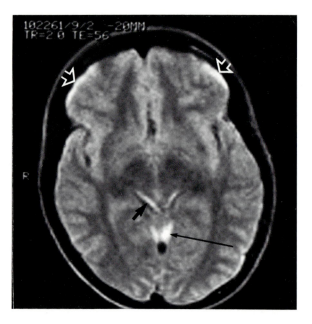

Figure 17.1 (SE 2000/56). Axial scan at the level of the cerebello-pontine angle.

Figure 17.2 (SE 2000/56). Axial scan 3 cm superior to Figure 17.1. (Reprinted with permission from Neurological Research (1984;6:91–106), Copyright © 1984, Butterworth Scientific Ltd.) from Magnetic Resonance Annual 1986 (p 106) with permission of Raven Press, © 1986.)

MR TECHNIQUES

a.	Coil	Head
b.	Centering point	CML
c.	Imaging plane	Axial
d.	Contrast	Mild to moderate T2W
e.	Slice thickness	Routine

This is the standard screening sequence with mild to moderate T2 weighting to maximize sensitivity. In this demonstration case, only the moderately T2-weighted second echo images are shown.

MR FINDINGS

Figure 17.1. Symmetric but abnormal linear high signal is seen along the lateral aspect of the cerebellar hemispheres (long white arrows) and the anterior aspect of the pons (short white arrows).

Figure 17.2. Similar bands of increased signal intensity are noted along the periphery of the frontal lobes (open white arrows) and also in the quadrigeminal plate cistern (short black arrow) and pineal cistern (long black arrow).

DIFFERENTIAL DIAGNOSIS

The findings are consistent with a diffuse meningeal or subarachnoid process. Subarachnoid hemorrhage could produce similar findings. However, the high intensity areas were less conspicuous on first echo images (not shown), indicating that T1 was not shortened and arguing against subacute bleeding. Both inflammation (meningitis) and neoplastic disease (leptomeningeal carcinomatosis) produce thickening and edema of the meninges, and either process could produce the findings in this case. There was no history of primary malignancy, and CSF analysis was consistent with an inflammatory process.

Final Diagnosis

Infectious meningitis.

SUMMARY OF MR FINDINGS FOR MENINGITIS[1]

1. Diffuse meningeal high intensity on T2-weighted images.
2. Complications include obstructive hydrocephalus, abscess formation, and deep infarcts related to spasm or occlusion of penetrating arteries of the skull base.

REFERENCE

1. Bradley WG: Review: Magnetic resonance imaging of the central nervous system. *Neurol Res* 1984;6:91–106.

CASE 18

HISTORY

A 25-year-old Hispanic man presented with a new onset of grand mal seizures. The patient was a frequent traveler to Mexico. The admitting contrast-enhanced CT is shown in Figure 18.1.

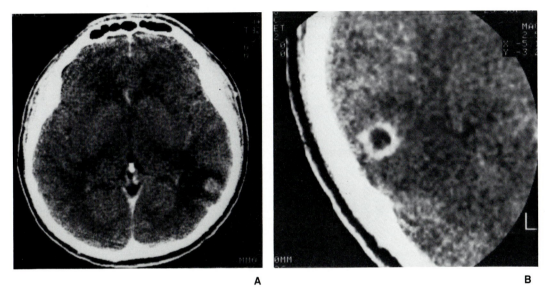

A   **B**

Figures 18.1A and **18.1B.** (A) Enhanced axial CT through the temporal lobes. (B) A magnified view from the same study 10 mm superior to Fig. 18.1A. (Courtesy of Michael Anselmo, MD, Glendale, CA.)

QUESTIONS

1. What are your differential considerations?

   _____

   _____

2. What MR techniques would you use?

	1	2	3
a. Coil	—	—	—
b. Centering point	—	—	—
c. Imaging planes	—	—	—
d. Contrast	—	—	—
e. Slice thickness	—	—	—

3. What do you expect to find?

   _____

   _____

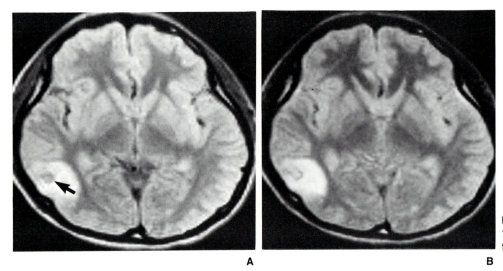

Figures 18.2A (SE 2000/28) and **18.2B** (SE 2000/56). Axial scans through the temporal lobes.

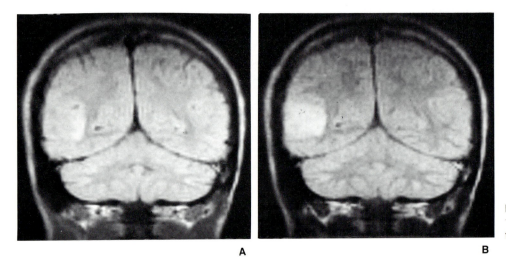

Figures 18.3A (SE 1000/28) and **18.3B** (SE 1000/56). Coronal scans through the region of interest.

MR TECHNIQUES

	1	2
a. Coil	Head	Head
b. Centering point	CML	Posterior cranium
c. Imaging planes	Axial	Coronal
d. Contrast	Mild to moderate T2W	Mild T1W/ mild T2W
e. Slice thickness	Routine	Routine

The first pulsing sequence is for routine cerebral screening. The second sequence provides additional localizing information and tissue characterization. In retrospect, greater T1 weighting may have yielded more information.

MR FINDINGS

Figure 18.1. The CT demonstrates a small, peripheral enhancing mass in the posterior right temporal lobe. The center of the mass is of low attenuation and probably fluid filled. There is surrounding white matter edema.

Figure 18.2. On the T2-weighted MR study, a well-defined area of increased signal intensity is noted in the corresponding area and is consistent with edema. Within this area is a low-signal central nidus that increases in intensity on the second echo (black arrow).

Figure 18.3. On the coronal images with more T1 weighting, abnormalities appear more homogeneous and the central nidus cannot be separated from the surrounding edema. If greater T1 weighting had been used, it is conceivable that the cyst may have had a lower signal intensity than the surrounding edema by virtue of differences in their respective T1 relaxation values.

The CT appearance of the central nidus is compatible with a cystic lesion. The differentiation of cystic and solid masses is more difficult on MR, although most cysts can be recognized by their typical intensity patterns[1]—prolonged T1 and T2 with CSF-like intensity (see arachnoid cyst, Case 2). However, the intensity of proteinaceous cysts is greater than that of CSF, primarily because of shorter T1 times. Therefore, distinguishing between a proteinaceous cyst and a solid lesion may not be straightforward.

The typical pattern of surrounding edema, producing low density on CT and increased signal on MR, is also seen.

DIFFERENTIAL DIAGNOSIS

The differential diagnosis of a solitary cystic mass would include both neoplastic and inflammatory processes. On the basis of MR findings alone, distinguishing between these entities may not be possible; therefore, the specificity of the findings in this instance is low. The CT and clinical history were helpful in this case. A diagnosis of cysticercosis was . made and confirmed by CSF titers.

Final Diagnosis

Parenchymal cysticercosis.

SUMMARY OF MR FINDINGS FOR PARENCHYMAL CYSTICERCOSIS[1–3]

1. The parenchymal form of cysticercosis accounts for approximately 80% of the cases.[1]
2. Pathologically, the cysts usually measure approximately 1 cm in diameter and contain clear fluid and a scolex. The signal intensity of such cysts is similar to that of CSF and reflects the low protein content.
3. Since the living cysticerci incite minimal host response, symptoms are not usually present until an inflammatory host reaction occurs following the death of the scolex. This stage is characterized by surrounding edema with mass effect (as seen in this case). Contrast enhancement on CT can be seen. The cyst fluid can become turbid and gel-like in consistency because of an increased protein content. As a result, on T2-weighted images the cyst's signal intensity will be greater than that of CSF. A well-defined, inflammatory fibrous capsule due to the host response may form. (An example of this capsule can be seen in another patient with surgically proven cysticercosis; see Figure 18.4).
4. The acute inflammatory stage of the illness will therefore have a central nidus with a high intensity peripheral zone of edema on T2-weighted images. On the basis of the MR findings alone, distinguishing this lesion from a primary or secondary tumor may be difficult.
5. Later the edema and host reaction are replaced by small (1 to 4 mm) punctate calcifications and gliosis. These calcifications may not be detectable on MR studies.
6. Other sites of involvement, including ventricular cysts (Figure 18.5) and basal cisternal (racemose) cysts (Figure 18.6), can also be seen.

REFERENCES

1. Byrd SE, Locke GE, Biggers S, et al: The computed tomographic appearance of cerebral cysticercosis in adults and children. *Radiology* 1982;144:819–823.
2. Handler LC, Mervis B: Cerebral cysticercosis with reference to the natural history of parenchymal lesions. *AJNR* 1983;4:709–712.
3. Suss RA, Maravilla KR, Thompson J: MR imaging of intracranial cysticercosis: Comparison with CT and anatomopathologic features. *AJNR* 1986;7:235–242.

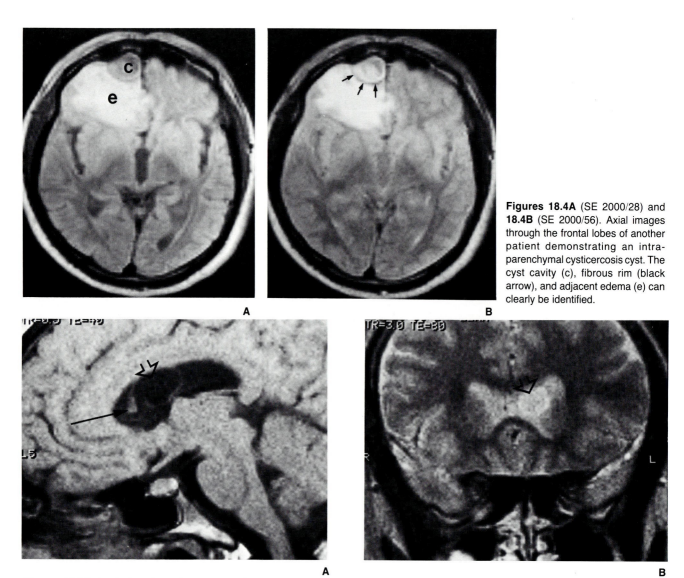

Figures 18.4A (SE 2000/28) and **18.4B** (SE 2000/56). Axial images through the frontal lobes of another patient demonstrating an intraparenchymal cysticercosis cyst. The cyst cavity (c), fibrous rim (black arrow), and adjacent edema (e) can clearly be identified.

Figures 18.5A (sagittal moderate T1-weighted, SE 500/40) and **18.5B** (coronal heavy T2-weighted, SE 3000/80). Images demonstrating an intraventricular cysticercosis cyst. The cyst contents (open arrow) are similar in intensity to CSF on all pulsing sequences. The sagittal view shows the scolex (closed arrow) and a more faintly seen cyst wall that extends into the body of the lateral ventricle.

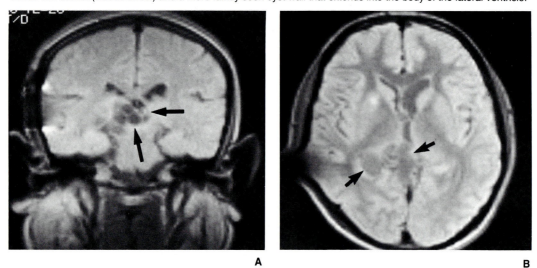

Figures 18.6A (coronal, SE 1000/28) and **18.6B** (axial, SE 2000/28). Multiple discrete proteinaceous cysts (arrows) can be seen throughout the quadrigeminal plate, supravermian, and pineal cisterns.

106

CASE 19

HISTORY

A 32-year-old man presented with a 5-month history of intermittent optic neuritis, extremity weakness, and numbness.

QUESTIONS

1. What are your differential considerations?

   _____

   _____

2. What MR techniques would you use?

	1	2	3
a. Coil			
b. Centering point			
c. Imaging planes			
d. Contrast			
e. Slice thickness			

3. What do you expect to find?

   _____

   _____

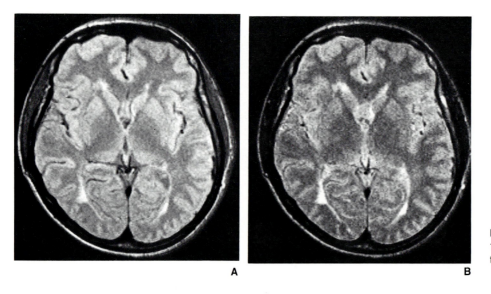

A   B

Figures 19.1A (SE 2000/40) and
19.1B (SE 2000/80). Axial scans
through the basal ganglia.

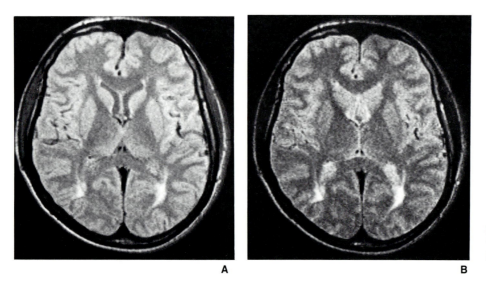

A   B

Figures 19.2A (SE 2000/40) and
19.2B (SE 2000/80). Axial scans
5 mm superior to Figure 19.1.

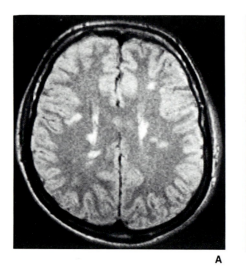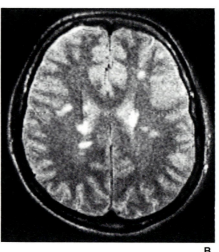

A   B

Figures 19.3A (SE 2000/40) and
19.3B (SE 2000/80). Axial scans
through the superior lateral ventricular bodies.

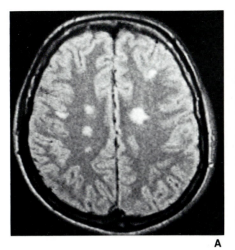
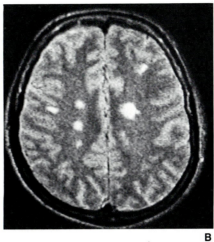

A   B

Figures 19.4A (SE 2000/40) and **19.4B** (SE 2000/80). Axial sections through the centrum semiovale.

MR TECHNIQUES

a.	Coil	Head
b.	Centering point	CML
c.	Imaging plane	Axial
d.	Contrast	Mild to moderate T2W
e.	Slice thickness	Thin

The axial plane is used as a standard imaging plane for screening most CNS abnormalities. Mild to moderate T2 weighting provides the best sensitivity for detecting demyelinating diseases.[1] Thin slices were used to minimize partial volume averaging of small lesions.

MR FINDINGS

Figures 19.1 through 19.4. There are multiple high intensity foci within the deep white matter. The pattern of involvement within the occipital poles is predominately confluent and extends to the region adjacent to the atria. Small punctate foci are seen adjacent to the frontal horn tips. Superiorly, the involvement in the periventricular white matter is predominately multifocal. All the lesions become more apparent with greater T2 weighting. Additional foci were noted in the brainstem (not shown).

DIFFERENTIAL DIAGNOSIS

Based upon the clinical history and the MR findings, the most likely diagnosis is MS. Other differential diagnostic considerations should include:

1. *Deep white matter infarcts.* These lesions are usually seen in patients who are elderly or have risk factors for cerebrovascular disease. Morphologically, these lesions are usually more confluent and less focal in the periventricular white matter, and there are fewer posterior fossa lesions[2] (see Cases 1 and 15). Other causes

of white matter infarcts include vasculitis and radiation therapy.

2. *Leukodystrophies.* Other forms of demyelinating or dysmyelinating disease may be considered. Clinical history may help to exclude these entities.[3]

3. Structural lesions: *foramen magnum masses, syringomyelia,* and/or *Arnold-Chiari malformations* may also present with these clinical symptoms, but these can easily be distinguished by MRI (see Case 3).

Final Diagnosis

Multiple sclerosis.

SUMMARY OF MR FINDINGS FOR MULTIPLE SCLEROSIS[1-4]

1. Multifocal high intensity lesions distributed in the periventricular white matter, brainstem, and cerebellum. There is a predilection for these lesions to involve the occipital poles and lateral atrial regions.[4]

2. The intensity of these lesions is characteristically greater on the second echo images, signifying a long T2.

3. Large acute lesions may produce mass effect.

4. The degree of involvement seen on MRI may correlate poorly with the severity of the clinical symptoms.

REFERENCES

1. Maravilla KR, Weinreb JC, Suss R, et al: Magnetic resonance demonstration of multiple sclerosis plaques in the cervical cord. *AJR* 1985;144:381–385.

2. Jackson JA, Leake DR, Schneiders NJ, et al: Magnetic resonance imaging in multiple sclerosis: Results in 32 cases. *AJNR* 1985;6:171–176.

3. Sheldon JJ, Siddharthan R, Tobias J, et al: MR imaging of multiple sclerosis: Comparison with clinical and CT examinations in 74 patients. *AJNR* 1985;6:683–690.

4. Kortman KE, Bradley WG, Rauch RA, et al: Multiple sclerosis versus cerebral vascular disease: Differentiation by MRI. *AJR*, publication pending.

CASE 20

HISTORY

A 42-year-old woman presented with internuclear ophthalmoplegia and an abnormal brainstem evoked response. The patient carried a clinical diagnosis of MS.

QUESTIONS

1. What MR techniques would you use?

		1	2	3
a.	Coil	____	____	____
b.	Centering point	____	____	____
c.	Imaging plane(s)	____	____	____
d.	Contrast	____	____	____
e.	Slice thickness	____	____	____

2. What do you expect to find?

_____

_____

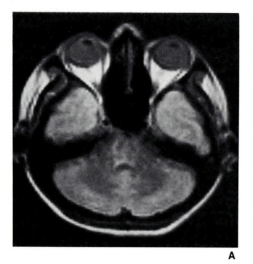
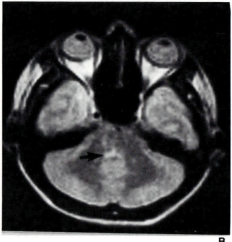

A

B

Figures 20.1A (SE 2000/28) and **20.1B** (SE 2000/56). Axial scans through the temporal lobes and brainstem.

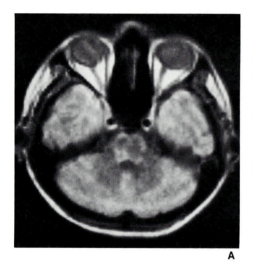
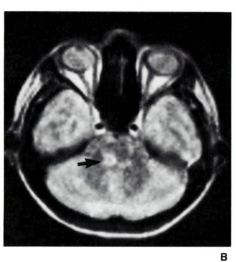

A

B

Figures 20.2A (SE 2000/28) and **20.2B** (SE 2000/56). Axial scans 1 cm superior to Figure 20.1.

MR TECHNIQUES

a. Coil — Head
b. Centering point — CML
c. Imaging plane — Axial
d. Contrast — Mild to moderate T2W
e. Slice thickness — Thin

The axial plane is used as a standard imaging plane for screening most CNS abnormalities. Mild to moderate T2 weighting provides the best sensitivity for detecting demyelinating diseases.[1,2] Thin slices are used to detect lesions that may be small (2 to 3 mm) but symptomatic by virtue of their position.

MR FINDINGS

Figures 20.1 and 20.2. There is a well-defined, discrete, high intensity lesion located in the right parasagittal posterior pons, in the expected position of the medial longitudinal fasciculus (MLF) (black arrows).

DIFFERENTIAL DIAGNOSIS

The appearance of the lesion is nonspecific and consistent with either an *MS plaque*, a *brainstem infarct*, or a small *tumor*. Given the clinical history and the presence of other lesions in the periventricular white matter (not shown), however, the lesion most likely represents a demyelinating plaque.

Final Diagnosis

Internuclear ophthalmoplegia secondary to MS involvement of the MLF.

SUMMARY OF MR FINDINGS FOR INTERNUCLEAR OPHTHALMOPLEGIA AND OTHER BRAINSTEM SYMPTOM COMPLEXES

The location of brainstem lesions may be closely correlated with clinical deficits. This requires a working knowledge of the position of major tracts and nuclei.[3,4] The MLF coordinates the oculomotor, trochlear, and abducens nuclei, which are essential for conjugate eye movements. It is located just off the midline near the floor of the fourth ventricle, extending from the medulla to the midbrain. This structure is often involved in patients with MS.

Comments

CT is limited in the evaluation of brainstem pathology, largely because of the presence of streak artifacts in the posterior fossa. Small lesions (infarcts, demyelinating plaques, focal hemorrhages) are readily demonstrated by MR, even in the absence of mass effect. The exact location of a lesion and its relation to specific nuclei and tracts are well demonstrated, allowing correlation with clinical signs and symptoms. Figure 20.3 is an example in another patient with MS who presented with trigeminal neuralgia. There are focal demyelinating plaques involving the trigeminal nuclei bilaterally. Additional focal plaques can also be seen within the cervical cord in Figure 20.4.[5]

REFERENCES

1. Bradley WG: Fundamentals of MR image interpretation, in Bradley WG, Adey WR, Hasso AN (eds): *Magnetic Resonance Imaging of the Brain, Head and Neck: A Text Atlas.* Rockville, Md, Aspen Systems, 1985, pp 6–12.

2. Brant-Zawadzki M, Norman D, Newton TH, et al: Magnetic resonance of the brain: The optimal screening technique. *Radiology* 1984; 152:71–77.

3. Flannigan BD, Bradley WG, Mazziotta JC, et al: Magnetic resonance imaging of the brainstem: Normal structure and basic functional anatomy. *Radiology* 1985;154:375–383.

4. Clark RG: Brain stem, in *Manter and Gatz's Essentials of Clinical Neuroanatomy and Neurophysiology*, ed 5. Philadelphia, FA Davis Co, 1975, pp 55–57.

5. Sheldon JJ, Siddharthan R, Tobias J, et al: MR imaging of multiple sclerosis: Comparison with clinical and CT examinations in 74 patients. *AJNR* 1985;6:683–690.

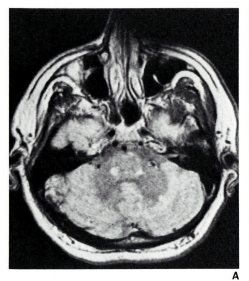
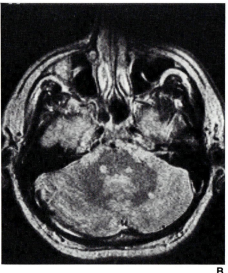

Figures 20.3A (SE 2000/40) and **20.3B** (SE 2000/80). Thin section through the pons demonstrating MS plaques within the trigeminal nuclei bilaterally.

A

B

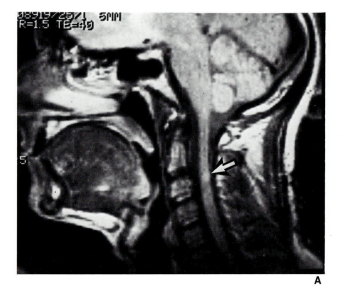
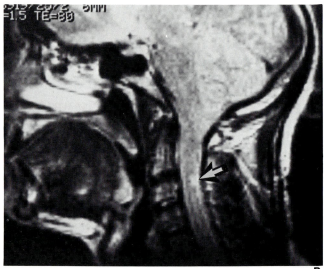

A

B

Figures 20.4A (SE 1500/40) and **20.4B** (SE 1500/80). Sagittal section of the cervical cord. The arrows indicate a focal MS plaque.

CASE 21

HISTORY

A 55-year-old man with progressive dementia.

QUESTIONS

1. What are your differential considerations?

   _____

   _____

2. What MR techniques would you use?

	1	2	3
a. Coil	___	___	___
b. Centering point	___	___	___
c. Imaging plane(s)	___	___	___
d. Contrast	___	___	___
e. Slice thickness	___	___	___

3. What do you expect to find?

   _____

   _____

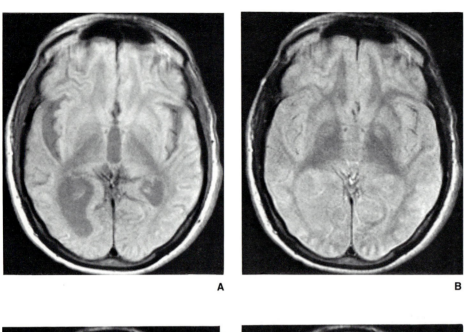

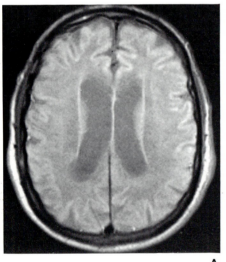
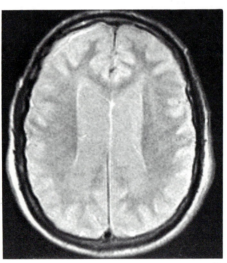

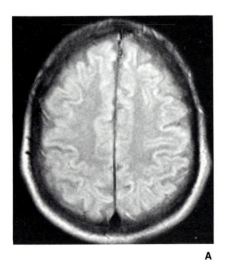
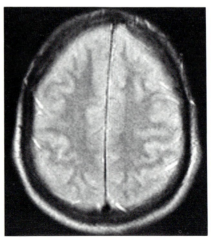

Figures 21.1A (SE 2000/30) and **21.1B** (SE 2000/60). Axial scans through the third ventricle.

A   B

Figures 21.2A (SE 2000/30) and **21.2B** (SE 2000/60). Axial scans through the bodies of the lateral ventricles.

A   B

Figures 21.3A (SE 2000/30) and **21.3B** (SE 2000/60). Axial scans through the parietal convexities.

A   B

116

MR TECHNIQUES

a. Coil — Head
b. Centering point — CML
c. Imaging plane — Axial
d. Contrast — Mild to moderate T2W
e. Slice thickness — Routine

This sequence is the routine screening exam for CNS diseases.

MR FINDINGS

Figures 21.1 through 21.3. There is evidence of cerebral atrophy, out of keeping with the patient's age, represented by the proportionate enlargement of the CSF spaces. Periventricular interstitial (transependymal) edema, which might be seen with elevated pressure hydrocephalus (see Case 33), is absent. There is also a paucity of parenchymal lesions, such as might be seen with extensive deep white matter infarction (see Cases 15 and 22) or cortical infarction (see Case 14).

The cortical sulci and ventricles are better defined on the first echo axial images than on the second echo images. This contrast pattern reflects the long T1 and T2 of CSF. CSF becomes isointense with the brain parenchyma on the second echo axial images because of the opposing effects of T1 and T2 prolongation. With heavy T2 weighting, the CSF will become more intense than the brain parenchyma (see Case 18).

DIFFERENTIAL DIAGNOSIS

The findings are characteristic of diffuse cortical atrophy. The causes of cortical atrophy are extensive and include trauma; ischemia; hypoxia; metabolic causes, such as chemotherapy and alcoholism; inflammation, including demyelinating diseases; infections such as encephalitis; and idiopathic causes such as Alzheimer's disease.[1] The lack of parenchymal lesions would exclude many of these etiologies. The findings described are consistent with but not specific for Alzheimer's disease. In our experience and that of others,[2,3] MR examination of these patients reveals atrophy without significant focal abnormalities such as periventricular white matter lesions. This is a helpful differentiating feature since patients with non-Alzheimer's dementia generally have increased periventricular white matter lesions when compared with age-matched controls.[4] Thus, MRI may be used to confirm a clinical diagnostic impression in patients with dementia. Obviously, clinical information must take precedence over imaging studies, as atrophy and deep white matter changes may be seen as "incidental" findings in non-demented elderly patients.

Final Diagnosis

Diffuse cortical atrophy consistent with Alzheimer's disease.

Comment

A generalized decrease in cerebral parenchyma is most often seen as an involutional change related to normal aging. Distinction between normal involutional change and clinically significant "atrophy" is a matter of judgment and/or semantics. Focal cerebral atrophy is most often due to a prior localized parenchymal insult, such as trauma, prior surgery, stroke, or inflammation. In addition to focal prominence of the adjacent CSF spaces, MRI frequently demonstrates alteration of normal parenchymal intensity, most often in a nonspecific pattern.

Cerebellar atrophy is frequently seen in conjunction with cerebral atrophy. Preferential or isolated cerebellar atrophy can be idiopathic but can also be seen in alcoholics, patients on diphenylhydantoin, and those affected by a paraneoplastic syndrome. There are a number of primary cerebellar degenerative diseases that may result in cerebellar atrophy. One of these is olivopontocerebellar degeneration, which results in striking atrophy of the pons and medulla in addition to the cerebellum.[5,6] An example is shown in Figures 21.4 through 21.6.

SUMMARY OF MR FINDINGS FOR ALZHEIMER'S DISEASE

1. Diffuse, proportionate cortical atrophy greater than expected for the patient's age.
2. The lack of parenchymal lesions may help in distinguishing this disease from other causes of dementia, such as normal pressure hydrocephalus or multi-infarct dementia.
3. Cortical atrophy may show rapid progression on serial examinations.

REFERENCES

1. Haughton VM: Hydrocephalus and atrophy, in Williams AL, Haughton VM (eds): *Cranial Computed Tomography. A Comprehensive Text.* St. Louis, CV Mosby Co, 1985, pp 240–256.
2. Friedland RP, Budinger TF, Brant-Zawadzki M, et al: The diagnosis of Alzheimer-type dementia: A preliminary comparison of PET and proton NMR imaging. *JAMA* 1985;252:2750–2752.
3. Erkinjuntti T, Sipponen JT, Iivanainen M, et al: Cerebral NMR and CT imaging in dementia. *J Comput Assist Tomogr* 1984;8:614–618.
4. Brant-Zawadzki M, Fein G, Van Dyke C, et al: MR imaging of the aging brain: Patchy white-matter lesions and dementia. *AJNR* 1985; 6:675–682.
5. Oppenheimer DR: Diseases of the basal ganglia, cerebellum and motor neurons, in Blackwood W, Corsellis J (eds): *Greenfields neuropathology.* London, Arnold, 1976, pp 622–632.
6. Rothman SLG, Glanz S: Cerebellar atrophy: The differential diagnosis by computerized tomography. *Neuroradiology* 1977;16:123–126.

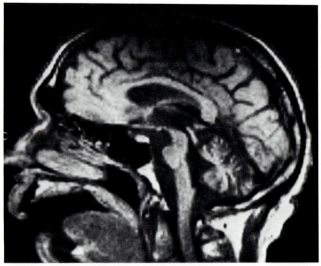

Figure 21.4 (SE 500/40). T1-weighted midsagittal section demonstrating striking atrophy of the brainstem and cerebellum.

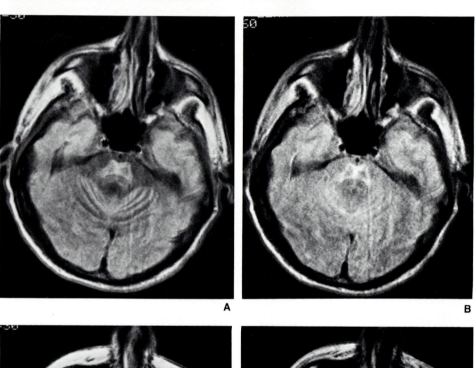

A   B

Figures 21.5A (SE 2000/30) and 21.5B (SE 2000/60). Axial sections through the pons demonstrating marked brainstem atrophy and prominence of the cerebellar sulci. The peripheral and midline pattern of pontine high intensity on the second echo image may reflect changes in water content related to neuronal degeneration.

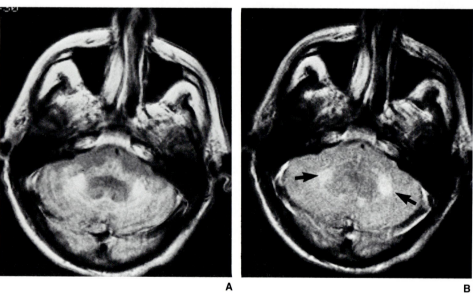

A   B

Figures 21.6A (SE 2000/30) and 21.6B (SE 2000/60). More inferiorly, there is a similar pattern of atrophy. Focal high intensity can be seen within the dentate nuclei bilaterally (arrows).

CASE 22

HISTORY

A 70-year-old man presenting with confusion and gait disturbance. A CT scan demonstrated prominent ventricles.

QUESTIONS

1. What are your differential considerations?
   _____
   _____

2. What MR techniques would you use?

	1	2	3
a. Coil	_____	_____	_____
b. Centering point	_____	_____	_____
c. Imaging plane(s)	_____	_____	_____
d. Contrast	_____	_____	_____
e. Slice thickness	_____	_____	_____

3. What do you expect to find?
   _____
   _____

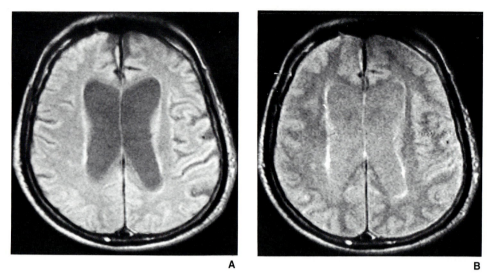

Figures 22.1A (SE 2000/30) and **22.1B** (SE 2000/60). Transaxial sections through the lateral ventricles.

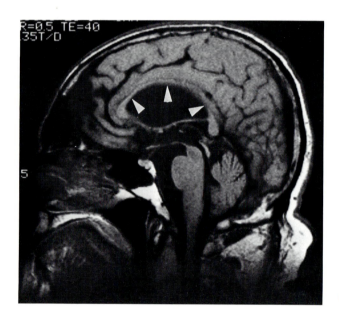

Figure 22.2 (SE 500/40). T1-weighted midsagittal section.

MR TECHNIQUES

	1	2
a. Coil	Head	Head
b. Centering point	Axial	Sagittal
c. Imaging planes	CML	Midsagittal plane
d. Contrast	Mild and moderate T2W	Moderate T2W
e. Slice thickness	Routine	Thin

The first sequence is a standard screening exam. The second sequence was used to evaluate the level of suspected ventricular obstruction.

MR FINDINGS

Figure 22.1A. The lateral ventricles are moderately and symmetrically enlarged. The degree of ventricular enlargement is out of proportion to the size of the cortical sulci.

Figure 22.1B. The more T2-weighted second echo image reveals a pattern of thin, symmetric, smooth and confluent high intensity bordering the lateral ventricles. There is a paucity of focal high intensity in the periventricular white matter.

Figure 22.2. The degree of lateral ventricular enlargement is graphically demonstrated on this T1-weighted midsagittal image. Note the thinning and stretching of the corpus callosum (arrowheads). The cerebral aqueduct and fourth ventricle are widely patent.

DIFFERENTIAL DIAGNOSIS

In the proper clinical setting—that is, gradual progression of dementia and gait disturbance—the MR findings are quite compatible with normal pressure hydrocephalus (NPH). This patient's symptoms resolved after placement of a ventriculoperitoneal shunt.

NPH is a relatively uncommon cause of dementia. Clinically, NPH is manifested as insidious and progressive dementia and gait disturbance. Urinary incontinence may be present, but this is a relatively late symptom. Affected patients may also present with parkinsonism and/or pseudobulbar palsies. These patients have dilated ventricles but normal CF/S pressures. Radionuclide cisternography may show delayed clearance and ventricular uptake, but the diagnostic accuracy of this modality is held in question. This disease is ultimately defined by a favorable response to ventricular shunting.[1]

The MR findings in this disease, as illustrated in this case, are ventricular dilatation and confluent periventricular high intensity.[2] These findings are relatively nonspecific. Obstructive hydrocephalus may have a similar appearance,

although the degree of periventricular high intensity noted in this case is less than that seen when ventricular pressures are significantly elevated. The patency of the ventricular axis and the inability to demonstrate an obstructing lesion are further evidence against this diagnosis.

Ventricular enlargement and periventricular high intensity can also be seen in elderly but normal individuals.[3,4] (See the discussion of Case 1.) The degree of ventricular and sulcal enlargement, however, is typically more proportionate.

Extensive deep white matter infarction may result in disproportionate ventricular enlargement. Since the periventricular white matter structures are involved, these patients may present with symptoms similar to those of patients with NPH. Making a distinction between the two conditions may be difficult with CT but can usually be accomplished with MR. An example of deep white matter infarction is shown in Figure 22.3.

MR is thus best used to confirm a diagnostic impression of NPH and to exclude other structural causes of dementia. A diagnosis of NPH should not be made on the basis of MR findings without correlative clinical information.

Final Diagnosis

Normal pressure hydrocephalus (NPH).

SUMMARY OF MR FINDINGS FOR NPH

1. There should be a correlative history of dementia and gait disturbance.
2. Lateral (and, to a lesser degree, third and fourth) ventricular enlargement out of proportion to the size of the cortical sulci.
3. T2-weighted images reveal a smooth and symmetric pattern of periventricular high intensity. The thickness of this high intensity band may vary considerably from patient to patient.
4. There should be a relative paucity of focal lesions in the periventricular white matter. A complete absence of such lesions is unusual in patients after the age of 70.

REFERENCES

1. Adams RO, Fisher CM, Hakim S, et al: Symptomatic occult hydrocephalus with normal cerebrospinal fluid pressure: A treatable syndrome. *N Engl J Med* 1965;273:117–126.
2. Kortman KE, Bradley WG: Magnetic resonance imaging of normal pressure hydrocephalus. Presented at the Annual Meeting of the American Society of Neuroradiology, New Orleans, Feb 18–23, 1985.
3. Bradley WG, Walluch V, Brant-Zawadzki M, et al: Patchy, periventricular white matter lesions in the elderly: A common observation during NMR imaging. *Noninvasive Medical Imaging* 1984;1:35–41.
4. Brant-Zawadzki M, Fein G, Van Dylee C, et al: MR imaging of the aging brain: Patchy white matter lesions and dementia. *AJNR* 1985; 6:675–682.

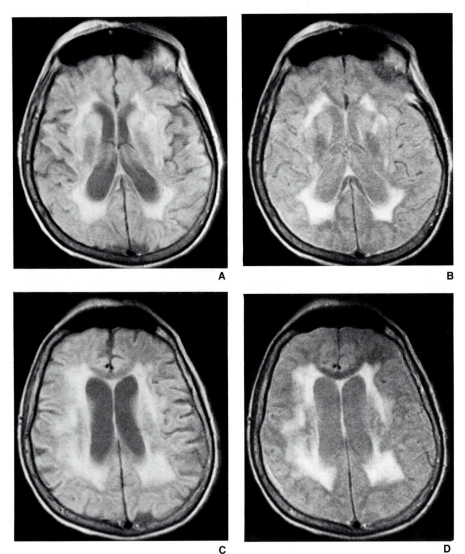

A

B

C

D

Figures 22.3A (SE 2000/30), **22.3B** (SE 2000/60), **22.3C** (SE 2000/30), and **22.3D** (SE 2000/60). This patient had a long history of poorly controlled hypertension. He presented with progressive dementia and frequent falls. The axial MR sections demonstrate slightly disproportionate lateral ventricular enlargement. There is an asymmetric and irregular pattern of primarily confluent, periventricular high intensity. Focal lesions were also seen in the basal ganglia. The pattern is consistent with deep white-matter infarction.

CASE 23

HISTORY

A 5-year-old boy presenting with progressive intellectual impairment and hyperpigmentation.

QUESTIONS

1. What are your differential considerations?
   _____
   _____

2. What MR techniques would you use?

	1	2	3
a. Coil	____	____	____
b. Centering point	____	____	____
c. Imaging plane(s)	____	____	____
d. Contrast	____	____	____
e. Slice thickness	____	____	____

3. What do you expect to find?
   _____
   _____

Source: Courtesy of Phillip Stanley, M.D., Los Angeles, CA.

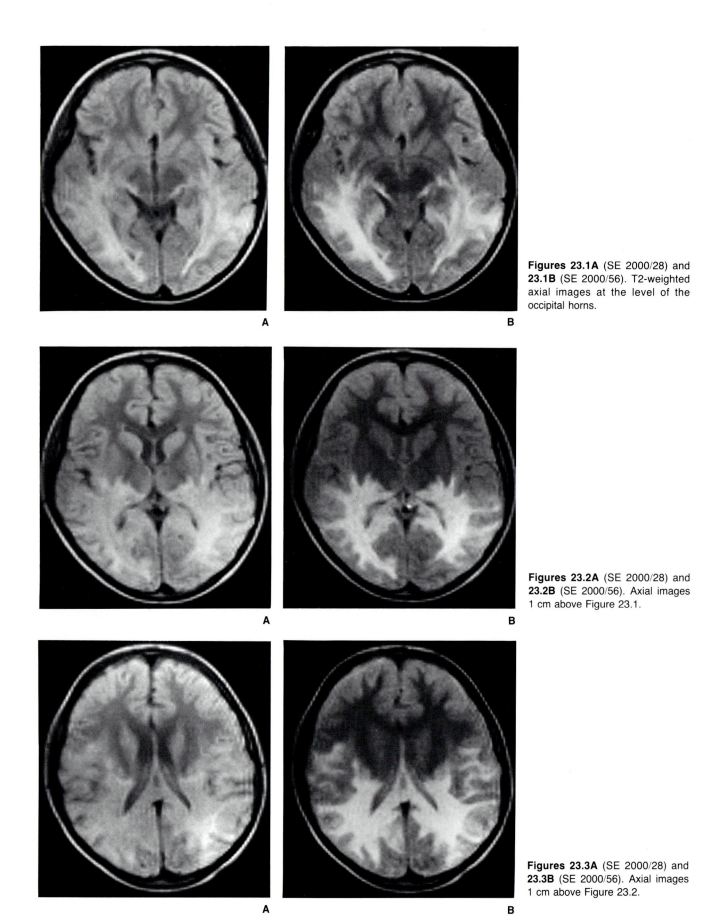

Figures 23.1A (SE 2000/28) and **23.1B** (SE 2000/56). T2-weighted axial images at the level of the occipital horns.

A

B

Figures 23.2A (SE 2000/28) and **23.2B** (SE 2000/56). Axial images 1 cm above Figure 23.1.

A

B

Figures 23.3A (SE 2000/28) and **23.3B** (SE 2000/56). Axial images 1 cm above Figure 23.2.

A

B

MR TECHNIQUES

   a. Coil   Head
   b. Centering point   CML
   c. Imaging plane   Axial
   d. Contrast   Mild to moderate T2W
   e. Slice thickness   Routine

This is a routine screening sequence.

MR FINDINGS

Figure 23.1. There is symmetric and extensive increased signal intensity involving the occipital and posterior temporal white matter. This hyperintensity is much more marked on the more T2-weighted second echo images. The gray matter is spared.

Figure 23.2. There is a similar pattern of posterior white matter involvement at the level of the lateral ventricular atria. Although there is no definite evidence of mass effect, the atria appear somewhat attenuated.

Figure 23.3. The high intensity abnormalities extend into the parietal white matter. Note the complete sparing of the frontal white matter.

DIFFERENTIAL DIAGNOSIS

The striking pattern of white matter disease in a patient of this age indicates an advanced demyelinating process. The increased signal intensity of the white matter reflects T2 prolongation related to a relative increase in water content. As with multiple sclerosis plaques, the alteration in water content can be attributed to both loss of myelin fat and reactive inflammatory edema.

The symmetric posterior distribution of this process is characteristic of adrenoleukodystrophy.[1] The patient's hyperpigmentation is secondary to adrenal insufficiency and elevated adrenocorticotropic hormone (ACTH). A prior conjunctival biopsy had confirmed the diagnosis, and a younger male sibling was similarly affected.

Adrenoleukodystrophy is a hereditary X-linked disease characterized by progressive central nervous system degeneration and adrenal insufficiency. Because of an enzyme deficit in fatty acid metabolism, the disease results in widespread demyelination and inflammatory reaction within the white matter. Symmetric involvement of the posterior white matter is the sine qua non of this disease and distinguishes it from other degenerative white matter disorders. CT exam-

ination of these patients reveals low density cerebral white matter and peripheral contrast enhancement.

The MR findings in this case are identical to those in the few cases described in the literature.[2] Mild mass effect, suggested in this case, is somewhat atypical but can be attributed to active inflammation and edema.

Other demyelinating/dysmyelinating disorders seen in this age group include subacute sclerosing panencephalitis (SSPE), metachromatic leukodystrophy, and globoid cell leukodystrophy. SSPE tends to be more focal and asymmetric in distribution. In globoid cell leukodystrophy, there is no predilection for the posterior white matter, while the lesions of metachromatic leukodystrophy are predominately anterior in location.

In recent years, leukodystrophy has been observed relatively frequently in leukemic children treated with intrathecal methotrexate and cranial irradiation. This has been termed diffuse necrotizing leukodystrophy (DNL).[3] In affected patients, there is extensive bilateral demyelination and inflammation, often leading to focal necrosis and eventual atrophy. The CT and MR findings in a patient with DNL are illustrated in Figures 23.4 and 23.5.

Similar MR findings of abnormal white matter intensity may be seen in adult patients treated with conventional doses of cranial irradiation. These findings may occur weeks to months after treatment and may present as clinical neurotoxicity.[4,5] The degree of radiation-induced white matter changes depends on the patient's age and the size of the radiation port.[6] An example is shown in Figure 23.6.

Final Diagnosis

Adrenoleukodystrophy.

SUMMARY OF MR FINDINGS IN ADRENOLEUKODYSTROPHY

1. Clinical presentation between 5 and 10 years of age, manifested by intellectual impairment, behavior disorder, visual and/or hearing disturbance, ataxia, pyramidal signs, and adrenal insufficiency.
2. T2-weighted MR images reveal symmetric high intensity within the posterior cerebral white matter.
3. The distribution of abnormalities allows distinction between adrenoleukodystrophy and other primary demyelinating/dysmyelinating disorders. This distinction is pertinent, as a small number of patients with adrenoleukodystrophy present without adrenal insufficiency.

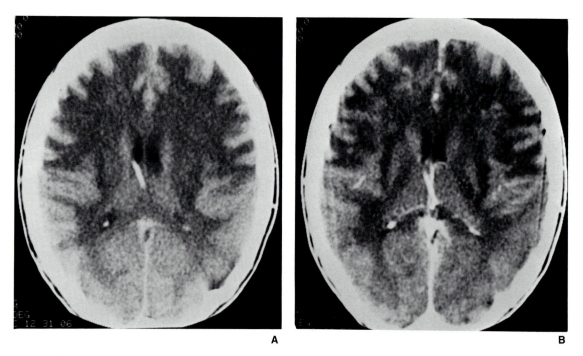

Figures 23.4A (nonenhanced) and **23.4B** (enhanced). This 10-year-old boy had received prophylactic cranial irradiation and intrathecal methotrexate for acute lymphocytic leukemia. He became progressively encephalopathic following treatment, prompting CT examination. There is extensive bilateral low attenuation within the periventricular white matter. (Courtesy of Phillip Stanley, MD, Los Angeles, CA.)

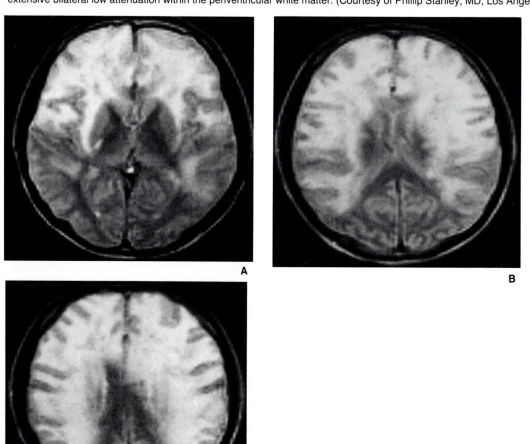

Figure 23.5A–C (SE 2000/56). T2-weighted axial images below (23.5A), at (23.5B), and above (23.5C) the level of the lateral ventricles reveal a strikingly symmetric and confluent pattern of high intensity involving the frontal and high parietal white matter and the gray–white junction. Biopsy revealed DNL.

126

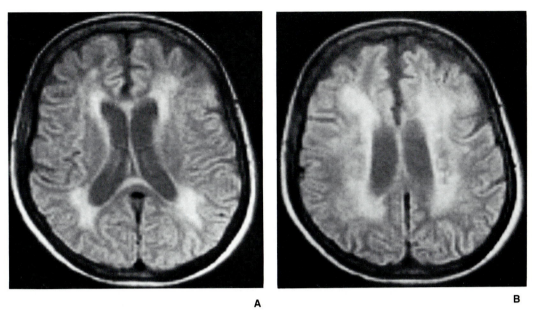

A

B

Figures 23.6A (SE 2000/28) and **23.6B** (SE 2000/28). A middle-aged patient treated with whole brain therapy with extensive, high intensity periventricular white matter lesions characteristic of radiation-related white matter changes.

REFERENCES

1. Aubour P, Diebler C: Adrenoleukodystrophy—Its diverse CT appearances and an evolutive or phenotypic variant: The leukodystrophy without adrenal insufficiency. *Neuroradiology* 1982;24:33–42.

2. Young IR, Randell CP, Kaplan PW, et al: Nuclear magnetic resonance (NMR) imaging in white matter disease of the brain using spin-echo sequences. *JCAT* 1983;7:290–294.

3. Peylan-Ramu N, Poplack DG, Pizzo PA, et al: Abnormal CT scans of the brain in asymptomatic children with acute lymphocytic leukemia after prophylactic treatment of the central nervous system with radiation and intrathecal chemotherapy. *N Engl J Med* 1978;298:815–818.

4. Curnes JT, Laster DW, Ball MR, et al: Magnetic resonance imaging of radiation injury to the brain. *AJNR* 1986;7:389–394.

5. Dooms GC, Hecht S, Brant-Zawadzki M, et al: Brain radiation lesions: MR imaging. *Radiology* 1986;158:149–155.

6. Tsuruda JS, Grossman I, Wheeler D, et al: Radiation effects on cerebral white matter: MR evaluation, submitted for publication.

CASE 24

HISTORY

A 75-year-old woman with Cushing's disease.

QUESTIONS

1. What are your differential considerations?

   _____

   _____

2. What MR techniques would you use?

	1	2	3
a. Coil	___	___	___
b. Centering point	___	___	___
c. Imaging plane(s)	___	___	___
d. Contrast	___	___	___
e. Slice thickness	___	___	___

3. What do you expect to find?

   _____

   _____

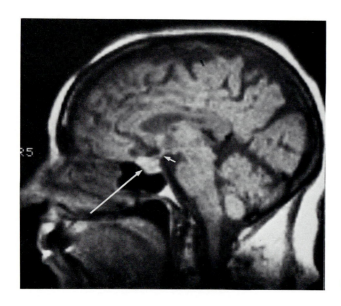

Figure 24.1 (SE 1000/28). Midsagittal section through the brain.

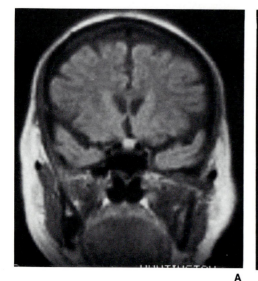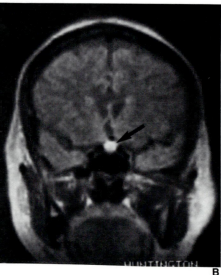

A

B

Figures 24.2A (SE 2000/28) and **24.2B** (SE 2000/56). Coronal scans through the sella.

MR TECHNIQUES

		1	2
a.	Coil	Head	Head
b.	Centering point	Midline	Midvertex
c.	Imaging planes	Sagittal	Coronal
d.	Contrast	Mild T1W	Mild to moderate T2W
e.	Slice thickness	Thin	Thin

The first sequence is used for all suspected midline lesions, such as pituitary adenomas and pineal tumors. Thin sections are required to determine the relationship of the lesion to contiguous structures. A mildly T1-weighted sequence yields good signal-to-noise, contrast between parenchymal structures and CSF, and enough T1 weighting to enable recognition of hemorrhage or fat. The coronal sequence permits evaluation of left/right symmetry (e.g., cavernous sinus invasion by pituitary tumors). Mild to moderate T2 weighting increases lesion conspicuousness by accentuating differences in T2 relaxation times.

With the increasing use of thinner sections and improved spatial resolution, we have altered our protocol for screening suspected pituitary lesions. We currently utilize 3- to 5-mm-thick, T1-weighted images through the sella in both the sagittal and coronal planes. These sequences are combined with a mildly to moderately T2-weighted sequence in the axial plane; the latter is used as a screening study of the remainder of the brain.

MR FINDINGS

Figure 24.1. A slightly hyperintense mass (long white arrow) is seen within the sella and extends into the suprasellar cistern. The pituitary infundibulum (short white arrow) can be seen extending to the posterosuperior aspect of the mass.

Figure 24.2. The tumor (black arrow) is markedly hyperintense on the more T2-weighted images, indicating T2 prolongation. There is no evidence of cavernous sinus extension.

DIFFERENTIAL DIAGNOSIS

In addition to pituitary adenoma, the differential diagnosis includes other sellar and parasellar lesions, including *meningioma, craniopharyngioma,* and *aneurysm.*

1. *Aneurysms* can be excluded on the basis of the MR findings—that is, lack of flow-related signal void or short T1 thrombus.
2. *Meningiomas* are typically isointense on moderately T1-weighted or T2-weighted sequences as used in this case. In addition, although meningiomas may extend into the sella, it would be unusual for such a lesion to be predominately intrasellar.
3. *Craniopharyngiomas,* while usually suprasellar, may be entirely intrasellar. Cystic craniopharyngiomas often contain enough cholesterol to cause marked T1 shortening (see Case 25). Cystic craniopharyngiomas without cholesterol appear less intense on T1-weighted images. A solid craniopharyngioma cannot be excluded on the basis of the MR findings alone. In this case, the clinical history is more consistent with a pituitary adenoma.

Final Diagnosis

Pituitary adenoma (basophilic by history and confirmed surgically).

SUMMARY OF MR FINDINGS FOR PITUITARY MACROADENOMAS

1. Usually hyperintense on T2-weighted images. Some adenomas may be isointense because of increased fibrous content.[1,2]
2. Isointense to slightly hypointense on moderately T1-weighted images.
3. Suprasellar extension is common and may produce optic chiasm compression.
4. Invasion of sphenoid or cavernous sinuses is seen less often.

Comments

While MRI can be useful to effectively evaluate suspected macroadenomas (i.e., those larger than 1 cm), it is relatively less sensitive in the detection of microadenomas when compared with high-resolution CT.[3] Limited spatial resolution and the variability of signal intensity within the tumor may make the detection of small microadenomas with MR difficult. For these reasons, we feel that patients with suspected microadenomas (i.e., those with amenorrhea, galactorrhea, and elevated prolactin levels) and no clinical evidence of extrasellar disease are better evaluated with CT than with MR. Occasionally, a microadenoma can be well demonstrated by MRI, as shown in Figure 24.3.

REFERENCES

1. Lee BCP, Deck MDF: Sellar and juxtasellar lesion detection with MR. *Radiology* 1985;157:143–147.
2. Bilaniuk LT, Zimmerman RA, Wehrli FW, et al: Magnetic resonance imaging of pituitary lesions using 1.0 to 1.5 T field strength. *Radiology* 1984;153:415–418.
3. Pojunas KW, Daniels DL, Williams AL, et al: MR imaging of prolactin-secreting microadenomas. *AJNR* 1986;7:209–213.

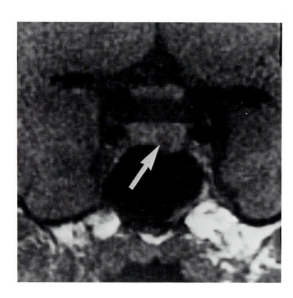

Figure 24.3 (SE 600/25). Coronal section through the sella demonstrating a pituitary microadenoma (arrow) in a patient with elevated prolactin levels. The signal is decreased compared with that of normal pituitary tissue, indicating a prolonged T1 relaxation time.

CASE 25

HISTORY

A 37-year-old woman with recent onset of headaches and left temporal vision loss. A CT examination showed a suprasellar mass (see Figure 25.1).

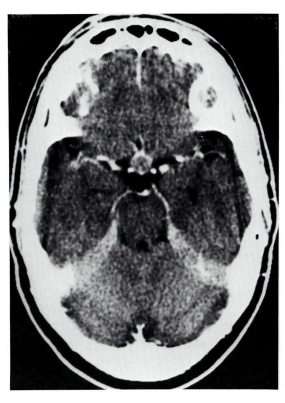

Figure 25.1. Contrast-enhanced axial CT scan through the suprasellar cistern.

QUESTIONS

1. What are your differential considerations?

_____

_____

2. What MR techniques would you use?

	1	2	3
a. Coil	___	___	___
b. Centering point	___	___	___
c. Imaging planes	___	___	___
d. Contrast	___	___	___
e. Slice thickness	___	___	___

3. What do you expect to find?

_____

_____

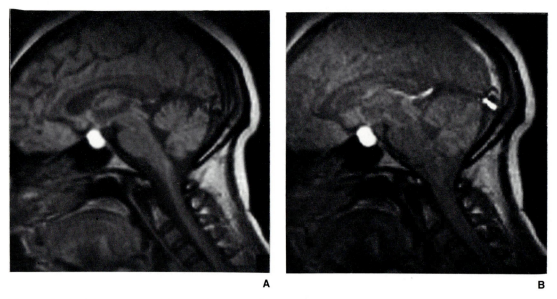

A   B

Figure 25.2A (SE 1500/28) and **25.2B** (SE 1500/56). Midsagittal scans.

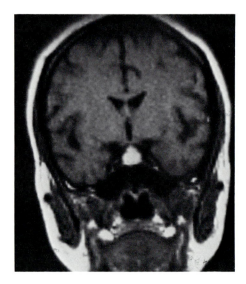

Figure 25.3 (SE 500/28). Coronal scan through the anterior aspect of the third ventricle.

MR TECHNIQUES

		1	2
a.	Coil	Head	Head
b.	Centering point	Midline	Midvertex
c.	Imaging planes	Sagittal	Coronal
d.	Contrast	Mild T2W	Moderate T1W
e.	Slice thickness	Thin	Thin

The extent of sellar and suprasellar lesions is best appreciated in the sagittal and coronal planes. In this case, the CT scan adequately demonstrated the lesion in the axial plane. Because of the proximity of the sella to adjacent structures (such as the cavernous sinuses and optic chiasm), slices measuring 5 mm or less are required to assess lesions in this area accurately. The repetition times of 1,500 and 500 mseconds provide sufficient T2 and T1 weighting, respectively, to characterize the lesion.

MR FINDINGS

Figure 25.1. The contrast-enhanced CT demonstrates a rounded, well-circumscribed soft tissue mass in the anterior aspect of the suprasellar cistern. Curvilinear high density along the anterior and posterior periphery of the mass could represent either calcification or contrast enhancement. Because of bone artifact, the inferior extent of the lesion was difficult to appreciate, as was the relationship of the mass to the optic chiasm.

Figures 25.2A and **25.2B.** These scans demonstrate a high intensity (long T2) suprasellar and intrasellar lesion that impinges on the inferior aspect of the optic chiasm and left optic nerve.

Figure 25.3. The mass remains intense on the T1-weighted coronal image, indicating significant T1 shortening. There is no evidence of hydrocephalus.

DIFFERENTIAL DIAGNOSIS

The differential diagnosis of masses in the sellar region is extensive. Primary considerations should include pituitary adenoma, aneurysm, meningioma, and craniopharyngioma.[1,2] Of these, meningioma and pituitary adenoma are unlikely because of the significant T1 shortening (see Cases 24 and 35). Pituitary adenomas may undergo spontaneous hemorrhage and thereby exhibit a short T1. A hemorrhage of this size, however, would be expected to produce acute symptoms of pituitary apoplexy.[3] Figure 25.4 demonstrates a focus of subacute hemorrhage within a macroadenoma in another patient. T1 shortening has also been noted within pituitary adenomas as a response to bromocriptine therapy.[4]

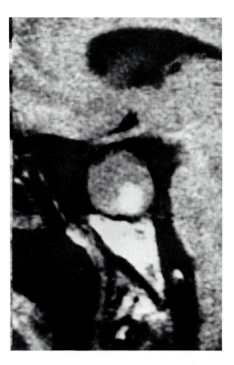

Figure 25.4 (SE 600/25). Sagittal section through a pituitary macroadenoma showing a hyperintense focus of subacute hemorrhage.

The absence of low intensity attributable to flowing blood makes an aneurysm unlikely. The possibility of a thrombosed aneurysm, however, cannot be completely excluded.

An unusual cause of T1 shortening in the region of the sella would be a fatty tumor, such as a dermoid or hamartoma of the tuber cinereum (see Figure 25.5).

Final Diagnosis

Craniopharyngioma.

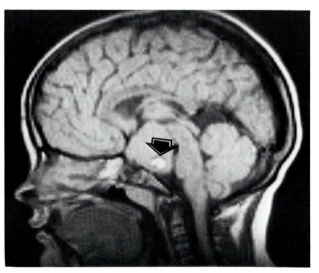

Figure 25.5 (SE 1000/28). Hamartoma of the tuber cinereum with a focus of fat intensity (arrow) within the mass.

SUMMARY OF MR FINDINGS FOR CRANIOPHARYNGIOMA[5]

1. In our experience, T1 shortening has been observed in more than 50% of all craniopharyngiomas. This may be due to the presence of either liquid cholesterol, proteinaceous fluid, or methemoglobin (if bleeding has occurred).

2. T2 prolongation is seen in the majority of cases.

3. Location
   a. Suprasellar
   b. Suprasellar and intrasellar
   c. Intrasellar (in less than 10% of cases)

4. Focal calcifications, although frequently present, are not generally well demonstrated on MRI.

REFERENCES

1. Price AC, Runge V, Allen JH, et al: Craniopharyngioma: Correlation of high resolution CT and MRI, abstracted. *AJNR* 1985;6:465.

2. Lee BCP, Deck MDF: Sellar and juxtasellar lesion detection with MR. *Radiology* 1985;157:143–147.

3. Reid RL, Quigley ME, Yen SSC: Pituitary apoplexy: A review. *Arch Neurol* 1985;42:712–719.

4. Weissbuch SS: Explanation and implications of MR signal changes within pituitary adenomas after bromocriptine therapy. *AJNR* 1986;7:214–216.

5. Kortman KE, Pusey E, Bradley WG, et al: MR imaging of craniopharyngiomas, publication pending.

CASE 26

HISTORY

A 55-year-old man with complaints of episodic numbness of the left side of his body and chronic headaches. A CT examination showed a mass near the foramen of Monro and is shown in Figure 26.1.

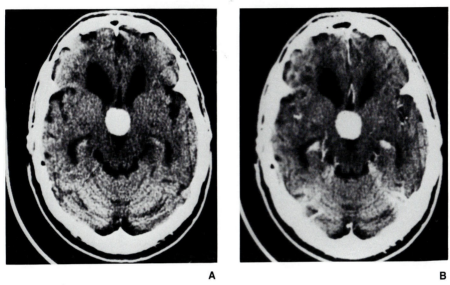

Figure 26.1A (unenhanced) and **26.1B** (enhanced). Axial CT section through the third ventricle.

QUESTIONS

1. What are your differential considerations?

_____

_____

2. What MR techniques would you use?

	1	2	3
a. Coil	___	___	___
b. Centering point	___	___	___
c. Imaging plane(s)	___	___	___
d. Contrast	___	___	___
e. Slice thickness	___	___	___

3. What do you expect to find?

_____

_____

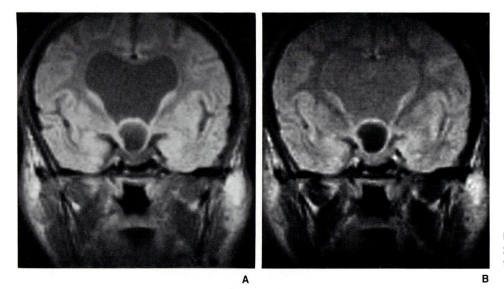

Figure 26.2A (SE 2000/28) and
26.2B (SE 2000/56). Coronal scan
through the anterior third ventricle.

A   B

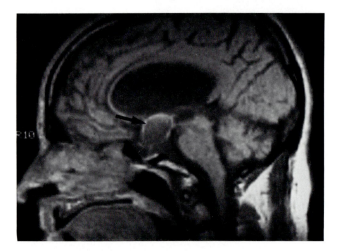

Figure 26.3 (SE 1000/28). Midline sagittal scan.

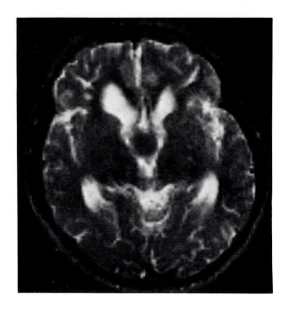

Figure 26.4 (SE 1500/150). Axial section through the region of interest.

MR TECHNIQUES

	1	2	3
a. Coil	Head	Head	Head
b. Centering point	Vertex	Midsagittal	CML
c. Imaging planes	Coronal	Sagittal	Axial
d. Contrast	Mild to moderate T2W	Mild T1W	Heavy T2W
e. Slice thickness	Routine	Thin	Routine

The first pulsing sequence is a variation of the routine screening sequence, performed in the coronal plane to provide better definition of the foramen of Monro. The second mildly T1-weighted sequence provides additional localizing definition and T1 information.

The third sequence is heavily T2 weighted and utilizes a TR of 1,500 mseconds and a TE of 150 mseconds. This was performed to confirm the impression of pathologic T2 shortening observed on the conventional sequences.

MR FINDINGS

Figure 26.1. There is a well-circumscribed and rounded high-density lesion located in the region of the foramen of Monro. There is no definite enhancement following contrast infusion, and moderate hydrocephalus is seen.

Figure 26.2. The mass is well depicted on these coronal MR images. On the mildly (first echo) T1-weighted image, the intensity of the mass is similar to that of CSF. On the moderately (second echo) T2-weighted image, however, the mass has a low intensity relative to that of CSF and adjacent brain parenchyma, indicating significant T2 shortening. The mass has a higher intensity capsule. Dilatation of the lateral ventricles is again noted. Note the absence of interstitial (transependymal) edema along the ventricular wall (compare with Case 33), indicating compensated hydrocephalus.

Figure 26.3. The midsagittal section shows the lesion (black arrow) within the anterior third ventricle. On this sequence, with more T1 weighting, the mass is noted to be intermediate in intensity with a homogeneous texture.

Figure 26.4. This image is from the multiecho, heavily T2-weighted sequence. Note the high intensity of the CSF within the ventricles and subarachnoid space. The mass has a shortened T2, with a very low intensity compared with CSF. The surrounding capsule is poorly identified. The apparent T2 shortening is discussed in greater detail later.

DIFFERENTIAL DIAGNOSIS

The most common mass lesions involving the anterior third ventricle and the foramen of Monro are colloid cysts and gliomas. In this example, the CT appearance is typical for a colloid cyst. The homogeneous high density on the unenhanced study probably represents a combination of dense proteinaceous material, calcium, and hemosiderin.[1] Occasional enhancement may be seen;[2] however, this is not definitely appreciated in this case. Gliomas, such as ependymomas or astrocytomas, are usually more infiltrative, with irregular and poorly defined margins. Either of these lesions may cause hydrocephalus.

The signal intensity of colloid cysts can vary on T2-weighted images. In a recent paper on cystic intracranial lesions,[3] three colloid cysts were described as having prolonged T2 and, therefore, as showing increased intensity on mildly to moderately T2-weighted images. In the preceding example, there is apparent T2 shortening, which may be secondary to the presence of hemosiderin (see Case 11). In our unpublished series of colloid cysts, we have noted that these cysts can have signal intensities on T2-weighted images ranging from low intensity (as in this case) to intermediate intensity (Figure 26.5) or high intensity (Figure 26.6). Thus, while MR is effective in detecting and localizing these lesions, they may be more specifically diagnosed on the basis of typical CT findings.

Final Diagnosis

Colloid cyst.

SUMMARY OF MR FINDINGS FOR COLLOID CYST

1. A rounded, well-circumscribed mass located in the anterior third ventricle.
2. The size of the mass may range from a few millimeters to several centimeters.
3. Obstructive hydrocephalus may be seen even with small lesions because of their strategic location near the foramen of Monro.
4. On a T2-weighted sequence, the intensity pattern is usually homogeneous, but the signal intensity may range from low (indicating a shortened T2) to high (indicating a prolonged T2), depending on the composition of the cyst.

REFERENCES

1. Latchaw RE: Primary tumors of the brain: Neuroectodermal tumors and sarcomas, in RE Latchaw (ed): *Computed Tomography of the Head, Neck and Spine.* Chicago, Year Book Medical Publishers, 1985, pp 220–223.

2. Michels LG, Rutz D: Colloid cysts of the third ventricle: A radiologic-pathologic correlation. *Arch Neurol* 1982;39:640–643.

3. Kjos BO, Brant-Zawadzki, Kucharzyk W, et al: Cystic intracranial lesions: Magnetic resonance imaging. *Radiology* 1985;155:363–369.

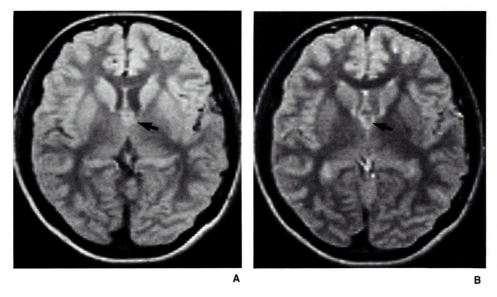

Figures 26.5A (SE 2000/28) and **26.5B** (SE 2000/56). Colloid cyst (black arrow) of intermediate intensity.

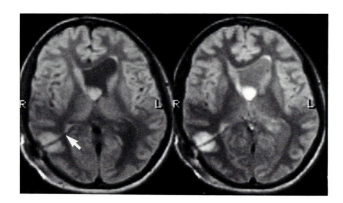

Figures 26.6A (SE 2000/28) and **26.6B** (SE 2000/56). Colloid cyst showing high intensity. Note the low intensity ventricular shunt (white arrow) and the surrounding parenchymal high intensity due to edema after shunt placement.

CASE 27

HISTORY

A 67-year-old woman with new onset of seizures and progressively worsening headaches, vomiting, and intellectual deterioration.

QUESTIONS

1. What are your differential considerations?

_____

_____

2. What MR techniques would you use?

	1	2	3
a. Coil	_____	_____	_____
b. Centering point	_____	_____	_____
c. Imaging plane(s)	_____	_____	_____
d. Contrast	_____	_____	_____
e. Slice thickness	_____	_____	_____

3. What do you expect to find?

_____

_____

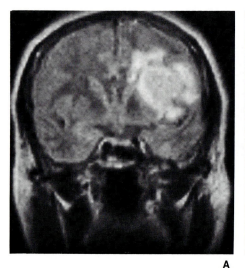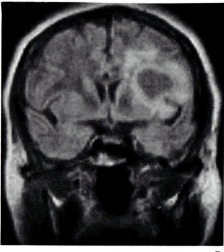

Figures 27.1A (SE 2000/28) and **27.2B** (SE 2000/56). Coronal images at the level of the foramen of Monro.

A   B

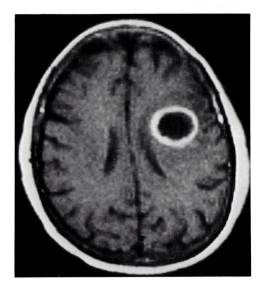

Figure 27.2 (SE 500/28). Axial image through the mass prior to the administration of gadolinium-DTPA.

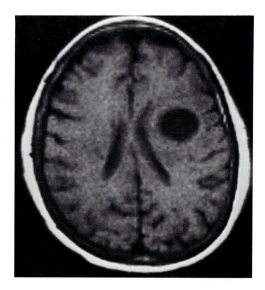

Figure 27.3 (SE 500/28). Axial image at the same level as Figure 27.2 after administration of gadolinium-DTPA.

MR TECHNIQUES

		1	2	3
a.	Coil	Head	Head	Head
b.	Centering point	Midvertex	Lateral ventricles	Lateral ventricles
c.	Imaging planes	Coronal	Axial	Axial
d.	Contrast	Mild to moderate T2W	Moderate T1W	Moderate T1W
e.	Slice thickness	Routine	Routine	Routine
f.	Contrast material	None	None	Gadolinium-DTPA

The first sequence is a variation of the standard screening study. The second sequence demonstrates T1 characteristics of the lesion and its anatomic relationships in the axial plane. The third sequence (post-gadolinium-DTPA) is designed to reveal areas of breakdown of the blood–brain barrier. The extravascular leakage of gadolinium-DTPA results in T1 shortening and increased signal intensity. This helps to grade the lesion and to guide biopsy.[1]

MR FINDINGS

Figure 27.1. A mass is seen in the deep left frontal lobe. It has a high intensity (long T2) rim and a medium intensity center. The lesion is surrounded by a moderate amount of edema, predominately distributed through the white matter and also increased in signal intensity. On the moderately T2-weighted (second echo) image, both the mass and the surrounding edema become more intense with respect to the normal brain.

Figure 27.2. In this coronal T1-weighted image, the mass has a central, probably necrotic area of decreased signal intensity (long T1) and a peripheral rim that is isointense with the surrounding edematous brain parenchyma because of similarities in the T1 relaxation values.

Figure 27.3. After the administration of gadolinium-DTPA, there is immediate, intense enhancement of the tumor, manifested as an increase in intensity, reflecting reduction of the T1 relaxation time.

DIFFERENTIAL DIAGNOSIS

The presence of a long-T1, long-T2 mass with contrast enhancement and surrounding edema is highly suggestive of a glioma. Other differential considerations should include:

1. *Abscess.* The lack of a clinical history of antecedent infection makes abscess unlikely. However, abscess cannot be excluded on the basis of MR findings alone.
2. *Metastasis.* Metastasis is less likely in the absence of known primary tumor or additional lesions. On the basis of MR findings alone, however, a glioma and an isolated metastasis may have identical appearances.
3. *Resolving hematoma.* The clinical history and the absence of T1 shortening virtually exclude hemorrhage (see Case 11).

Final Diagnosis

Glioblastoma multiforme.

SUMMARY OF MR FINDINGS FOR GLIOBLASTOMA MULTIFORME[2,3]

1. Mass effect.
2. Surrounding edema.
3. Prolonged T1, shown as decreased signal intensity on T1-weighted images.
4. Prolonged T2, shown as increased signal intensity on T2-weighted images.
5. Contrast (gadolinium-DTPA) enhancement seen as increased signal intensity on T1-weighted images.

REFERENCES

1. Carr DH, Brown J, Leung AWL, et al: Iron and gadolinium chelates as contrast agents in NMR imaging: Preliminary studies. *J Comput Assist Tomogr* 1984;8:385–389.
2. Brant-Zawadzki M, Badami JP, Mills CM, et al: Primary intracranial tumor imaging: A comparison of magnetic resonance and CT. *Radiology* 1984;150:435–440.
3. Kortman KE, Bradley WG: MRI of intracranial neoplasms, in Mettler FA, Muroff LR (eds): *Practical Nuclear Magnetic Resonance*. New York, Churchill Livingstone Inc., in press.

CASE 28

HISTORY

A 48-year-old woman presenting with extremity weakness and numbness.

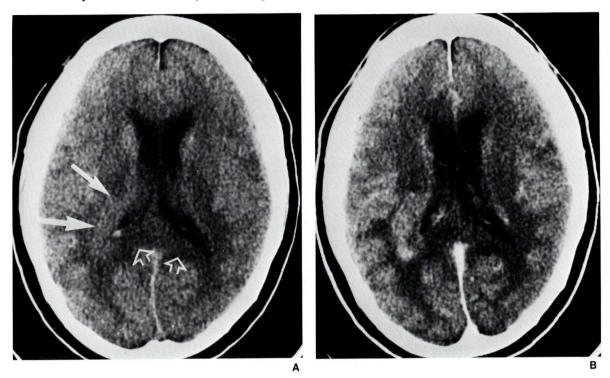

Figure 28.1. Axial CT sections through the lateral ventricles. (A) Non-contrast-enhanced and (B) contrast enhanced.

QUESTIONS

1. What are your differential considerations?

   _____

   _____

2. What MR techniques would you use?

	1	2	3
a. Coil	_____	_____	_____
b. Centering point	_____	_____	_____
c. Imaging plane(s)	_____	_____	_____
d. Contrast	_____	_____	_____
e. Slice thickness	_____	_____	_____

3. What do you expect to find?

   _____

   _____

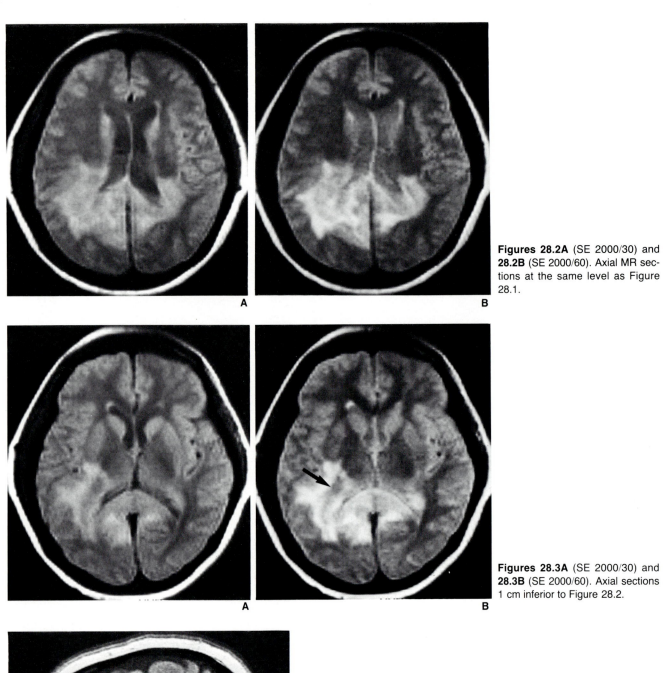

Figures 28.2A (SE 2000/30) and **28.2B** (SE 2000/60). Axial MR sections at the same level as Figure 28.1.

Figures 28.3A (SE 2000/30) and **28.3B** (SE 2000/60). Axial sections 1 cm inferior to Figure 28.2.

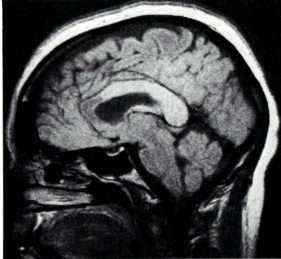

Figure 28.4 (SE 1000/40). Midsagittal MR image.

MR TECHNIQUES

	1	2
a. Coil	Head	Head
b. Centering point	CML	Midsagittal plane
c. Imaging planes	Axial	Sagittal
d. Contrast	Mild to moderate T2W	Mild T1W
e. Slice thickness	Routine	Thin

The first sequence is a standard screening study. The second sequence was added to define midline pathology more accurately.

MR FINDINGS

Figure 28.1A. The non-contrast-enhanced CT section demonstrates asymmetric truncation of the right atrium. There is a subtle mass (closed arrows) isodense with gray matter along the lateral aspect of the atrium. The splenium of the corpus callosum (open arrows) appears thickened.

Figure 28.1B. The right periatrial mass enhances mildly and somewhat heterogeneously. No other abnormal enhancement can be identified.

Figure 28.2. Corresponding T2-weighted MR sections demonstrate an extensive high intensity lesion with mass effect involving the right periatrial white matter and extending posteriorly and medially to involve the corpus callosum and left periatrial white matter. The area that was enhanced on CT is slightly less intense than the surrounding white matter.

Figure 28.3. On a slightly more inferior section, thickening of the corpus callosum and splaying of the occipital horns are more apparent. On the second echo image, the intensity of the enhancing lesion on CT (arrow) is less than that of surrounding edema, indicating less T2 prolongation.

Figure 28.4. There is marked thickening of the posterior corpus callosum.

DIFFERENTIAL DIAGNOSIS

The most likely lesion to present as a solitary mass extending across the midline through the corpus callosum is a primary brain neoplasm. In this case, a stereotactic biopsy was performed, yielding a diagnosis of grade 2 astrocytoma.

A solitary metastasis should be considered. In this case, there was no history of primary malignancy. The absence of additional lesions and the relative lack of contrast enhancement are additional factors that argue against this diagnosis. Furthermore, involvement of midline white matter structures is not characteristic of metastases.

Primary intracranial lymphoma often involves midline structures. This diagnosis cannot be excluded on the basis of MR findings alone but is statistically unlikely in a patient with normal immunity. The relative lack of contrast enhancement also militates against this diagnosis.

Inflammatory disease—that is, cerebritis—should be considered. Involvement of midline structures has not been stressed in the CT literature. We have observed, however, a number of patients with extensive midline (especially brainstem) involvement, including mass effect, whose presenting history or therapeutic response was most compatible with inflammatory disease. Many of these patients had multifocal disease demonstrated by MR, making a primary intracranial neoplasm unlikely.

The history and location of the lesion are incompatible with either trauma or vaso-occlusive disease.

Final Diagnosis

Grade 2 astrocytoma.

SUMMARY OF MR FINDINGS FOR GLIOMA[1-3]

1. Nonspecific alteration in signal intensity. T2 prolongation produces increased signal intensity on T2-weighted images. T1 prolongation produces less conspicuous decreased intensity on moderately or heavily T1-weighted images.
2. Application of heavy T2 or T1 weighting may allow separation of tumor (relatively hypointense) from edema (relatively hyperintense). In most cases, however, this distinction is not as conspicuous as that achieved by contrast-enhanced CT.
3. Mass effect varies and is more pronounced with higher grade lesions. Mass effect is most conspicuous on T1-weighted images that maximize contrast between tumor and CSF-containing structures.
4. Extension across the corpus callosum is quite characteristic of gliomas. This is much more readily demonstrated with MRI than with CT.

REFERENCES

1. Bydder GM, Steiner RO, Young IR, et al: Clinical NMR imaging of the brain: 140 cases. *AJR* 1982;139:215–236.
2. Brant-Zawadzki M, Badami P, Mills CM, et al: Primary intracranial tumor imaging: A comparison of magnetic resonance and CT. *Radiology* 1984;150:435–440.
3. Kortman KE, Bradley WG: MRI of intracranial neoplasms, in Mettler FA, Muroff LR (eds): *Practical Nuclear Magnetic Resonance*. New York, Churchill Livingstone Inc, in press.

CASE 29

HISTORY

A 55-year-old woman with a history of breast carcinoma now presenting with headaches, dizziness, and aphasia.

QUESTIONS

1. What are your differential considerations?

   _____

   _____

2. What MR techniques would you use?

	1	2	3
a. Coil	_____	_____	_____
b. Centering point	_____	_____	_____
c. Imaging plane(s)	_____	_____	_____
d. Contrast	_____	_____	_____
e. Slice thickness	_____	_____	_____

3. What do you expect to find?

   _____

   _____

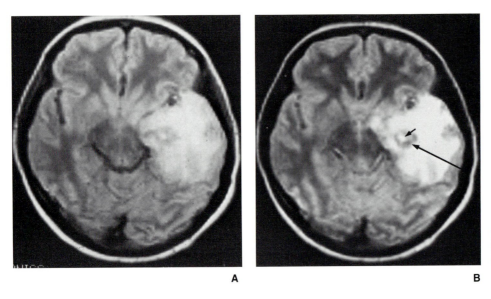

A B

Figures 29.1A (SE 2000/28) and **29.1B** (SE 2000/56). Axial scans through the temporal fossa.

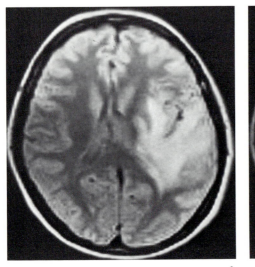 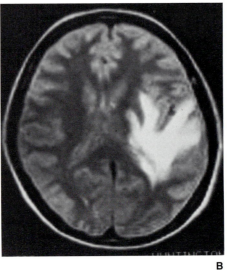

A B

Figures 29.2A (SE 2000/28) and **29.2B** (SE 2000/56). Axial scans through the bodies of the lateral ventricles.

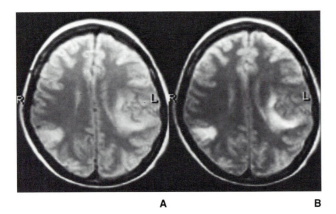

A B

Figures 29.3A (SE 2000/28) and **29.3B** (SE 2000/56). Axial scans 1 cm superior to Figure 29.2.

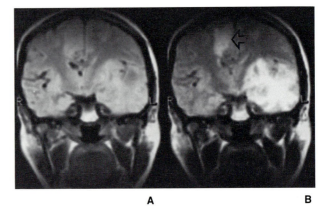

A B

Figures 29.4A (SE 1000/28) and **29.4B** (SE 1000/56). Coronal scans through the frontoparietal region.

MR TECHNIQUES

	1	2
a. Coil	Head	Head
b. Centering point	CML	Midvertex
c. Imaging planes	Axial	Coronal
d. Contrast	Mild to moderate T2W	Mild T1W/ mild T2W
e. Slice thickness	Routine	Routine

The first pulsing sequence is the standard screening sequence for most CNS abnormalities. The second sequence with an intermediate TR provides additional localizing information and tissue characterization.

MR FINDINGS

Figure 29.1. There is extensive edema and mass effect in the left temporal lobe, with a 1-cm, low intensity nidus in the hippocampus (long black arrow). Within this low intensity nidus, there is a punctate high intensity focus (short black arrow) with an increased T2 that may represent central necrosis.

Figure 29.2. Note the "fingerlike" distribution of vasogenic edema in the white matter.

Figure 29.3. A smaller lesion is seen at the gray-white junction within the right parietal lobe.

Figure 29.4. A third focus is demonstrated in the right parasagittal area (open black arrow).

DIFFERENTIAL DIAGNOSIS

The history of breast carcinoma and the presence of multiple high intensity lesions associated with edema are consistent with metastatic disease. The patient's aphasia can be explained by involvement of Wernicke's area (posterior left temporal lobe). Other differential diagnostic considerations may include:

1. *Multiple abscesses.* This disease entity cannot be distinguished from metastases by MR findings alone. Clinical history is an important distinguishing feature, but biopsy is required for definitive diagnosis.
2. Infarcts secondary to *vasculitis* or *thromboembolism*. The extensive edema and mass effect, especially in the left temporal lobe, would be unusual for infarcts. In addition, the clinical history is not supportive of this diagnosis.
3. *Multifocal gliomas.* This is a relatively uncommon entity but cannot be distinguished from metastases on the basis of MR findings alone.

Final Diagnosis

Brain metastases from breast carcinoma.

SUMMARY OF MR FINDINGS FOR METASTASES[1,2]

1. Multifocal lesions usually centered in the gray–white junction. Extensive vasogenic edema commonly extends into the white matter with fingerlike projections. In general, MR reveals more lesions than does CT; signal intensity patterns, however, are nonspecific.
2. On T2-weighted images, the tumor nidus may be less intense than the surrounding edema because of its slightly shorter T2. This is not a consistent finding, however.
3. On T1-weighted images, the tumor nidus (with a slightly longer T1) may be distinguished from edema by its lower signal.

REFERENCES

1. Kortman KE, Bradley WG: MRI of intracranial neoplasms, in Mettler FA, Muroff LR (eds): *Practical Nuclear Magnetic Resonance.* New York, Churchill Livingstone, in press.
2. Lee BCP, Kneeland JB, Cahill PT, et al: MR recognition of supratentorial tumors. *AJNR* 1985;6:871–878.

CASE 30

HISTORY

A 28-year-old man presented with headaches. Physical examination revealed paralysis of upward gaze (Parinaud's syndrome). CT (not shown) demonstrated a pineal region tumor.

QUESTIONS

1. What are your differential considerations?

   _____

   _____

2. What MR techniques would you use?

	1	2	3
a. Coil	___	___	___
b. Centering point	___	___	___
c. Imaging plane(s)	___	___	___
d. Contrast	___	___	___
e. Slice thickness	___	___	___

3. What do you expect to find?

   _____

   _____

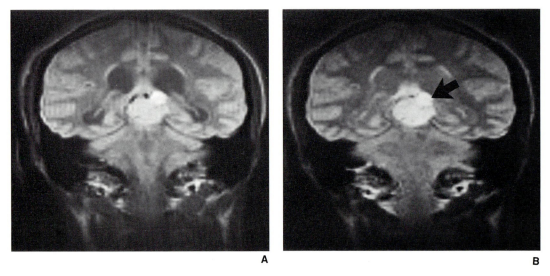

A B

Figures 30.1A (SE 2000/28) and **30.1B** (SE 2000/56). Coronal scans through the pineal region.

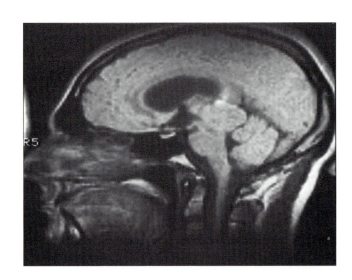

Figure 30.2 (SE 1000/28). Sagittal scan through the midline.

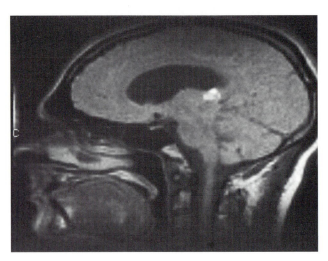

Figure 30.3 (SE 1000/28). Sagittal section 5 mm to the left of Figure 30.2.

MR TECHNIQUES

		1	2
a.	Coil	Head	Head
b.	Centering point	CML	Midline sagittal
c.	Imaging planes	Coronal	Sagittal
d.	Contrast	Mild to moderate T2W	Mild T1W
e.	Slice thickness	Routine	Thin

The first sequence is a variation of the standard sequence protocol. Coronal sections were utilized, as the prior CT had shown the location of the tumor in the axial plane. Sagittal images are utilized in the evaluation of all midline lesions. A TR of 1000 provides good brain-CSF contrast and enough T1-weighting to define hemorrhagic or fatty components of the tumor.

MR FINDINGS

Figure 30.1. There is a high intensity (long T2) mass in the pineal region, with a focus of even greater intensity along the left superolateral aspect of the lesion.

Figure 30.2. The sagittal image demonstrates obliteration of the tectal plate and the cerebral aqueduct. Obstructive hydrocephalus is shown on both sagittal and coronal sections.

Figure 30.3. The left parasagittal image demonstrates a markedly hyperintense focus along the posterosuperior aspect of the isointense mass.

Note the distortion of the images. This is due to dysfunction of a gradient coil power supply.

DIFFERENTIAL DIAGNOSIS

The differential diagnosis of a pineal region tumor includes germ cell tumors (e.g., dysgerminoma), tumors of pineal cell origin (e.g., pinealocytoma, pinealoblastoma), gliomas of the posterior hypothalamus and tectum, epidermoids, arachnoid cysts, and teratomas. As with CT, MRI seldom permits a specific histologic diagnosis of a pineal tumor.[1,2] However, nonaxial scanning capability and MR signal characteristics may add some specificity in differentiating "pineal" tumors from gliomas, epidermoids, and arachnoid cysts. Marked intratumoral variations in signal intensity may suggest the diagnosis of a teratoma containing fat, hair, and/or dental elements. Unfortunately, these changes may be mimicked by other lesions containing foci of calcium and/or hemorrhage. As calcification is an important

differentiating feature of the tumor, CT may provide additional useful information.[2] In this case, the high intensity component seen at the periphery of the lesion was hyperdense on CT, consistent with focal hemorrhage.

Dysgerminoma is statistically the most common pineal tumor, particularly in young males. In this case, the diagnosis was established by excisional biopsy.

A word of caution: normal pineal glands generally have T1 and T2 signal intensity characteristics similar to those of normal gray matter. In some cases, normal glands may have prolonged T1 and T2 relaxation values that overlap with those seen with pineal tumors. Alternatively, these may represent benign cysts.[3] We are therefore cautious in reporting a definite pineal tumor on the basis of signal intensity changes alone in a normal size gland.

Final Diagnosis

Pineal dysgerminoma.

SUMMARY OF MR FINDINGS FOR PRIMARY PINEAL TUMORS AND DYSGERMINOMAS

1. A pineal gland greater than 1.5 cm in diameter.
2. Prolonged T2.
3. May contain foci of hemorrhage (increased intensity) or calcium (decreased intensity).
4. Mass effect on adjacent tectum, which is responsible for the paralysis of the upward gaze (Parinaud's syndrome).[4]
5. Other lesions within the hypothalamic axis—the "multiple midline tumor syndrome"—are seen almost exclusively with dysgerminomas.
6. "Drop" metastases to the ventricular system and spinal canal may be seen with pinealoblastoma and dysgerminoma.

REFERENCES

1. Futrell NN, Osborn AG, Cheson BD: Pineal region tumors: Computed tomographic-pathologic spectrum. *AJR* 1981;137:951–956.
2. Holland BA, Brant-Zawadzki M, Norman D, et al: Magnetic resonance of pineal region tumors. Presented at the 24th Annual Meeting of the American Society of Neuroradiology, San Diego, January 1986.
3. Riley HK, Maravilla KR, Sory C: MR appearance of the pineal gland. Presented at the 24th Annual Meeting of the American Society of Neuroradiology, San Diego, January 1986.
4. Flannigan BD, Bradley WG, Maziotta JC, et al: Magnetic resonance imaging of the brainstem: Normal structure and basic functional anatomy. *Radiology* 1985;154:375–383.

CASE 31

HISTORY

A 29-year-old man presenting with unexplained bilateral papilledema, auditory disturbance, and dizziness.

QUESTIONS

1. What are your differential considerations?

   _____

   _____

2. What MR techniques would you use?

	1	2	3
a. Coil	___	___	___
b. Centering point	___	___	___
c. Imaging plane(s)	___	___	___
d. Contrast	___	___	___
e. Slice thickness	___	___	___

3. What do you expect to find?

   _____

   _____

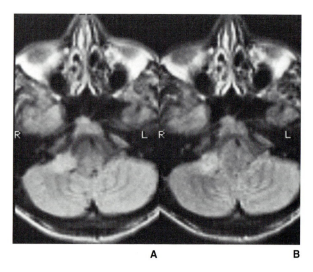

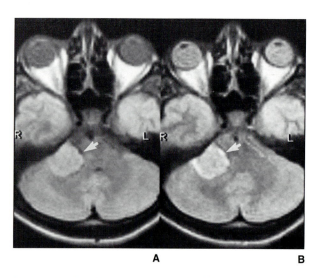

Figures 31.1A (SE 2000/28) and **31.1B** (SE 2000/56). Axial scans through the posterior fossa.

Figures 31.2A (SE 2000/28) and **31.2B** (SE 2000/56). Axial scans 1 cm superior to Figure 31.1.

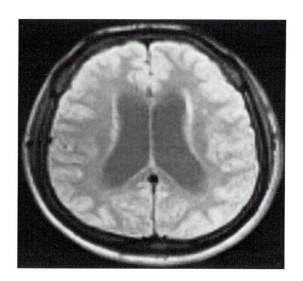

Figure 31.3 (SE 2000/28). Axial scan through the bodies of the lateral ventricles.

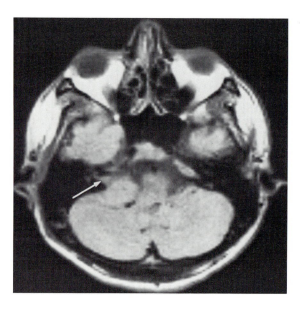

Figure 31.4 (SE 1000/28). Axial scan at the same level as Figure 31.2.

MR TECHNIQUES

	1	2
a. Coil	Head	Head
b. Centering point	CML	CML
c. Imaging planes	Axial	Axial
d. Contrast	Mild to moderate T2W	Mild to moderate T2W
e. Slice thickness	Routine	Thin

Our usual sequence for evaluating acoustic neuromas includes contiguous, thin-slice axial sections with mild to moderate T2 weighting. We have also found that moderately T1-weighted images with thin to very thin contiguous slices may provide sufficient anatomic detail to enable detection of subtle intracanalicular tumors, provided the imaging unit is capable of producing an MR image with adequate signal-to-noise and sufficient spatial resolution.[1] In this case, an acoustic neuroma was not suspected clinically; the history of auditory disturbance was obtained after the fact. Therefore, a general screening sequence with routine slice thickness and a 25% gap between slices was performed. After reviewing the sequence and discovering a right cerebellopontine angle (CPA) mass, a second sequence with thinner slices was performed to evaluate the internal auditory canal. We have not found coronal images to be as helpful as axials in the evaluation of internal auditory canal (IAC) pathology; this imaging plane should be used, however, if the axial study is equivocal.

MR FINDINGS

Figures 31.1 and 31.2. There is a well-circumscribed and relatively homogeneous mass involving the right CPA in the region of the porus acousticus. We considered this to be an extra-axial mass in light of the medial displacement of superficial cortical vessels. Even-echo rephasing[2] (white arrow) within the vessels is shown on Figure 31.2. The low intensity rim outlining the mass on the first echo image increases markedly in intensity on the second echo image.

Figure 31.3 Hydrocephalus is noted and is due to compression of the fourth ventricle by the right CPA mass. The smooth periventricular high intensity indicates transepen-dymal spread of CSF (interstitial edema). The hydrocephalus correlates with the clinical finding of papilledema.

Figure 31.4. On thinner slices, the intracanalicular extension of the tumor is demonstrated (white arrow). This was not seen on the thicker, noncontiguous slices of the first sequence.

DIFFERENTIAL DIAGNOSIS

1. *Acoustic neuroma.* This is the most likely diagnosis. (See MR characteristics later.)
2. *Meningioma.* The intracanalicular extension of the tumor and the relative hyperintensity compared with adjacent cortex on moderately T2-weighted images are not characteristic of meningioma.[3] (See Case 35.)
3. *Epidermoid.* These tumors are characteristically heterogeneous[4] and of low intensity on T1-weighted images (long T1). (See Case 33.)

Final Diagnosis

Right acoustic neuroma.

SUMMARY OF MR FINDINGS FOR ACOUSTIC NEUROMA

In general, neuromas have a prolonged T2 and are uniform in texture. More importantly, they occur at characteristic sites, which aids in diagnosing these lesions.[5,6] Small, totally intracanalicular tumors can be demonstrated by MRI (Figure 31.5).[1]

REFERENCES

1. Daniels DL, Schenck JF, Foster T, et al: Surface-coil magnetic resonance imaging of the internal auditory canal. *AJR* 1985; 145:469–472.
2. Waluch V, Bradley WG: NMR even echo rephasing in slow laminar flow. *J Comput Assist Tomogr* 1984;8:594–598.
3. Bucon KA, Bradley WG, Kortman KE: MR imaging and meningiomas with and without paramagnetic contrast. Submitted for publication.
4. Kortman KE, Van Dalsem W, Bradley WG: MRI of intracranial epidermoid tumors. *AJNR,* submitted for publication.
5. New PFJ, Bachow TB, Wismer GL, et al: MR imaging of the acoustic nerves and small acoustic neuromas at 0.6 T: Prospective study. *AJR* 1985;144:1021–1026.
6. Waluch V, Bradley WG, Whitaker SG, et al: MRI of acoustic neuromas and other temporal bone diseases. *AJNR,* in press.

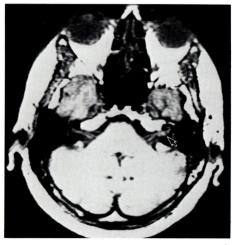

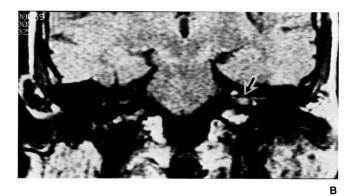

Figures 31.5A (axial, SE 600/25) and **31.5B** (coronal, SE 600/25). Magnified view of the posterior fossa demonstrating a small left intracanalicular acoustic neuroma (arrows) with subtle soft tissue thickening within the internal auditory canal. Note that the individual components, the seventh and eighth nerve bundles, are beginning to be resolved (see reference 1 for a more detailed description of the anatomic findings in this region). The study was photographed at a narrow window setting to accentuate the contrast differences between the low-signal petrous bone and soft tissues. (Courtesy of Washington MR Center, Whittier, CA.)

CASE 32

HISTORY

A 53-year-old man presenting with occipital headaches and ataxia. CT demonstrated a cystic posterior fossa mass (Figure 32.1).

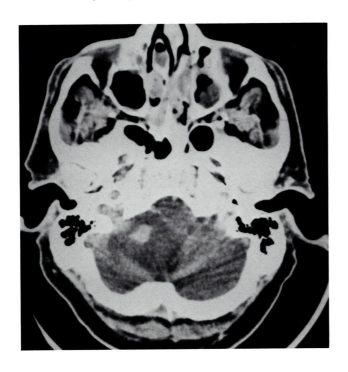

Figure 32.1 Contrast-enhanced CT scan through the posterior fossa.

QUESTIONS

1. What are your differential considerations?

_____

_____

2. What MR techniques would you use?

	1	2	3
a. Coil	___	___	___
b. Centering point	___	___	___
c. Imaging plane(s)	___	___	___
d. Contrast	___	___	___
e. Slice thickness	___	___	___

3. What do you expect to find?

_____

_____

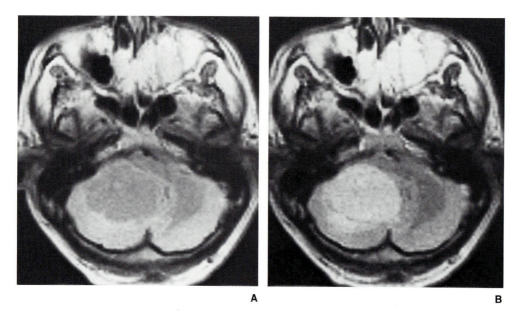

Figures 32.2A (SE 2000/28) and **32.2B** (SE 2000/56). Axial MR scans at a comparable level.

A   B

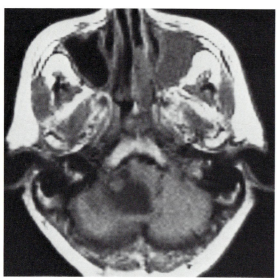

Figure 32.3 (SE 500/28). Axial scan at a slightly lower level.

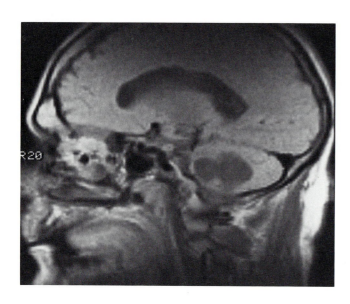

Figure 32.4 (SE 1000/28). Right parasagittal scan.

MR TECHNIQUES

	1	2	3
a. Coil	Head	Head	Head
b. Centering point	CML	Lower EAC*	Midsagittal
c. Imaging planes	Axial	Axial	Sagittal
d. Contrast	Mild to moderate T2W	Moderate T1W	Moderate T1W
e. Slice thickness	Routine	Routine	Routine

The first pulsing sequence is the routine screening sequence for CNS abnormalities. The second sequence was performed to define T1 characteristics. The third sequence was performed to determine the relationship of the lesion to adjacent brainstem structures and the foramen magnum.

MR FINDINGS

Figure 32.1. The contrast-enhanced CT scan demonstrates a large, well-defined and apparently intra-axial cystic mass in the right cerebellar hemisphere. A hyperdense (presumably contrast-enhancing) nodule is seen in the right anterolateral aspect of the cyst.

Figures 32.2A and 32.2B. The intensity of this cystic mass is greater than that of CSF on the first echo image. This difference is more pronounced on the second echo image. This intensity pattern reflects a relatively short T1 and prolonged T2 characteristic of proteinaceous solutions.[1] The tumor nodule is at a slightly lower level and therefore is not seen on this scan.

Figure 32.3 On this T1-weighted image, the cyst is clearly shown to be intra-axial, being surrounded on all sides by brain parenchyma. The tumor nodule is conspicuously demonstrated. On T2-weighted images at this level, the high intensity (long T2) nodule was difficult to distinguish from high intensity cyst fluid.

Figure 32.4. The sagittal scan again demonstrates the cystic mass and inferior tumor nodule.

DIFFERENTIAL DIAGNOSIS[2]

1. *Hemangioblastoma*. Morphologically, the MR appearance may be similar to that of a cystic astro-

---

*External auditory canal

cytoma. The history of a slowly growing cerebellar neoplasm in a middle-aged patient is helpful.
2. *Cystic astrocytoma*. Typically, this is a tumor of childhood and adolescence.
3. *Medulloblastoma*. This is seen almost exclusively in children and is typically a more solid lesion.
4. *Cystic schwannoma*. The intra-axial location of the mass excludes this possibility.

Final Diagnosis

Hemangioblastoma of the cerebellum.

SUMMARY OF MR FINDINGS FOR HEMANGIOBLASTOMA

1. The majority are intra-axial and involve the posterior fossa.
2. The mass is predominately cystic; the cyst's T1 and T2 relaxation times are between those of brain parenchyma and CSF.
3. The mass is generally well circumscribed with minimal surrounding edema.[3]
4. If present, the tumor nodule measures from 1 to 2 cm in diameter. The intensity of the tumor nodule is greater than that of the cyst on T1-weighted images and mildly T2-weighted images. In some instances we have noted focal areas of decreased signal within the tumor nodule (Figure 32.5) that may represent enlarged vascular channels noted on angiography.
5. Differentiation from cystic astrocytomas may be difficult. The patient's age and an angiographic blush may differentiate these lesions.

REFERENCES

1. Bradley WG: Fundamentals of magnetic resonance image interpretation, in Bradley WG, Adey WR, Hasso AN (eds): *Magnetic Resonance Imaging of Brain, Head, and Neck: A Text Atlas*. Rockville, Md, Aspen Publishers, Inc., 1985, pp 1–16.

2. Kjos BO, Brant-Zawadzki M, Kucharzyk W, et al: Cystic intracranial lesions: Magnetic resonance imaging. *Radiology* 1985;155:363–369.

3. Kortman KE, Bradley WG: MRI of intracranial neoplasms, in Mettler FA, Muroff LR (eds): *Practical Nuclear Magnetic Resonance*. New York, Churchill Livingstone, in press.

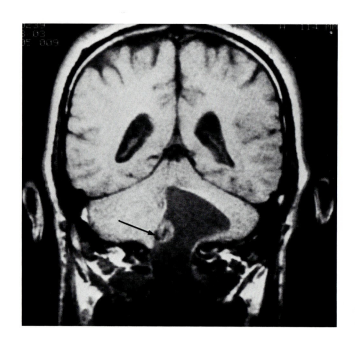

Figure 32.5. (SE 600/25). Coronal section through a posterior fossa hemangioblastoma demonstrating a cyst and mural nodule. Note the curvilinear focus of low intensity (arrow), probably representing an enlarged vascular channel.

CASE 33

HISTORY

A 62-year-old woman with headaches and loss of balance. CT examination revealed enlargement of the lateral and third ventricles. A low density, non-enhancing lesion in the region of the quadrigeminal cistern was thought to be a cyst.

QUESTIONS

1. What are your differential considerations?

   _____

   _____

2. What MR techniques would you use?

	1	2	3
a. Coil	____	____	____
b. Centering point	____	____	____
c. Imaging plane(s)	____	____	____
d. Contrast	____	____	____
e. Slice thickness	____	____	____

3. What do you expect to find?

   _____

   _____

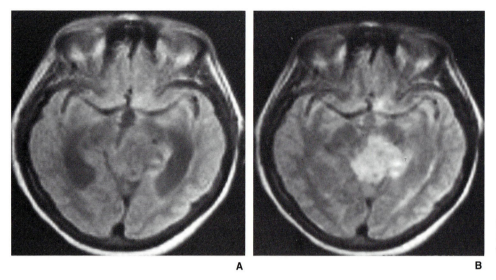

Figures 33.1A (SE 2000/28) and **33.1B** (SE 2000/56). Axial scans at the level of the quadrigeminal plate.

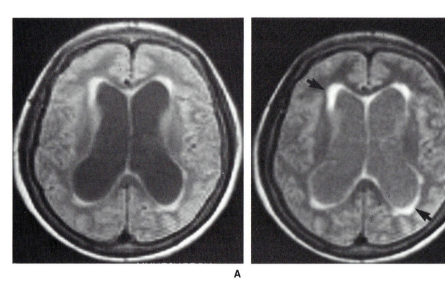

Figures 33.2A (SE 2000/28) and **33.2B** (SE 2000/56). Axial scans at the level of the bodies of the lateral ventricles.

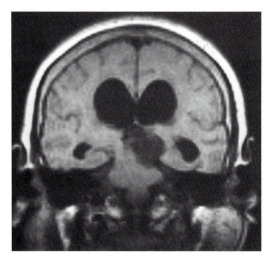

Figure 33.3 (SE 500/28). Coronal scan posterior to the third ventricle.

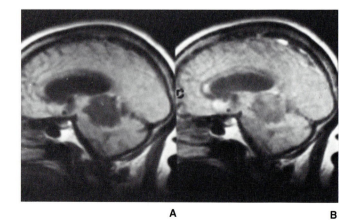

Figures 33.4A (SE 1000/28) and **33.4B** (SE 1000/56). Midsagittal sections.

MR TECHNIQUES

	1	2	3
a. Coil	Head	Head	Head
b. Centering point	CML	Midvertex	Midsagittal
c. Imaging planes	Axial	Coronal	Sagittal
d. Contrast	Mild to moderate T2W	Moderate T1W	Mild T1W/ mild T2W
e. Slice thickness	Routine	Routine	Routine

Multiple imaging planes with both T1 and T2 weighting were obtained for tissue characterization and anatomic localization.

MR FINDINGS

Figure 33.1. There is a heterogeneous, well-defined, high intensity mass located posterior to the third ventricle. It is difficult to determine whether this mass is intra-axial or extra-axial in the transverse plane.

Figure 33.2. There is hydrocephalus with smooth, periventricular interstitial edema (black arrows).

Figure 33.3. This coronal T1WI provides greater localizing information. The mass is shown to be extra-axial because of its transtentorial extension and extrinsic compression of both the brainstem and left medial temporal lobe. The low intensity of the mass indicates a long T1.

Figure 33.4. With an intermediate TR, the lesion is shown to be heterogeneous, with an intermediate intensity between that of CSF and brain parenchyma.

DIFFERENTIAL DIAGNOSIS

The extra-axial location of this mass, its heterogeneous texture, and particular intensity pattern are typical of an epidermoid tumor.[1] Other extra-axial lesions, however, should be considered:

1. *Arachnoid cyst.* This is unlikely since the signal intensity of this lesion is heterogenous and different from that of CSF (see Case 2).
2. *Pineal region tumors (e.g., germ cell tumors, tumors of pineal cell origin, and gliomas).* The marked hetero-geneity and infiltration along natural tissue planes seen in this case would be atypical for pineal region tumors (see Case 30).
3. *Meningioma.* Meningiomas are characteristically homogeneous and isointense with brain parenchyma on most pulsing sequences.[2,3] (See Case 35.) *Note:* The fact that the mass was of low density and non-enhancing on CT argues against either pineal region tumor or meningioma.
4. *Dermoid tumor or lipoma.* These fatty tumors have a short T1 and should have a high intensity on T1-weighted images.

Final Diagnosis

Epidermoid tumor.

SUMMARY OF MR FINDINGS FOR EPIDERMOID TUMOR[1]

1. Extra-axial location.
2. Heterogeneous intensity pattern on all pulsing sequences, reflecting the heterogeneity of the tumor elements.
3. Mass effect may be detectable if the tumor is of sufficient size but is usually mild relative to tumor volume. Cisternal infiltration and insinuation are characteristic.
4. These tumors typically have a long T1 and a long T2. Therefore, on T1-weighted images, they are of low intensity, but they become more intense with greater T2 weighting. The lack of T1 shortening is interesting, as these lesions invariably contain cholesterol, which produces T1 shortening when found in craniopharyngiomas. Intensity differences are thought to relate to differences in the physical state of the cholesterol. Epidermoids are solid, waxy tumors, while craniopharyngiomas are typically cystic. The lack of hydrolyzed cholesterol in epidermoids renders the fat "MR-invisible."[1]

REFERENCES

1. Kortman KE, Van Dalsem W, Bradley WG: MRI of intracranial epidermoid tumors. Submitted for publication.
2. Zimmerman RD, Fleming CA, Saint-Louis LA, et al: Magnetic resonance imaging of meningiomas. *AJNR* 1985;6:149–158.
3. Bucon KA, Bradley WG, Kortman KE: MR imaging of meningiomas with and without paramagnetic contrast. submitted for publication.

CASE 34

HISTORY

A 38-year-old man presents with recurrent left-sided facial numbness and hearing loss. He had undergone previous surgery for resection of a left fifth nerve neuroma.

QUESTIONS

1. What are your differential considerations?

   _____

   _____

2. What MR techniques would you use?

	1	2	3
a. Coil	___	___	___
b. Centering point	___	___	___
c. Imaging plane(s)	___	___	___
d. Contrast	___	___	___
e. Slice thickness	___	___	___

3. What do you expect to find?

   _____

   _____

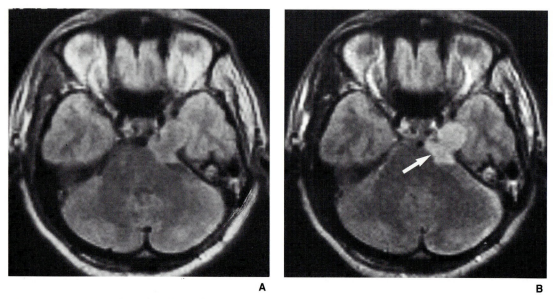

Figures 34.1A (SE 2000/28) and **34.1B** (SE 2000/56). Axial scans through the parasellar region.

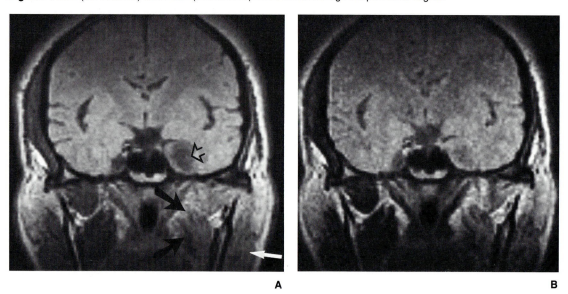

Figures 34.2A (SE 1000/28) and **34.2B** (SE 1000/56). Coronal scans through the parasellar region.

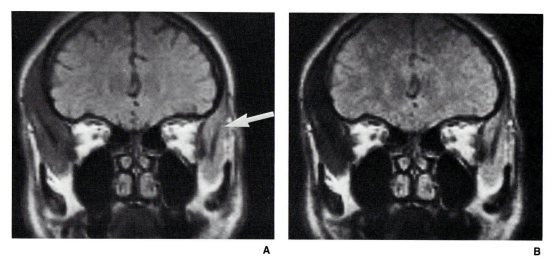

Figures 34.3A (SE 1000/28) and **34.3B** (SE 1000/56). Coronal scans through the frontal lobes.

MR TECHNIQUES

	1	2
a. Coil	Head	Head
b. Centering point	CML	Midvertex
c. Imaging planes	Axial	Coronal
d. Contrast	Mild to moderate T2W	Mild T1W/ mild T2W
e. Slice thickness	Thin	Thin

The first pulsing sequence is the routine screening sequence. Because of the proximity of critical structures in the parasellar region, thin slices are required to accurately assess lesions in this area. The second sequence was performed in the coronal plane with greater T1 weighting to provide additional localizing information and tissue characterization.

MR FINDINGS

Figure 34.1. There is a well-circumscribed, homogeneous, high intensity mass with a bilobed configuration located in the left cavernous sinus and the region of Meckel's cave. The mass causes displacement of the adjacent gray and white matter of the medial temporal lobe, and there is inferior and posterior extension (white arrow) of the mass into the posterior fossa, producing mild displacement of the brainstem. These findings indicate an extra-axial mass. The intensity of the mass increases on the second echo image, indicating a prolonged T2.

Figure 34.2. On this mildly T1-weighted image, the tumor (open black arrow) has a low signal intensity relative to the brain parenchyma, reflecting a slightly prolonged T1.

Compared with the right, the left pterygoid (black arrow) and masseter (white arrow) muscles are slightly thinner and higher in signal intensity on both the first and second echo images, indicating a slightly shortened T1 and a prolonged T2. This is consistent with fatty replacement of the muscle due to denervation atrophy.[1]

Figure 34.3. Marked atrophy of the left temporalis muscle (white arrow) is well demonstrated on this image.

DIFFERENTIAL DIAGNOSIS

The findings of a well-defined, homogeneous, high intensity extra-axial lesion located in Meckel's cave and associated denervation atrophy of the muscles of mastication are characteristic of a trigeminal neuroma. Other extra-axial lesions that could be considered are as follows.

1. *Meningioma*. The prolonged T2 is less characteristic of a meningioma, which usually is isointense with brain parenchyma because of similar T2 values (see Case 35).
2. *Epidermoid*. These tumors are usually more heterogeneous in intensity pattern, and the muscle atrophy would be atypical (see Case 33).
3. *Arachnoid cyst*. These lesions have a signal intensity similar to that of CSF (see Case 2).

Final Diagnosis

Left trigeminal neuroma.

SUMMARY OF MR FINDINGS FOR NEUROMAS[2,3]

1. These masses are extra-axial in location and are well circumscribed and homogeneous.
2. Prolonged T2 results in increased signal intensity on T2WI.
3. There may be secondary fatty atrophy of muscles innervated by the affected nerve.
4. Associated osseous erosions may be difficult to detect on MRI.

REFERENCES

1. Harnsberger HR, Dillon WP: Major motor atrophic patterns in the face and neck: CT evaluation. *Radiology* 1985;155:665–670.
2. New PFJ, Bachow TB, Wismer GL, et al: MR imaging of the acoustic nerves and small acoustic neuromas at 0.6 T: Prospective study. *AJR* 1985;144:1021–1026.
3. Waluch V, Bradley WG, Whitaker SG, et al: MRI of acoustic neuromas and other temporal bone diseases. *AJNR*, in press.

CASE 35

HISTORY

A 50-year-old woman presenting with frontal headaches and dizziness. Decreased visual acuity in the left eye was noted. A CT examination is shown in Figure 35.1.

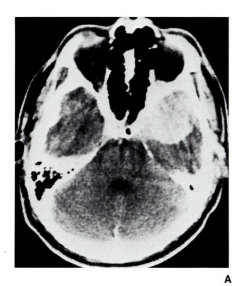 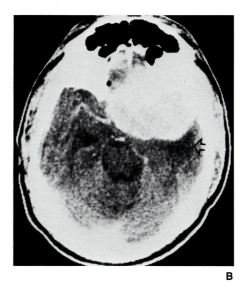

A **B**

Figures 35.1A and **35.1B.** Enhanced axial CT images through the left sphenoid wing.

QUESTIONS

1. What are your differential considerations?

_____
_____

2. What MR techniques would you use?

	1	2	3
a. Coil	___	___	___
b. Centering point	___	___	___
c. Imaging plane(s)	___	___	___
d. Contrast	___	___	___
e. Slice thickness	___	___	___

3. What do you expect to find?

_____
_____

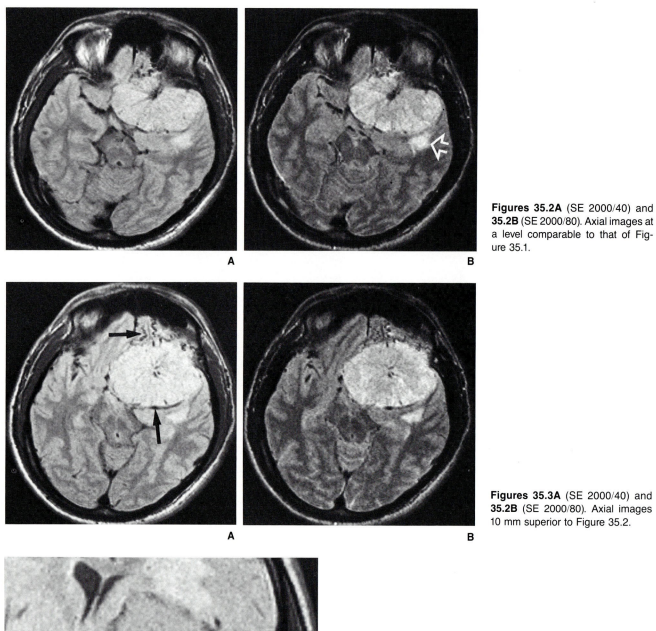

Figures 35.2A (SE 2000/40) and **35.2B** (SE 2000/80). Axial images at a level comparable to that of Figure 35.1.

Figures 35.3A (SE 2000/40) and **35.2B** (SE 2000/80). Axial images 10 mm superior to Figure 35.2.

Figure 35.4 (SE 1000/40). Enlarged coronal section through the region of interest.

MR TECHNIQUES

	1	2
a. Coil	Head	Head
b. Centering point	CML	Anterior cranium
c. Imaging plane	Axial	Coronal
d. Contrast	Mild to moderate T2W	Mild T1W
e. Slice thickness	Thin	Thin

The first sequence was a general screening study. Thin sections were used for anatomic detail. The second sequence was used to evaluate the relationship of the cavernous sinus to the mass and to provide T1 information.

MR FINDINGS

Figure 35.1. There is a dense, presumably enhancing, well-circumscribed homogeneous mass projecting from the left sphenoid wing. The mass extends to the cavernous sinus, and edema (open arrow) within the compressed left temporal lobe can be identified. There is hyperostosis of the left sphenoid wing. The findings are consistent with a meningioma.

Figures 35.2 and 35.3. The mass is noted to have increased intensity on both the first and second echo T2-weighted images. Similar findings of edema (open arrow— Figure 35.2B) can be seen. The tumor has an inhomogeneous appearance, which is not shown by the CT study. Fine low intensity striations produce a "sunburst" or "spoke-wheel" pattern. Such a pattern is classically seen within meningiomas on angiography and is due to fine, radially oriented, small arterial branches. Although not proven, the MR findings are thought to reflect this type of vascular distribution. Low intensity structures (arrows— Figure 35.3A) noted in the periphery of the mass represent enlarged draining veins, displaced cortical vessels, and the left middle meningeal artery. As on CT, the exact relationship of the mass to the cavernous sinus could not be determined on the axial study.

Figure 35.4. On this mildly T1-weighted image, the mass is isointense with normal brain parenchyma and can be seen invaginating the adjacent compressed temporal and frontal lobes. The inferolateral border of the mass is indicated by arrows. The left cavernous sinus does not appear to be invaded although the tumor extends medially into the suprasellar cistern.

DIFFERENTIAL DIAGNOSIS

The CT findings are typical of a meningioma. The MR findings are also characteristic, with the following exceptions. First, the majority of meningiomas are usually isointense with brain parenchyma on mildly T1- and T2-weighted images.[1] Two examples of isointense meningiomas appear in Figures 35.5 and 35.6. Second, the "spoke-wheel" pattern has not been a consistent finding, and most meningiomas have a homogeneous to slightly heterogeneous pattern on MRI.

The differential diagnosis should include all extra-axial lesions, such as:

1. *Neuromas.* The size and location would be atypical of a neuroma.
2. *Arachnoid cyst.* The intensity of an uncomplicated arachnoid cyst should exactly follow CSF on all pulsing sequences. The mass in this case clearly has a signal intensity different from that of CSF (see Case 2).
3. *Epidermoid.* Characteristically, epidermoids have prolonged T1 and T2 values and are heterogeneous. A typical example is discussed in Case 33.
4. *Metastasis.* The extra-axial location would be very atypical of a metastasis.

Final Diagnosis

Left sphenoid wing meningioma.

SUMMARY OF MR FINDINGS FOR MENINGIOMAS

1. Extra-axial location with a predilection for certain sites, including the sphenoid wing, the parasellar region, the parasagittal convexity, and the cerebellopontine angle. Displaced cortical vessels and white matter "buckling" indicate an extra-axial location.[1,2]
2. The majority of meningiomas are isointense with brain parenchyma except on heavily T1- and T2-weighted images. This makes the detection of small tumors difficult. Surrounding edema may help to define the boundary of the tumor.[2]
3. Calcifications within meningiomas that are readily seen on CT scans are generally not well demonstrated by MRI.[1,2] Adjacent bony changes, while apparent in this case, are generally better appreciated on CT than MRI.
4. In the future, gadolinium-DTPA infusion may aid in the diagnosis of meningioma, a pattern of dense and homogeneous enhancement being characteristic.[2,3] (See Figure 35.7.)

REFERENCES

1. Bucon KA, Bradley WG, Kortman KE: MR imaging of meningiomas with and without paramagnetic contrast. Submitted for publication.
2. Zimmerman RD, Fleming CA, Saint-Louis LA, et al: Magnetic resonance imaging of meningiomas. *AJNR* 1985;6:149–158.
3. Felix R, Schorner W, Laniado M, et al: Brain tumors: MR imaging with gadolinium-DTPA. *Radiology* 1985;156:681–688.

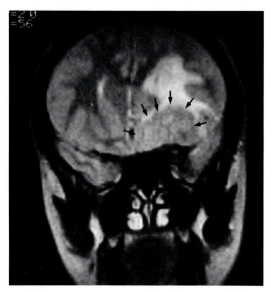

Figure 35.5 (SE 2000/56). This sphenoid wing meningioma (arrows) is isointense with normal brain parenchyma on a moderately T2-weighted image.

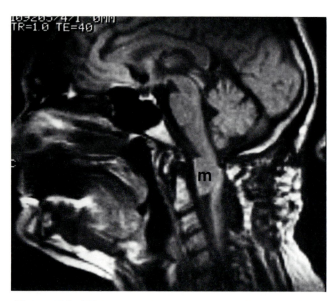

Figure 35.6. (SE 1000/28). An isointense, partially resected meningioma anterior to the upper cervical cord (m) can be seen on the mildly T1-weighted image. A cleavage plane between the mass and the compressed cervical cord is not evident.

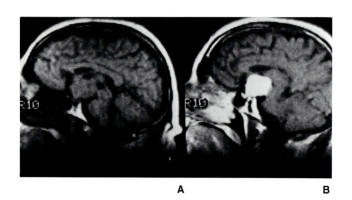

A   B

Figures 35.7A (precontrast, SE 500/28) and **35.7B** (postcontrast, SE 500/28). Sagittal scans of a diaphragm meningioma showing marked enhancement following administration of gadolinium-DTPA.

CASE 36

HISTORY

A 36-year-old woman presenting with headaches and diplopia.

QUESTIONS

1. What are your differential considerations?

_____

_____

2. What MR techniques would you use?

		1	2	3
a.	Coil	___	___	___
b.	Centering point	___	___	___
c.	Imaging plane(s)	___	___	___
d.	Contrast	___	___	___
e.	Slice thickness	___	___	___

3. What do you expect to find?

_____

_____

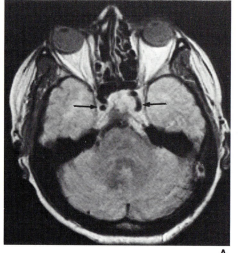

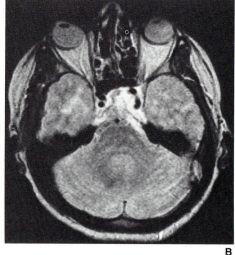

A **B**

Figures 36.1A (SE 2000/40) and **36.1B** (SE 200/80). Axial images at the level of the internal auditory canals.

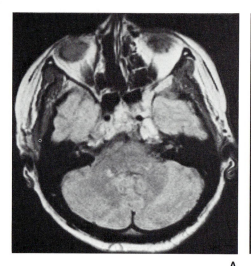

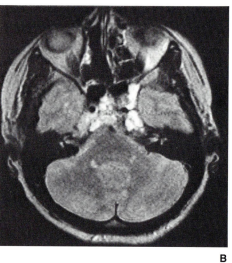

A **B**

Figures 36.2A (SE 2000/40) and **36.2B** (SE 2000/80). Axial images 5 mm superior to Figure 36.1.

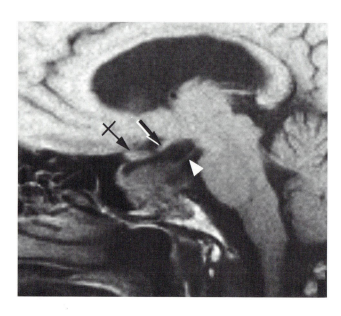

Figure 36.3 (SE 500/40). T1-weighted midsagittal image.

MR TECHNIQUES

	1	2
a. Coil	Head	Head
b. Centering point	CML	Midsagittal plane
c. Imaging planes	Axial	Sagittal
d. Contrast	Mild and moderate T2W	Moderate T1W
e. Slice thickness	Thin	Thin

The first sequence is a variation of the routine screening study. Because of the history of diplopia, thin slices were used for a more detailed examination of the cavernous sinuses and brainstem. The second sequence was added for additional localizing information and tissue characterization.

MR FINDINGS

Figure 36.1. There is a heterogeneous high intensity mass extending from the region of the upper clivus into the sphenoid sinus and the left and right cavernous sinuses. The hyperintensity is more pronounced on the second echo image, indicating T2 prolongation.

Figure 36.2. At a slightly higher level, the mass can be seen surrounding tubular low intensity structures (arrows). These are the internal carotid arteries within the cavernous sinuses.

Figure 36.3. On the T1-weighted midsagittal section, the mass is slightly hypointense with respect to brain parenchyma. The mass is clearly extra-axial in location. It has eroded the anterosuperior aspect of the clivus, expanded the sella, and extended anteriorly into the sphenoid sinus. Superiorly, the tumor extends into the suprasellar cistern and abuts the third nerve (arrowhead). The optic tracts (closed arrow) and chiasm (crossed arrow) are not displaced or compressed by the lesion.

DIFFERENTIAL DIAGNOSIS

Differential diagnostic considerations include all sellar and parasellar region tumors, including chordoma, chondroma, meningioma, pituitary adenoma, pituitary carcinoma, metastasis, sphenoid sinus carcinoma, and craniopharyngioma. The heterogeneity and aggressive nature of the lesion, although somewhat nonspecific, are characteristic of chordoma, and this diagnosis was established by transphenoidal excisional biopsy.

Chordomas are the most common tumors arising from the clivus. These tumors may also be sellar or parasellar in location. They arise from notochordal remnants and produce symptoms via local invasion. Pain and cranial nerve palsies are common presenting symptoms.

On CT examination, tumor calcification and clival destruction/erosion are typical findings.[1] MRI is insensitive to calcification, and tumor heterogeneity is a more characteristic MR finding.[2] Anterior extension into the sphenoid sinus and nasopharynx is readily appreciated on direct sagittal images, as is posterior or superior extension into the prepontine and suprasellar cisterns, respectively.

The intensity pattern of this lesion militates against either meningioma or craniopharyngioma. The aggressive nature of the tumor, indicated by clival destruction and cavernous sinus invasion, would be atypical for a chondroma, pituitary adenoma, or craniopharyngioma. Carcinoma of the pituitary or sphenoid sinus would be unusual but cannot be excluded on the basis of MR findings alone. There was no history of primary malignancy in this patient. These findings, however, could certainly be produced by metastatic disease, as illustrated in Figure 36.4.

Final Diagnosis

Chordoma.

SUMMARY OF MR FINDINGS FOR CHORDOMA

1. Aggressive soft tissue mass arising from the clivus and/or sellar region.
2. These tumors appear hyperintense on T2-weighted images and isointense to hypointense on T1-weighted images.
3. The extent of local invasion is better appreciated on sagittal sections.
4. Tumor heterogeneity may relate to a combination of focal calcification and necrosis.

REFERENCES

1. Krol G, Sundareson N, Deck M: Computed tomography of axial chordomas. *JCAT* 1983;7:286–289.
2. Sze GK, Uichanco LS III, Brant-Zawadzki M, et al: Magnetic resonance imaging of craniocervical chordomas. Presented at the 24th Annual Meeting of the American Society of Neuroradiology, San Diego, January 1986.

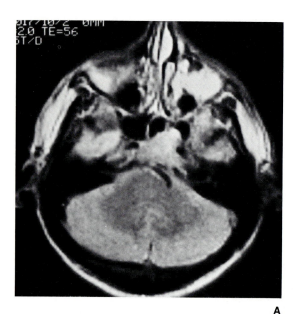

A

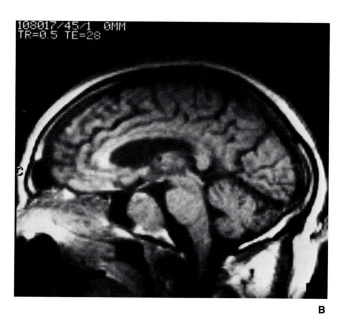

B

Figure 36.4A (SE 2000/56). This 70-year-old man had known metastatic prostate carcinoma. He presented with occipital pain and diplopia. A T2-weighted axial section at the skull base demonstrates a slightly hyperintense midline mass extending into the sella.

Figure 36.4B (SE 500/28). On a T1-weighted sagittal image, the mass is isointense with brain parenchyma and can be seen eroding the superior aspect of the high intensity clivus. A biopsy confirmed the diagnosis of metastatic prostate carcinoma.

4

HEAD AND NECK IMAGING

Unlike cross-sectional imaging performed elsewhere in the body, imaging of the extracranial head and neck is largely employed as an adjunct to physical and endoscopic examination. A histologic diagnosis is typically determined at the time of endoscopy or via fine needle aspiration. Thus, the lack of imaging specificity is relatively less disadvantageous, and imaging sensitivity assumes greater importance. The role of head and neck imaging is to determine exact tumor location, submucosal extent, and the presence of nodal metastases.

X-ray computed tomography (CT) has had a major impact on the staging of head and neck tumors in several ways: it allows evaluation of mucosal surfaces that may be hidden to the endoscopist, provides an accurate method of determining deep extension of tumor, depicts invasion of bone and/or cartilaginous structures, and is a reliable and reproducible method of evaluating nodal metastases. Magnetic resonance imaging (MRI) offers several other advantages. It is less invasive than CT, requiring no ionizing radiation or injection of contrast material. Greater imaging flexibility is afforded by multiplanar scanning capability and the ability to vary sequence parameter times that accentuate differences in proton density and the T1 and T2 relaxation times of various tissues. When appropriate pulsing parameters are used, the contrast resolution of MR imaging is markedly greater than that of CT. In addition, MR is less sensitive to artifacts from beam hardening or dental fillings.

CT currently retains a number of advantages over MRI. These include greater spatial resolution, better depiction of cortical bone and calcified cartilage, and more accurate determination of nodal disease.[1] CT is also less sensitive to patient motion, which may produce significant MR image degradation. The nontechnical advantages of CT include a lesser incidence of claustrophobia, greater scanner availability, and lower cost per examination.

SIGNAL INTENSITIES OF NORMAL AND PATHOLOGIC TISSUES

On spin echo images, signal intensity I can be approximated as $I = Hf(v)(1 - e^{-TR/T1})(e^{-TE/T2})$ where H is the proton density, $f(v)$ is a function of flow, e is the base of the natural logarithm, TR is the repetition time, TE is the echo delay time, and T1 and T2 are the relaxation times. Thus, the intensity of normal and pathologic tissues varies depending on the sequence parameters used—that is, on the degree of T1- or T2-weighting. A simplified description of signal intensities appears in Tables 4–1 and 4–2.

181

EXAMINATION PLANNING

The MR examination should be tailored in an effort to optimize lesion conspicuity and to determine accurately the local extent of a pathologic process. With respect to neoplastic disease, tumor and fat are best differentiated on T1-weighted (short TR, short TE) sequences, while tumor and muscle are best distinguished on T2-weighted (long TR, long TE) sequences. Within the temporal bone or the paranasal sinuses, tumor mass can often be separated from associated inflammatory exudates or mucus on moderately T2-weighted images.

Most lymph nodes are bordered by fat within fascial planes; thus T1-weighted sequences are the most sensitive in evaluating suspected lymphadenopathy. However, central necrosis within a node—usually indicative of metastatic invasion—is best depicted on T2-weighted sequences. With these observations in mind, an MR examination should include both T1- and T2-weighted sequences and, if possible, should be obtained in two different orthogonal planes.

Axial sections are obtained routinely, as they are the most familiar to imaging physicians and clinicians and allow the evaluation of left to right symmetry. The longitudinal extent of a pathologic process is best assessed in the coronal plane, while sagittal imaging is used in the evaluation of midline structures, such as the pre-epiglottic space and anterior com-

Table 4–1. Signal Intensities of Normal Tissues in the Extracranial Head and Neck

Tissue	Intensity on Mild to Moderate T1W Image[1]	Intensity on Mild to Moderate T2W Image[1]	Basis of Intensity Pattern
Cortical bone	Low	Low	Decreased proton density
Calcified cartilage	Low	Low	Decreased proton density
Air	Very low	Very low	Decreased proton density
Flowing blood	Very low[2]	Very low	Flow void
Muscle	Intermediate low	Intermediate low	Long T1, short T2
Ligament	Intermediate low	Intermediate low	Long T1, short T2 Decreased proton density
Fibrocartilage	Intermediate low	Intermediate low	Long T1, short T2 Decreased proton density
Lymphatic/ glandular tissue	Intermediate	Intermediate high	Long T2
Fat/bone marrow	High	Intermediate high	Short T1

[1]See Appendix B.
[2]Exceptions to the pattern are frequently observed because of other flow-related phenomena.

Table 4–2. Signal Intensity of Pathologic Tissues

Tissue	Intensity on Mild to Moderate T1W Image[1]	Intensity on Mild to Moderate T2W Image[1]	Basis of Intensity Pattern
Solid neoplasms	Intermediate low	Intermediate high	Long T1, long T2
Granulation tissue	Intermediate low	Intermediate high	Long T1, long T2
Chronic fibrosis	Intermediate low	Intermediate low	Decreased proton density
Cyst with pure fluid	Low	Very high	Very long T1, very long T2
Cyst with proteinaceous fluid	Intermediate low	High	Long T1, long T2
Mucus	Intermediate low	High	Long T1, long T2
Subacute-subchronic hemorrhage	Very high	High	Very short T1, long T2

[1]See Appendix B.

missure. Slice thickness may vary depending on the clinical indication. In general, contiguous 5-mm sections are utilized and currently offer the best compromise between anatomic detail and time efficiency.

Surface coils may be used to examine superficial structures such as the temporomandibular joint (TMJ) and the larynx.[2] These coils yield significant increases in signal to noise but restrict the effective field of view and require proportionately greater radiologist/technologist input. Solenoidal surface coils offer a number of advantages over circular (round) or rectangular (''license plate'') coils, but they are applicable only to systems that use permanent or resistive magnets in which the main magnetic field is oriented vertically (perpendicular to the axis of the solenoid). Many of the limitations of surface coil imaging will be eliminated with further improvements in the design of conventional ''volume'' coils (e.g., quadrature detection).

CLINICAL IMAGING

Skull Base

CT and MRI may be considered complementary modalities in the evaluation of lesions at the skull base.[3] CT is far superior in demonstrating bony detail and, because of its greater spatial resolution, remains the modality of choice in the evaluation of congenital anomalies and inflammatory processes within the middle and inner ear. CT depiction of soft tissue abnormalities at the skull base is often hampered by beam-hardening artifacts. Axial CT scanning is also limited by partial volume averaging. While direct coronal CT scanning can be performed in many patients, such exams are often degraded by spray artifacts from dental fillings.

MRI is not limited by beam-hardening artifacts from bone or dental fillings. Axial, coronal, and/or sagittal images can be obtained in all patients with the neck held in a comfortable, neutral position. Because cortical bone at the skull base yields little MR signal, bony erosion or destruction cannot be visualized directly but can be inferred by the extent and contour of the corresponding soft tissue lesion, which is conspicuous. Intracranial and extracranial extension of these lesions is often best depicted on coronal and/or sagittal images.

On T2-weighted images, glomus tumors appear as irregular, high intensity masses in characteristic locations, most often the jugular fossa or middle ear. Thrombosis or slow flow within the jugular vein or dural sinuses may result in a high intraluminal signal. Normal positional variations in flow patterns, however, may also result in loss of expected flow void. Thus, in the evaluation of vascular lesions at the skull base, specific diagnosis depends on demonstration of a soft tissue mass with bone destruction and on additional confirmation by angiography.

Nasopharynx, Parapharyngeal Space, Infratemporal Fossa

Within the nasopharynx, as in other regions of the extracranial head and neck, mucosal alterations and tissue diagnoses are most often determined endoscopically. Imaging goals are to determine the extent of submucosal disease and the presence of nodal metastases. MRI is ideally suited to evaluation of this region, since its superior contrast resolution allows ready distinction between fat, muscle, and tumor.[4] Extension of tumor beyond the pharyngobasilar fascia markedly decreases the likelihood of surgical cure and is easily recognized on T1-weighted axial sections. Retropharyngeal nodal metastases are difficult to detect with CT but can be shown accurately with either T1- or T2-weighted pulsing sequences. Superior tumor extension to the skull base is best depicted on T2-weighted coronal images.

Lesions in the parapharyngeal space and/or infratemporal fossa are also easily recognized on T1-weighted or moderately T2-weighted images. Displacement or invasion of the carotid artery and jugular vein can be demonstrated without using intravenous contrast materials. In the assessment of extensive lesions, the vector of vascular displacement may suggest the site of tumor origin.

At our institution, MRI is the modality of choice in evaluating lesions in the nasopharynx, parapharyngeal space, or infratemporal fossa. Routine examination consists of a T1-weighted axial sequence, followed by a moderately T2-weighted sequence in the coronal plane.

Oropharynx, Tongue, Floor of Mouth

MRI and CT are complementary in the evaluation of lesions within the oral cavity, and both modalities are used routinely at our institution. Each is effective in determining tumor extent within the oral cavity and the floor of the mouth, although CT better demonstrates invasion of the hard palate and mandible. Tongue tumors are best evaluated with MRI, particularly when T2-weighted images are used. Axial sections demonstrate tumor extension across the midline of the tongue and allow accurate assessment of the status of the hypoglossal nerves and lingual arteries. Coronal sections effectively show inferior extension of an oral cavity lesion into the hypopharynx and supraglottic larynx. In our experience, CT is more effective than MRI in the evaluation of associated cervical adenopathy.

Hypopharynx and Larynx

Hanafee and Lufkin have used solenoidal surface coils in a vertically directed main field to demonstrate graphically tumors of the larynx and hypopharynx.[5] In our own experience, however, CT has remained the more effective modality in this region. Thin CT sections can be obtained with preservation of a high level of signal to noise. More importantly, the short CT scan times (3 to 5 seconds per slice) minimize artifacts related to coughing or swallowing. The longer (5 to 15 minutes) MR imaging times result in significant image degradation when such motion occurs. As previously mentioned, many investigators feel MRI is less effective in evaluating cervical adenopathy. For these reasons, at our institution CT remains the modality of choice in the evaluation of laryngeal or hypopharyngeal malignancies, and MRI is used as an adjunct study when indicated. Longitudinal extension of a tumor may be accurately depicted with T1-weighted coronal images, and T1-weighted sagittal images demonstrate tumor involvement of the pre-epiglottic space.

Benign and/or congenital neck lesions, such as branchial cleft cysts and laryngoceles, may be evaluated effectively with either modality. MRI is particularly effective in evaluating midline abnormalities, such as thyroglossal duct cysts.

Salivary Glands

In contrast to other regions of the extracranial head and neck, where squamous cell carcinomas predominate, pathology of the salivary glands is relatively varied and includes both benign and malignant neoplasms and various inflammatory lesions. With respect to neoplastic disease, a tissue diagnosis can occasionally be suggested by CT or MR findings but is almost always verified or predetermined by fine needle aspiration. Cross-sectional imaging is used prior to surgical excision to determine accurately tumor location and extent—that is, intraparotid vs. extraparotid, deep lobe vs. superficial lobe. While both CT and MRI permit accurate localization of parotid pathology, MRI may be slightly more effective in defining tumor location with respect to the facial nerve, which can frequently be recognized as a linear and branching, low intensity structure within the higher intensity parotid tissue. With CT, the location of the facial nerve is approximated by the position of the slightly deeper retromandibular vein; therefore, lesions between the vein and nerve may be falsely localized to the superficial lobe.

The specificity of MRI, similar to that of CT, is relatively low in this region, as the signal intensities of various salivary gland tumors and inflammatory lesions overlap. MRI is also insensitive in the detection of calcification, thus it may be difficult to recognize inflammatory changes related to sialolithiasis.

Axial imaging is used almost exclusively in evaluating salivary gland pathology. Both T1- and T2-weighted sequences are routinely employed.

Paranasal Sinuses

Mass lesions within the paranasal sinuses may be effectively evaluated with either CT or MRI. The modalities often yield complementary information. CT demonstrates bone erosion and/or destruction more effectively, while MRI better characterizes soft tissue abnormalities within the sinus (e.g., tumor vs. mucus within an obstructed sinus). Soft tissue extension into an adjacent sinus, the nasal cavity, or the orbit is well shown with either modality, as both yield good contrast between tumor and air or fat. Intracranial tumor extension is better depicted by MRI than by CT.

T1-weighted or moderately T2-weighted axial images are obtained routinely in evaluation of the paranasal sinuses. Coronal sections are obtained when appropriate.

Thyroid and Parathyroid Glands

Most thyroid lesions are best evaluated by a combination of radionuclide scintigraphy and ultrasound. CT and MRI have limited roles in evaluation of the thyroid gland, with the possible exception of malignant tumor staging. Tumor extension outside the thyroid gland can be demonstrated with either modality, but inferior/intrathoracic extension is better demonstrated by MRI. T1-weighted sections are obtained in the axial plane and, when indicated, additional T2 sections are obtained in the coronal or sagittal plane.

Cervical lymph nodes and parathyroid glands are better evaluated with CT than with MRI because of CT's greater spatial resolution.

Thoracic Inlet

Cervical lesions that extend below the thoracic inlet are difficult to evaluate with CT because of the attenuation of the x-ray beam by overlying shoulders. MRI is not limited in this regard and also yields a high degree of contrast between mediastinal fat, thoracic musculature, blood vessels, and soft tissue abnormalities. Thus, patients with symptoms of airway obstruction, vascular compromise, and/or brachial plexopathy are best studied with MRI.

Cervical Adenopathy

The relative efficacy of CT and MRI in evaluation of cervical lymphadenopathy is the subject of considerable debate. In our experience, MRI's relatively limited spatial resolution is not compensated by its greater contrast resolution. As a result, CT more effectively demonstrates small nodes and necrosis within normal size nodes. The spatial resolution of MRI may be significantly increased with the application of surface coils but, except for solenoidal coils, such techniques are cumbersome and inefficient in time use. Vascular encasement and/or fixation by tumor limits the feasibility of curative lymph node dissection and may be better appreciated with MRI because of the natural contrast between flowing blood and tumor. For these reasons, we feel that CT is the imaging modality of choice in evaluating cervical adenopathy and use MRI as an adjunct study when vascular encasement and/or fixation is suspected. In that setting, T1-weighted axial images are used exclusively.

Temporomandibular Joint (TMJ)

MRI has already become the imaging modality of choice in the evaluation of temporomandibular (TMJ) dysfunction and degenerative disease.[6] Thin-slice, T1-weighted sagittal images obtained with a surface coil can be used to determine accurately the location of the disk with the jaw in the closed and open positions; thus disk displacement with or without reduction can be determined confidently in a completely noninvasive manner. Secondary considerations include bone erosions and disk perforation, and these are best studied with conventional tomography and arthrography, respectively.

SUMMARY

In a short period of time, MRI has already proven effective in the evaluation of a wide variety of head and neck pathologies. While the number of well-controlled comparison studies is limited, MRI appears to be the modality of choice in evaluation of the skull base, the nasopharynx, and the temporomandibular joint. In other regions, such as the oropharynx, salivary glands, and paranasal sinuses, MRI and CT offer comparable and/or complementary information. The role of MR imaging in the evaluation of laryngeal tumors and cervical lymphadenopathy is more limited but is expected to increase with continued technologic advances.

REFERENCES

1. Dooms GC, Hricak H, Crooks LE, et al: Magnetic resonance imaging of the lymph nodes: Comparison with CT. *Radiology* 1984;153:719–728.

2. Lufkin RB, Hanafee WN: Application of surface coils to MR anatomy of larynx. *AJNR* 1985;6:491–497.

3. Hans JS, Huss RG, Benson JE, et al: MR imaging of the skull base. *J Comput Assist Tomogr* 1984;8:944–952.

4. Dillon WP, Mills CM, Kjos B, et al: Magnetic resonance imaging of the nasopharynx. *Radiology* 1984;152:731–738.

5. Lufkin RB, Hanafee WN, Wortham D, et al: Larynx and hypopharynx: MR imaging with surface coils. *Radiology* 1986;158:747–757.

6. Katzberg RW, Bessette RW, Tallents RH, et al: Normal and abnormal temporomandibular joint: MR imaging with surface coils. *Radiology* 1986;158:183–189.

CASE 37

HISTORY

A 60-year-old man presents with a mass in the upper neck. The patient complains of some difficulty in swallowing but denies pain associated with the mass. There is no previous history of surgery or radiation.

QUESTIONS

1. What are your differential considerations?

   _____

   _____

2. What MR techniques would you use?

	1	2	3
a. Coil	_____	_____	_____
b. Centering point	_____	_____	_____
c. Imaging plane(s)	_____	_____	_____
d. Contrast	_____	_____	_____
e. Slice thickness	_____	_____	_____

3. What do you expect to find?

   _____

   _____

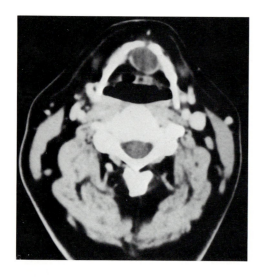

Figure 37.1. Enhanced axial CT at the level of the hyoid bone.

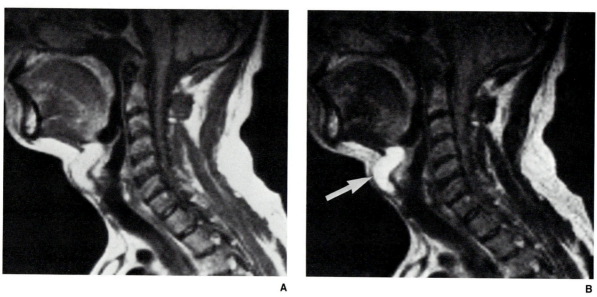

A   B

Figures 37.2A (SE 1000/28) and **37.2B** (SE 1000/56). Midline sagittal scans through the neck.

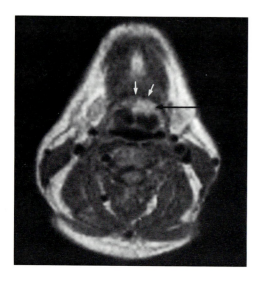

Figure 37.3. (SE 2000/28). Axial scan at the level of the hyoid bone.

MR TECHNIQUES

		1	2
a.	Coil	Neck	Neck
b.	Centering point	Midline	Tongue
c.	Imaging planes	Sagittal	Axial
d.	Contrast	Mild T1W and mild T2W	Mild and moderate T2W
e.	Slice thickness	Thin	Routine

The first pulsing sequence with mild T1 weighting and thin-slice thickness was performed to provide good anatomic detail of the neck structures. The second sequence was performed to demonstrate the anatomic relationship of the lesion in the transverse plane, as well as to provide T2 information.

MR FINDINGS

Figure 37.1. There is a well-defined, low-density mass located in the middle of the pre-epiglottic space. There is slight enhancement of the wall of the mass.

Figure 37.2. A tortuous tubular mass (white arrow) is seen in the midline, extending from the base of the tongue to the anterior aspect of the thyroid cartilage. The mass has a homogeneous high intensity on both the first and second echo images. The increased intensity reflects a combination of a prolonged T2 and a relatively short T1 (compared with the long T1 of pure fluids, such as CSF and urine). The appearance is consistent with a proteinaceous fluid collection. T1 shortening, when pronounced, may also be attributed to the presence of methemoglobin from previous hemorrhage.

Figure 37.3. On this axial image, the lesion (black arrow) is shown to be in the pre-epiglottic space posterior to the hyoid bone (white arrow), which is seen as a curved, low-intensity structure. Erosion of the inner cortex of the hyoid bone seen on CT (Figure 37.1) is poorly seen on MRI because cortical bone is suboptimally depicted.

DIFFERENTIAL DIAGNOSIS

The most common entity in the midline of the neck, extending from the base of the tongue to the region of the thyroid, is a thyroglossal duct cyst. This would be an unusual location for other common neck masses, including adenopathy, branchial cleft cyst, or salivary gland tumor.[1] Rarely, a lingual thyroid may be seen in this location. Differentiation between a solid mass and a cyst would provide more specificity; this differentiation could not be made on the MR study alone, however, since a complicated cyst (i.e., one with elevated protein or subacute hemorrhage) may have high signal on both T1- and T2-weighted images. In this case, the CT scan showed the lesion to be of low density, consistent with a cystic mass (Figure 37.3).

One advantage MRI has over CT is its ability to display the anatomy in the sagittal plane, which is helpful for preoperative planning.

At surgery, a thyroglossal duct cyst was found and resected. The cyst content was noted to be turbid, with a red-brown color indicating previous hemorrhage.

Final Diagnosis

Thyroglossal duct cyst.

SUMMARY OF MR FINDINGS FOR THYROGLOSSAL DUCT CYST

1. Anterior triangle midline location.
2. Intimate association with the hyoid bone anterior to, posterior to, or within the body of the bone.
3. The majority of such cysts extend below the level of the hyoid bone in the region of the thyrohyoid membrane.
4. Generally presents before the age of 10.
5. The relatively short T1 reflects the proteinaceous fluid and/or methemoglobin content of these lesions.

REFERENCE

1. Reede DL, Whelan MA, Bergeron RT: CT of the soft tissue structures of the neck, in Potter GD (ed): *The Radiologic Clinics of North America.* Philadelphia, WB Saunders, 1984, pp 239–264.

CASE 38

HISTORY

A 44-year-old male with right Eustachian tube dysfunction. Axial CT scan through the nasopharynx is shown in Figure 38.1.

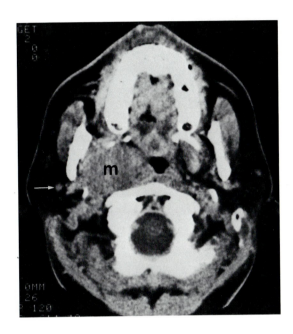

Figure 38.1 Contrast-enhanced axial CT scan through the nasopharynx.

QUESTIONS

1. What are your differential considerations?

_____

_____

2. What MR techniques would you use?

	1	2	3
a. Coil	___	___	___
b. Centering point	___	___	___
c. Imaging plane(s)	___	___	___
d. Contrast	___	___	___
e. Slice thickness	___	___	___

3. What do you expect to find?

_____

_____

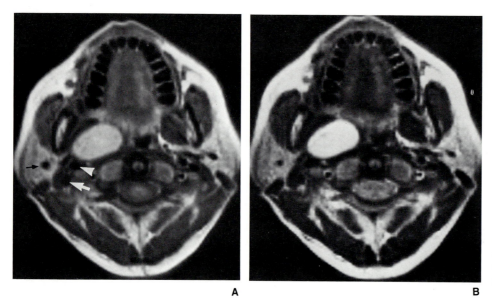

Figures 38.2A (SE 2000/28) and **38.2B** SE (2000/56). Axial scans through the same level as Figure 38.1.

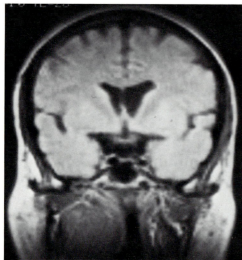

Figure 38.3 (SE 1000/28). Coronal image through the pharynx.

MR TECHNIQUES

	1	2
a. Coil	Neck	Neck
b. Centering point	Mandibular angle	Mandibular angle
c. Imaging planes	Axial	Coronal
d. Contrast	Mild and moderate T2W	Mild T1W and mild T2W
e. Slice thickness	Routine	Routine

The first echo axial scans provide sufficient T1 weighting to define tumor extent, manifested by alterations of normal fat planes. The second echo images allow T2 characterization of the mass. The coronal images allow greater T1 characterization and definition of longitudinal tumor extent.

MR FINDINGS

Figure 38.1. The contrast-enhanced CT demonstrates a large right parapharyngeal mass (m). The contours of the mass and its relation to adjacent parapharyngeal musculature are not well defined. Despite an adequate contrast dose, the positions of the right carotid artery and jugular vein are poorly demonstrated. Note the enhancement of the retromandibular vein (white arrow) within the right parotid gland.

Figure 38.2. This axial MR image confirms the presence of a rounded, right parapharyngeal mass. The mass is conspicuous by virtue of its increased signal intensity (long T2). The contours of the mass are smooth and well defined, indicative of a benign process. The mass is separate from the low intensity carotid artery (white arrowhead) and jugular vein (white arrow) and displaces these structures posteriorly. Note the retromandibular vein (black arrow) with flow void.

Figure 38.3. The superior extent of the mass is shown to be well below the skull base.

DIFFERENTIAL DIAGNOSIS

By MR criteria,[1-3] this is a benign lesion. In addition to tumors of salivary gland origin, the differential diagnosis would include neurogenic tumor (e.g., hypoglossal neuroma) or neurenteric cyst. The absence of fatty atrophy of the intrinsic musculature makes a neuroma unlikely. An uncomplicated cyst, even one with a slightly elevated protein level, would be likely to appear less intense on the mild T1-weighted images.

Final Diagnosis

Mixed-cell tumor (pleomorphic adenoma) of an accessory salivary gland.

SUMMARY OF MR FINDINGS FOR BENIGN SALIVARY GLAND TUMOR

1. Well-defined, rounded contours.
2. Prolongation of T2, which is shown as increased intensity on T2WI (also seen in malignant neoplasms).
3. Lack of adenopathy.

REFERENCES

1. Stark DD, Moss AA, Gamsu G, et al: Magnetic resonance imaging of the neck. Part I: Normal anatomy. *Radiology* 1984;150:447–454.
2. Stark DD, Moss AA, Gamsu G, et al: Magnetic resonance imaging of the neck. Part II: Pathologic findings. *Radiology* 1984;150:455–461.
3. Dillon WP, Mills CM, Kjos B, et al: Magnetic resonance imaging of the nasopharynx. *Radiology* 1984;152:731–738.

CASE 39

HISTORY

A 60-year-old woman presented with facial pain, dysarthria, dysphagia, and diplopia. Physical examination revealed paralysis of right lateral gaze, a depressed corneal reflex, paresis of the right tongue and palate, and right scapular winging.

QUESTIONS

1. What are your differential considerations?

_____

_____

2. What MR techniques would you use?

	1	2	3
a. Coil	___	___	___
b. Centering point	___	___	___
c. Imaging plane(s)	___	___	___
d. Contrast	___	___	___
e. Slice thickness	___	___	___

3. What do you expect to find?

_____

_____

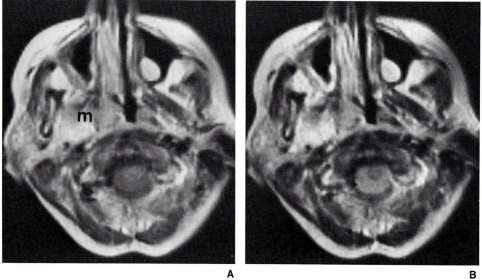

Figures 39.1A (SE 2000/30) and **39.1B** (SE 2000/60). Axial scans through the superior nasopharynx.

A

B

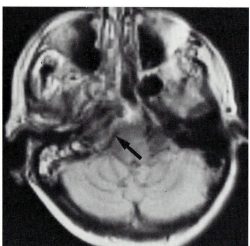

Figure 39.2 (SE 2000/30). Axial section 2 cm superior to Figure 39.1.

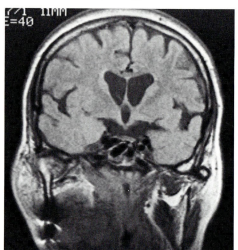

Figure 39.3 (SE 1000/40). Coronal section through the nasopharynx and cavernous sinus.

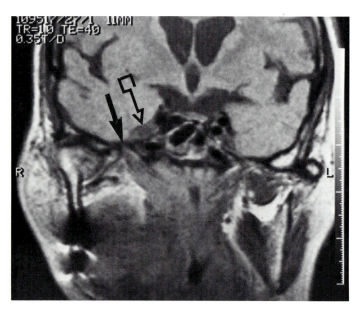

Figure 39.4 (SE 1000/40). Magnification of Figure 39.3.

MR TECHNIQUES

	1	2
a. Coil	Head	Head
b. Centering point	EAC	EAC
c. Imaging planes	Axial	Coronal
d. Contrast	Mild and moderate T2W	Mild T1W
e. Slice thickness	Routine	Thin
f. Spatial resolution	High	High

The first sequence was used as a screening study of the brain, skull base, and nasopharynx. The second sequence was obtained for additional tissue characterization and localizing information. Thin slices were used specifically to examine the skull base and cavernous sinus region.

MR FINDINGS

Figure 39.1A. There is a large soft tissue mass (m) in the right nasopharynx, extending laterally into the infratemporal fossa. There is mild distortion of the right nasopharyngeal airway. Incidental note is made of a small mucous retention cyst in the left maxillary sinus.

Figure 39.1B. The intensity of the mass increases on the second echo image, indicating T2 prolongation.

Figure 39.2. The mass extends into the petrous apex (arrow). More anterior involvement of the skull base is suspected but cannot be confidently identified. Inflammatory fluid is seen within the mastoid air cells, relating to Eustacian tube obstruction by the mass.

Figure 39.3. The coronal image verifies the presence of a bulky right nasopharyngeal mass with infratemporal extension. Metallic clips from previous right mandibular surgery produce focal, mixed low and high intensity artifacts.

Figure 39.4. The magnified coronal image shows superior tumor extension through the skull base via the foramen ovale (arrow). Tumor can also be seen within the inferior right cavernous sinus (boxed arrow).

DIFFERENTIAL DIAGNOSIS

The findings are consistent with an aggressive neoplastic process. Statistically squamous cell carcinoma of the nasopharynx is most likely, and this was confirmed by surgical biopsy. The extension into the skull base and cavernous sinus is a well-recognized pathway of tumor spread.

Differential diagnostic considerations in an adult would include adenocystic carcinoma and lymphoma. In the pediatric age group, the most common malignancy in the nasopharynx is rhabdomysarcoma.

Final Diagnosis:

Nasopharyngeal carcinoma.

SUMMARY OF TYPICAL MR FINDINGS FOR NASOPHARYNGEAL CARCINOMA[1,2]

1. A mass of intermediate and inhomogeneous intensity producing soft-tissue asymmetry within nasopharynx.
2. The pharyngobasilar fascia is often breached.
3. The lateral pharyngeal recess (fossa of Rosenmuller) and the Eustachian tube opening are often obliterated.
4. Infiltration of the parapharyngeal space is a reliable sign of malignancy. This is seen on MR as a pattern of inhomogeneous intermediate signal intensity within the involved parapharyngeal space.
5. The involved muscles (eg, tensor and levator palati and pterygoid and pharyngeal muscles) often have higher signal intensity than normal striated muscle.
6. Skull base and cavernous sinus extension are best appreciated on thin slice coronal images.
7. These tumors may spread to the lateral retropharyngeal, internal jugular, and spinal accessory nodes. Approximately 50% of patients have bilateral nodes.

REFERENCES

1. Mancuso AA, Hanafee WN: Nasopharynx and parapharyngeal space. In *Computed Tomography and Magnetic Resonance Imaging of the Head and Neck*. Baltimore, Williams & Wilkins, 1985, pp 428–497.
2. Dillon WP, Mills CM, Kjos B, et al: Magnetic resonance imaging of the nasopharynx. *Radiology* 1984;152:731.

CASE 40

HISTORY

A 62-year-old woman presenting with sinus pain and epistaxis.

QUESTIONS

1. What are your differential considerations?

   _____

   _____

2. What MR techniques would you use?

	1	2	3
a. Coil	_____	_____	_____
b. Centering point	_____	_____	_____
c. Imaging plane(s)	_____	_____	_____
d. Contrast	_____	_____	_____
e. Slice thickness	_____	_____	_____

3. What do you expect to find?

   _____

   _____

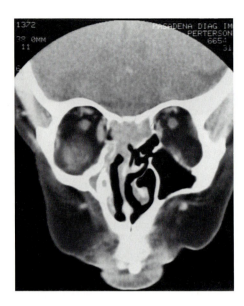

Figure 40.1. Direct coronal CT through the paranasal sinuses and the nasal cavity.

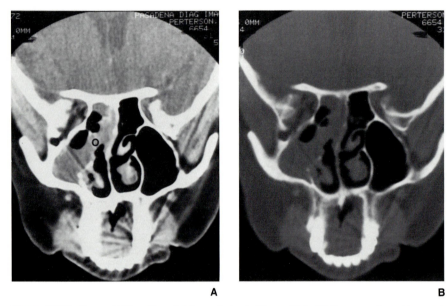

A   B

Figure 40.2A Coronal CT section slightly posterior to Figure 40.1. (B) Same section at bone window settings.

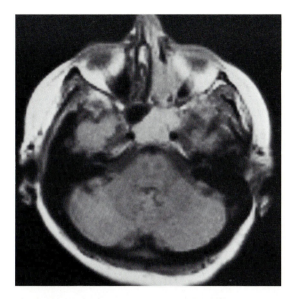

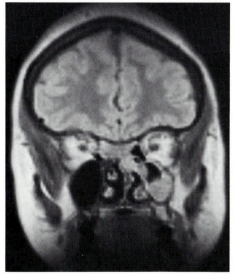

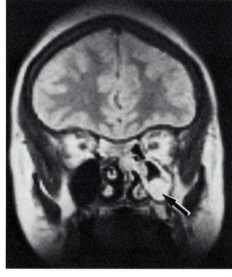

Figure 40.3 (SE 1000/28). Mildly T1-weighted axial MR image through the sphenoid, ethmoid, and superior maxillary sinuses.

Figures 40.4A (SE 2000/28) and **40.4B** (SE 2000/56). T2-weighted coronal MR images corresponding to CT sections.

A

B

MR TECHNIQUES

	1	2
a. Coil	Head	Head
b. Centering point	Orbital floor	Pterygoid plates
c. Plane	Axial	Coronal
d. Contrast	Mild T1W	Mild and moderate T2W
e. Slice thickness	Thin	Thin

The first sequence is similar to that used for routine head and neck imaging. The axial plane is the most familiar to clinicians and imaging physicians. It allows evaluation of left–right symmetry and serves as a reference plane for additional coronal and/or sagittal sequences. Mild T1 weighting yields good signal-to-noise and contrast between fat, muscle, and tumor. An additional T2-weighted coronal sequence was obtained for localizing information and to separate tumor from reactive inflammatory changes within the sinuses.

MR FINDINGS

Figure 40.1. The CT section demonstrates a soft tissue mass involving the ethmoid sinuses and destroying the sinus walls.

Figure 40.2. More posteriorly, the mass involves the sphenoid sinus. Soft tissue density extends to the ostium of the left maxillary sinus (O). Additional soft tissue within the sinus is noted inferiorly and laterally. The density of this tissue is similar to that seen within the sphenoid and ethmoid sinuses.

Figure 40.3. The axial T1-weighted MR image demonstrates a homogeneous soft tissue density filling the sphenoid sinus and extending anteriorly to involve the posterior ethmoid air cells and the superior left antrum.

Figure 40.4. T2-weighted coronal MR images verify extension of the tumor to the ostium of the left maxillary sinus. The intensity of the soft tissue elsewhere in the antrum (arrow), however, is higher than that at the ostium. This intensity difference is only apparent on the more T2-weighted second echo image.

DIFFERENTIAL DIAGNOSIS

The bone destruction and tumor extension demonstrated in this case are indicative of an aggressive neoplasm. The most common sinus malignancy is squamous cell carcinoma.[1] Less common malignancies include lymphoma, adenocystic carcinoma, adenocarcinoma, and metastases. None of these diagnoses can be excluded on the basis of the CT or MR findings. Surgical exploration and biopsy in the patient yielded a diagnosis of adenocarcinoma.

Final Diagnosis

Adenocarcinoma of the sphenoid sinus.

Comment:

CT and MR can be considered complementary modalities in the evaluation of paranasal sinus pathology. As in this case, CT is usually more effective in demonstrating bone erosion or destruction. MRI is more effective in characterizing soft tissue abnormalities. In this example, surgical exploration of the maxillary sinus revealed tumor obstructing the ostium and mucus filling the sinus. The T2-weighted coronal MR images allowed accurate distinction between medium intensity tumor and higher intensity mucus, while CT failed to distinguish these tissues.

SUMMARY OF MR FINDINGS FOR SINUS CARCINOMA

1. Soft tissue mass with bone expansion or destruction.
2. The tumor will have an intensity between that of fat and muscle on mildly to moderately T1- and T2-weighted sequences.
3. On T2-weighted images, mucus and/or inflammatory tissue will typically appear more intense than tumor.
4. Lymph node metastases occur in approximately 10% of sinus malignancies and are best appreciated on T1-weighted axial scans.

REFERENCES

1. Hasso AN: CT of tumors and tumor-like conditions of the paranasal sinuses. *Radiol Clin North Am* 1984;22:119–130.

CASE 41

HISTORY

This 61-year-old man presents with an ulcerating mass in the anterior aspect of the tongue and a palpable node in the right submental area. The patient has a significant smoking history.

QUESTIONS

1. What are your differential considerations?

_____

_____

2. What MR techniques would you use?

	1	2	3
a. Coil	___	___	___
b. Centering point	___	___	___
c. Imaging plane(s)	___	___	___
d. Contrast	___	___	___
e. Slice thickness	___	___	___

3. What do you expect to find?

_____

_____

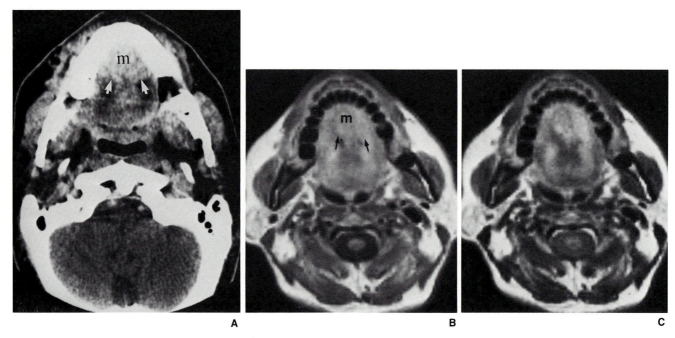

Figures 41.1A (enhanced CT), **41.1B** (SE 1000/28), and **41.1C** (SE 1000/56). Axial scans through the mobile portion of the tongue.

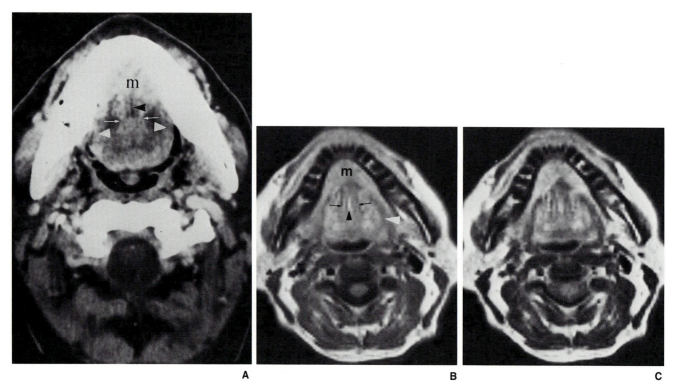

Figures 41.2A (enhanced CT), **41.2B** (SE 1000/28), and **41.2C** (SE 1000/56). Axial scans 1 cm inferior to Figure 41.1.

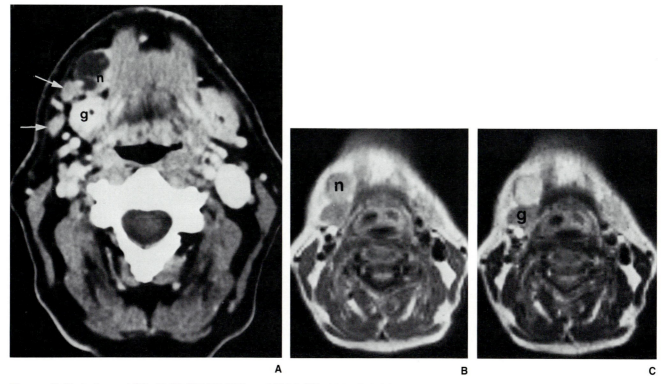

Figures 41.3A (enhanced CT), **41.3B** (SE 1000/28), and **41.3C** (SE 1000/56). Axial scans at the level of the hyoid bone.

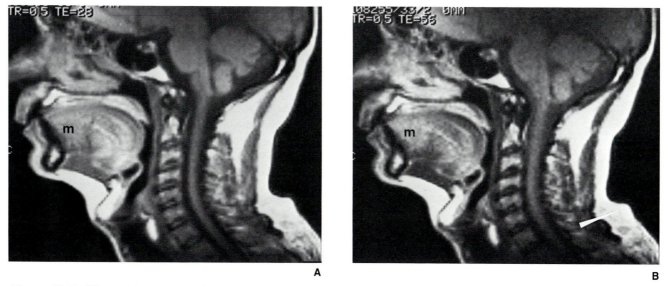

Figures 41.4A (SE 500/28) and **41.4B** (SE 500/56). Midsagittal scans through the tongue.

MR TECHNIQUES

	1	2	3
a. Coil	Neck	Neck	Neck
b. Centering point	Mandible	Mandible	Mandible
c. Imaging planes	Axial	Coronal	Sagittal
d. Contrast	Mild T1W and mild T2W	Mild T2W	Moderate T1W
e. Slice thickness	Thin	Thin	Thin

The first sequence was performed with mild T1 weighting designed to provide anatomic distinction between muscle and the fat within fascial planes of the tongue. The second sequence (not shown) was performed with greater T2 weighting to improve sensitivity in the detection of tumors, which generally have a prolonged T2. The third sequence was designed to provide additional anatomic details in the sagittal plane.

FINDINGS

Figure 41.1. There is an ill-defined, infiltrating, enhancing mass (m) involving the anterior one third of the tongue. The lesion encroaches upon sublingual spaces (arrows) bilaterally.

Figure 41.2. The mass (m) also involves the anterior portion of the paired genioglossus muscles (small arrows), the mylohyoid muscles (white arrowheads), and the lingual septum (black arrowheads). In this case, the soft tissue involvement is better demonstrated on MRI than on CT.

Figure 41.3. There is a 2-cm lymph node (n) with a necrotic center located anterior to the right submandibular gland (g). In addition, there are two slightly enlarged lymph nodes (arrows) seen only on the CT scan.

Figure 41.4. This T1WI demonstrates the three normal layers of intrinsic muscle (superior longitudinal, transverse, inferior longitudinal fibers)[1] within the posterior two thirds of the tongue. Anteriorly, these fibers are interrupted by the high intensity mass (m).

Because the tumor is located anteriorly and involves both sides of the tongue, the coronal images (not shown) were not helpful in determining the extent of the lesion. In general, coronal images are useful in detecting slight asymmetry of the musculature, especially in the posterior two thirds of the tongue.

DIFFERENTIAL DIAGNOSIS

The preceding findings are quite characteristic of a primary neoplasm of the tongue with metastases to the regional lymph nodes. The primary roles of both CT and MRI are to define the extent of the lesion and to detect nodal involvement. Because of the higher contrast resolution and the multiplanar imaging capabilities of MRI, we have found MRI slightly superior to CT in determining the degree of primary tumor involvement in cooperative patients. In uncooperative patients, however, MRI is plagued by significantly more motion artifacts than CT because of the longer scanning times employed.

In our experience, nodal involvement is more difficult to detect with MRI than CT. The abnormal nodes may have intensity ranging from intermediate to high, and they are difficult to separate from the subcutaneous tissues.

A more remote differential consideration in this case would be an inflammatory lesion, such as cellulitis of the tongue. This is less common, and one might expect a more generalized involvement of the tongue.

Final Diagnosis

Carcinoma of the anterior portion of the tongue with involvement of the regional lymph nodes.

SUMMARY OF MR FINDINGS FOR CARCINOMA OF TONGUE[1,2]

1. High intensity mass with distortion of the musculature of the tongue.
2. High tendency to infiltrate deeply, sometimes with little evidence of mucosal disease.
3. Tend to begin laterally and remain on one side until advanced.
4. Mandibular destruction is unusual except in the most advanced cases. Mandibular involvement is generally better detected on CT than MRI, as MRI depicts cortical bone poorly.
5. Approximately 75% of patients have palpable neck nodes at presentation; 30% have bilateral nodes.

REFERENCES

1. Lufkin RB, Larsson SG, Hanafee WN: Work in progress: NMR anatomy of the larynx and tongue base. *Radiology* 1983;148:173–175.
2. Mancusso AA, Hanafee WN: Oral cavity and oropharynx including tongue base, floor of the mouth and mandible, in *Computed Tomography and Magnetic Resonance Imaging of the Head and Neck,* ed 2. Baltimore, Williams & Wilkins, 1985, pp 358–375.

CASE 42

HISTORY

A 42-year-old woman presenting with pulsatile tinnitus. The CT is shown in Figure 42.1.

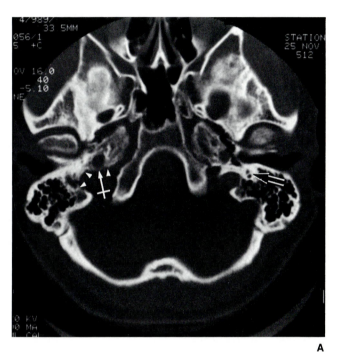
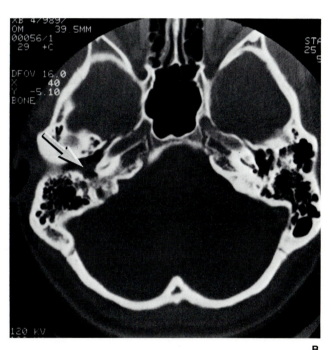

A

B

Figures 42.1A and **42.1B.** Axial CT sections through the temporal bone. A and B are at the level of the middle ear and the jugular bulb, respectively. (Courtesy of Edward Helmer, MD, Los Angeles, CA.)

QUESTIONS

1. What are your differential considerations?

_____

_____

2. What MR techniques would you use?

	1	2	3
a. Coil	___	___	___
b. Centering point	___	___	___
c. Imaging plane(s)	___	___	___
d. Contrast	___	___	___
e. Slice thickness	___	___	___

3. What do you expect to find?

_____

_____

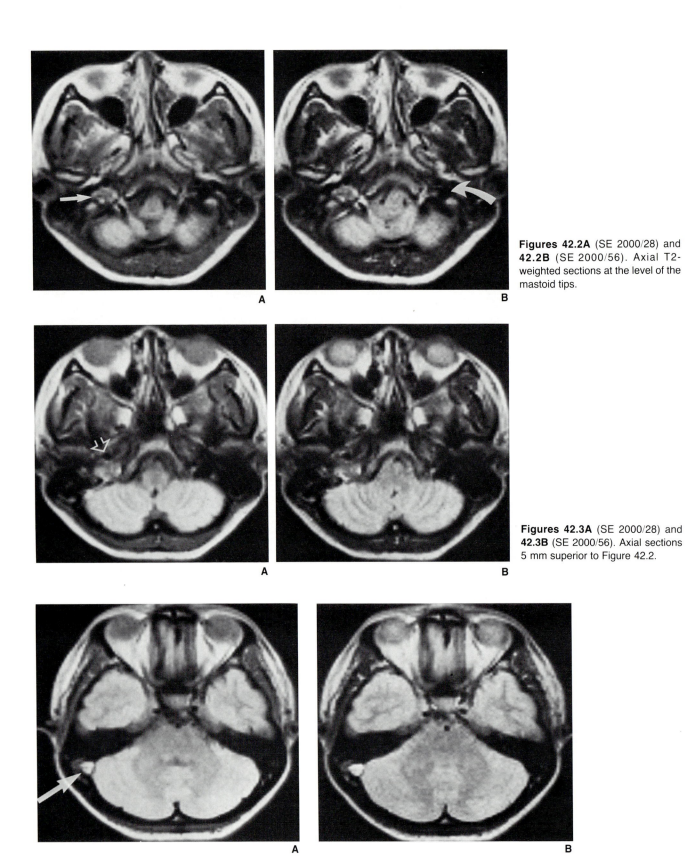

Figures 42.2A (SE 2000/28) and **42.2B** (SE 2000/56). Axial T2-weighted sections at the level of the mastoid tips.

Figures 42.3A (SE 2000/28) and **42.3B** (SE 2000/56). Axial sections 5 mm superior to Figure 42.2.

Figures 42.4A (SE 2000/28) and **42.4B** (SE 2000/56). Axial sections 15 mm superior to Figure 42.3.

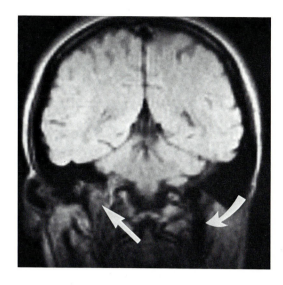

Figure 42.5 (SE 1000/28). Coronal section through the petrous bones.

MR TECHNIQUES

a. Coil	Head	Head
b. Centering point	CML	EAC*
c. Imaging planes	Axial	Coronal
d. Contrast	Mild to moderate T2W	Mild T1W
e. Slice thickness	Thin	Thin

The first sequence is a variation of the routine screening study. Thin slices were used to yield a more detailed examination of the temporal bone. The second sequence was obtained for additional localizing information and tissue characterization.

MR FINDINGS

Figure 42.1. Image 42.1A demonstrates irregular enlargement with osseous destruction of the jugular bulb (arrowheads) and the vertical facial nerve canal (compare with the normal left side, arrow). The osseous crest between the jugular and carotid canal is thinned (crossed arrow). In Figure 42.1B, the superior extent of the mass is seen in the middle ear cavity (arrow). When compared with the normal contralateral side, bony destruction is again noted.

Figure 42.2. There is a medium intensity, somewhat heterogeneous mass in the right jugular fossa (arrow). Note the low intensity flow void within the normal left jugular vein (curved arrow).

Figure 42.3. The mass is slightly larger on this more superior section. A patent internal carotid artery (open arrow) can be seen anterior to the mass.

Figure 42.4. Asymmetric high signal intensity can be seen at the junction of the right transverse and sigmoid sinuses (arrow). This increased intensity is equally pronounced on the first and second echoes. This lack of change is more consistent with sinus thrombosis than slowed flow, since even-echo rephasing would be expected with the latter condition.[1]

Figure 42.5. The lesion (arrow) appears slightly hypointense with respect to brain on this mildly T1-weighted coronal image. It extends longitudinally along the course of the jugular vein. Note the patient's low intensity jugular vein on the left side (curved arrow). Superomedially, the mass extends toward the flocculus of the cerebellum.

---

*external auditory canal

DIFFERENTIAL DIAGNOSIS

The history and MR/CT findings are most consistent with a glomus jugulare tumor or chemodectoma.[1,2] Other considerations include primary and metastatic skull base neoplasms and jugular fossa neuroma. The coronal MR demonstration of mass intrinsic to the jugular vein is pathognomonic of a glomus jugulare tumor. Additional confirmation of the nature of the mass was provided by an angiogram (Figure 42.6). During surgery, the tumor was noted to involve the jugular foramen with extension into the facial nerve canal.

Neuromas of the ninth, tenth, and eleventh cranial nerves may occur within the jugular fossa but are typically more rounded in contour and homogeneous. An example is shown in Figure 42.7.

Occasionally, asymmetric but normal flow phenomena may simulate a jugular fossa vascular tumor. An example appears in Figure 42.8. Because of the pitfall, we consider high-resolution CT and confirmatory angiography the diagnostic procedures of choice in the evaluation of suspected glomus tumors.

Final Diagnosis

Glomus jugulare tumor.

SUMMARY OF MR FINDINGS FOR JUGULOTYMPANIC GLOMUS TUMORS[3]

1. Intrapetrous irregular soft tissue mass involving the jugular foramen (glomus jugulare) or tympanic cavity (glomus tympanicum).
2. T2 prolongation results in increased signal intensity on T2-weighted images.
3. Signal alterations in the adjacent dural sinuses may reflect slowed flow or thrombosis.
4. Normal flow phenomena may produce similar findings. CT and/or angiography is required for confirmation.

REFERENCES

1. Koenig H, Lenz M, Sauter R: Temporal bone region: High resolution MR imaging using surface coils. *Radiology* 1986;159:191–194.
2. Som PM, Reede DL, Bergeron RT, et al: Computer tomography of glomus tympericum tumors. *JCAT* 1983;7:14–17.
3. Curtin HO: CT of acoustic neuromas and other tumors of the ear. *Radiol Clin North Am* 1984;22:77–105.

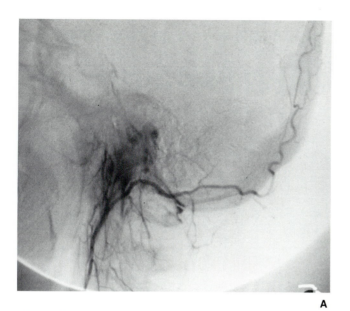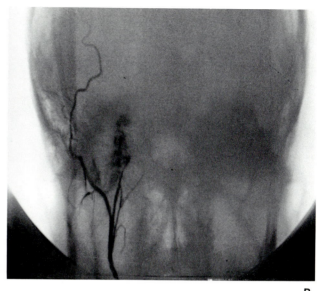

A

B

Figures 42.6A (Lateral projection) and **42.6B** (AP projection). Selected films from the arterial phase of an external carotid angiogram. A tumor blush can be identified within the jugular foramen consistent with a glomus tumor. (Courtesy of Edward Helmer MD, Los Angeles, CA.)

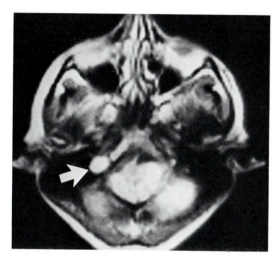

Figure 42.7 (SE 2000/28). Axial view showing a glossopharyngeal neuroma (arrow) within the jugular foramen.

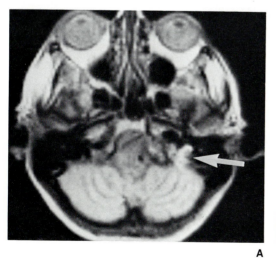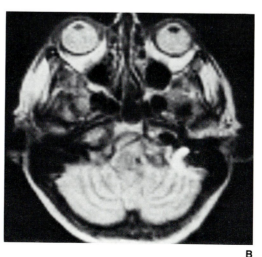

A

B

Figures 42.8A (SE 2000/28) and **42.8B** (SE 2000/56). Flowing blood within a jugular foramen (arrow) simulating a tumor. Because of this finding and the patient's symptoms, an angiogram was performed (not shown) and demonstrated a normal jugular bulb.

CASE 43

HISTORY

A 35-year-old man presenting with hoarseness. Laryngoscopy revealed a large mass in the pre-epiglottic space, apparently limited to the supraglottis. Biopsy revealed squamous cell carcinoma. A partial laryngectomy with resection to the level of the true cord was initially planned. MRI was requested to define further the extent of the lesion.

QUESTIONS

1. What MR techniques would you use?

	1	2	3
a. Coil	———	———	———
b. Centering point	———	———	———
c. Imaging plane(s)	———	———	———
d. Contrast	———	———	———
e. Slice thickness	———	———	———

2. What do you expect to find?

_____

_____

Source: Courtesy of William Hanafee, MD, and Robert Lufkin, MD, UCLA.

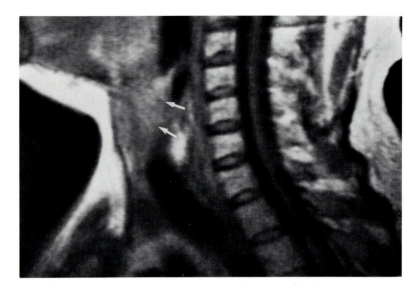

Figure 43.1 (SE 500/28). Midsagittal scan through the larynx and hypopharynx.

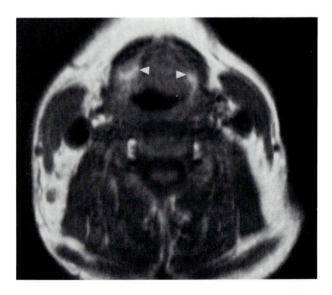

Figure 43.2 (SE 700/28). Axial scan at the level of the hypopharynx.

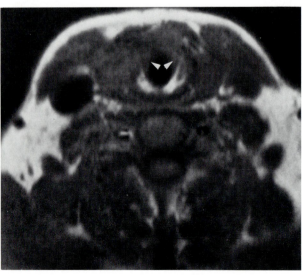

Figure 43.3 (SE 700/28). Axial scan at the level of the cricoid cartilage.

MR TECHNIQUES

	1	2	3
a. Coil	Surface	Surface	Surface
b. Centering point	Midsagittal plane	Thyroid cartilage	Thyroid cartilage
c. Imaging planes	Sagittal	Axial	Coronal
d. Contrast	Moderate T1W	Moderate T1W	Moderate T1W
e. Slice thickness	Thin	Thin	Thin

This is the standard imaging protocol for examining the larynx at UCLA Medical Center, using a 0.3 T permanent magnet. A specially designed laryngeal solenoid surface coil is used. A seven-section sagittal image is initially performed to localize the lesion. This is followed by seven axial sections centering directly over the lesion as shown by the sagittal images. Finally, coronal sections are obtained through the area of abnormality localized by the sagittal and axial images.[1]

MR FINDINGS

Figure 43.1. There is an ill-defined mass (arrows) with intermediate intensity invading the epiglottis and the pre-epiglottic space. The pre-epiglottic space usually has homogeneous high signal intensity due to its fat content. Compare the appearance of the pre-epiglottic space of this patient with that of a normal patient, as shown in Figure 43.4.

Figure 43.2. The lateral border (arrowheads) of this mass is relatively well defined on this axial image. Note the residual high intensity fat within the pre-epiglottic space. Compare this axial image with that of a normal patient shown in Figure 43.5.

Figure 43.3. There is abnormal tumor tissue (arrowheads) within the lumen of the airway at the subglottic level. The anterior ring of the cricoid cartilage has been destroyed.

DISCUSSION

One of the primary goals in laryngeal surgery is the preservation of natural speech. This requires some form of conservation surgery, with minimal resection of the laryngeal skeleton if possible. Accurate knowledge of the full extent of the tumor is essential in determining the feasibility of conservation surgery. An intact cricoid cartilage is required in any type of conservation surgery. Direct extension of the tumor to the tongue base indicates the need for partial glossectomy in addition to the primary surgery. Extralaryngeal spread may render the tumor unresectable. In addition, lymph node involvement influences the staging of the tumor, prognosis, and surgical planning.[1]

Neither MRI nor CT shows mucosal detail well, but both are extremely accurate in defining deep extension of disease. Hence, they are complementary to clinical examination. Compared with CT, MRI has the advantages of direct coronal and sagittal imaging and superior soft tissue contrast resolution. These factors allow better visualization of the intrinsic laryngeal musculature and permit more accurate tumor staging.

In this case, MRI demonstrated tumor spread to the subglottic space and destruction of the cricoid cartilage; therefore, conservation surgery would not be effective. The patient underwent a total laryngectomy.

Final Diagnosis

Transglottic laryngeal carcinoma.

SUMMARY OF MR FINDINGS FOR LARYNGEAL CARCINOMA[1,2]

1. Mass of intermediate signal intensity on T1-weighted images.
2. Replacement of the normal high signal intensity fat in the pre-epiglottic space and the paralaryngeal space.
3. The mass may project into the luminal portion of the larynx. There should not be any tissue within the lumen of the airway at the subglottic level.
4. Cartilage invasion may be detected as a defect in the normal low signal of calcified cartilages and/or as a loss of high signal within the central marrow. Normal variation in patterns of cartilage calcification, however, may simulate destruction.
5. Adenopathy (intracapsular and extracapsular) may be detected. Extracapsular disease is recognized by a lack of distinct margins and spread beyond the lymph node capsule; it is associated with an extremely poor prognosis.

REFERENCES

1. Lufkin RB, Hanafee WN, Wortham D, et al: Larynx and hypopharynx: MR imaging with surface coils. *Radiology* 1986;158:747–754.
2. Mancuso AA, Hanafee WN: Larynx and hypopharynx, in *Computed Tomography and Magnetic Resonance Imaging of the Head and Neck*, ed 2. Baltimore, Williams & Wilkins, 1985, pp 241–357.

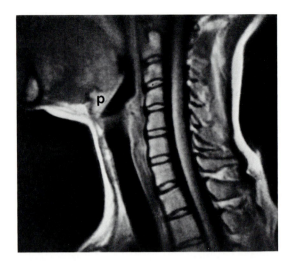

Figure 43.4 (SE 500/28). Midsagittal scan of a normal larynx and hypopharynx. Note the normal homogeneous high intensity of the pre-epiglottic space (p).

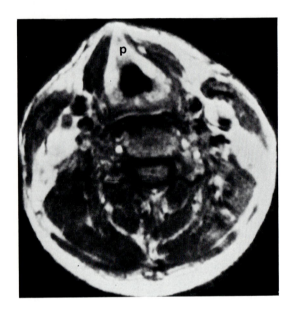

Figure 43.5 (SE 700/28). Axial scan through the supralarynbgeal level of a normal patient. The pre-epiglottic space (p) is again shown to have a homogeneous high intensity pattern.

CASE 44

HISTORY

An 88-year-old woman with a history of breast carcinoma presented with difficulty breathing. On physical examination, a large neck mass was discovered. On a cine esophagram, the cervical esophagus was displaced to the left.

QUESTIONS

1. What are your differential considerations?

   _____

   _____

2. What MR techniques would you use?

	1	2	3
a. Coil	___	___	___
b. Centering point	___	___	___
c. Imaging plane(s)	___	___	___
d. Contrast	___	___	___
e. Slice thickness	___	___	___

3. What do you expect to find?

   _____

   _____

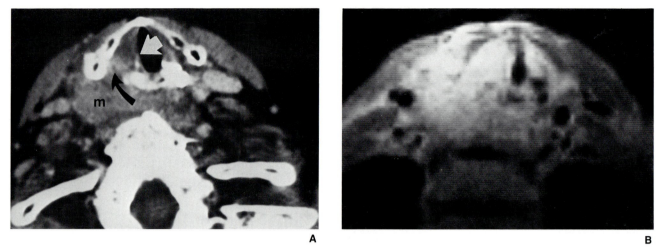

Figures 44.1A (enhanced CT) and **44.1B** (SE 2000/28). Axial scans through the level of the true vocal cords.

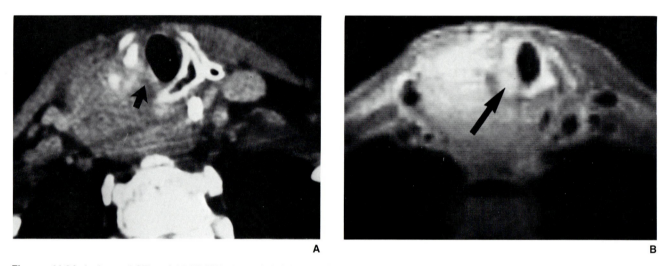

Figures 44.2A (enhanced CT) and **44.2B** (SE 2000/28). Axial scans through the level of cricoid cartilage.

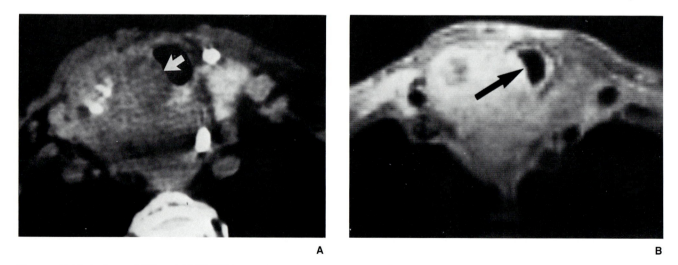

Figures 44.3A (enhanced CT) and **44.3B** (SE 2000/28). Axial scans at the subglottic level.

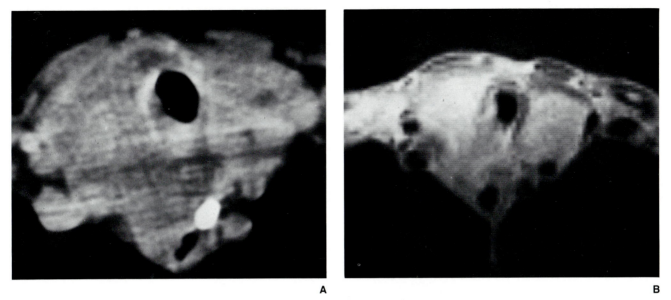

A   B

Figures 44.4A (enhanced CT) and **44.4B** (SE 2000/28). Axial scans at the level of the thyroid bed.

MR TECHNIQUES

	1	2
a. Coil	Surface	Surface
b. Centering point	Thyroid cartilage	Thyroid cartilage
c. Imaging planes	Axial	Coronal
d. Contrast	Mild to moderate T2W	Moderate T1W
e. Slice thickness	Thin	Thin

Axial scans were performed to allow direct comparison with CT scans. A mildly to moderately T2-weighted pulsing sequence was used to distinguish between the tumor mass and normal adjacent tissue. Thin slices were chosen to evaluate the detailed anatomy of the neck more accurately. A surface coil was used to improve anatomic definition by enhancing the signal to noise in this small area of interest.

The second pulsing sequence was performed with more T1 weighting in the coronal plane (not shown) to define better the superior and inferior extent of the tumor relative to the glottis.

MR FINDINGS

Figure 44.1. There is a large infiltrating mass (m) obliterating the right pyriform sinus and fixating the right vocal cord (arrow). There is splaying of the right cricothyroid joint as compared with the normal joint on the left (curved arrow).

Figure 44.2. There is erosion of the right cricoid cartilage (arrows) by the mass.

Figure 44.3. Subglottic extension of the mass (arrows) is seen. A low-density/intensity area centrally represents tumor necrosis.

Figure 44.4. More inferiorly, the mass is shown encircling and compressing the airway. A normal thyroid gland was not found on CT or on MR. The mass also extended inferiorly into the superior mediastinum (not shown).

DIFFERENTIAL DIAGNOSIS

The finding of a large infiltrating tumor with transglottic extension and obliteration of the right pyriform sinus sug- gests that this is a primary *laryngeal* or *paralaryngeal tumor*. In fact, the splaying or splitting of the right cricothyroid joint is a characteristic finding of a *pyriform sinus tumor*. The bulk of the mass is in the thyroid bed, however, where it extends in a circumferential fashion around the trachea into the superior mediastinum. This would suggest thyroid origin, either an aggressive primary *thyroid neoplasm* or *metastases*. On the basis of both the MR and CT findings, differentiating between these latter two entities is not possible. Although *lymphoma* or an extensive *inflammatory process* might considered, both are unlikely in view of the pattern of spread and the degree of destruction of surrounding structures.

Final Diagnosis

Anaplastic thyroid carcinoma.

SUMMARY OF MR FINDINGS FOR ANAPLASTIC THYROID CARCINOMA[1,2]

1. Approximately 5% to 30% of all thyroid carcinomas are of the anaplastic type.
2. This tumor has an aggressive local pattern of spread with invasion and/or destruction of the trachea, esophagus, and various other soft structures of the neck, which accounts for its poor prognosis.
3. Posterior and medial spread may involve the recurrent laryngeal nerve. This causes vocal cord paralysis, which may be appreciated on either CT or MRI.
4. The T2 relaxation time of the tumor is prolonged in this case. This is seen in most pathologic processes and is a nonspecific finding. Depending on the tumor size, necrosis may be demonstrated.

REFERENCES

1. Mancuso AA: Thyroid cancer, in Bragg DG, Rubin P, Youker JE (eds): *Oncologic Imaging*. New York, Pergamon Press Inc, 1985, pp 137–144.
2. Mancuso AA, Hanafee WN: The neck, in *Computed Tomography and Magnetic Resonance Imaging of the Head and Neck*, ed 2. Baltimore, Williams & Wilkins, 1985, pp 169–191.

CASE 45

HISTORY

A 72-year-old man presents with bilateral cervical adenopathy by physical examination.

QUESTIONS

1. What are your differential considerations?

_____

_____

2. What MR techniques would you use?

	1	2	3
a. Coil	____	____	____
b. Centering point	____	____	____
c. Imaging plane(s)	____	____	____
d. Contrast	____	____	____
e. Slice thickness	____	____	____

3. What do you expect to find?

_____

_____

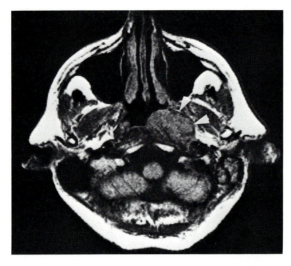

Figure 45.1 (SE 500/40). Axial scan at the nasopharyngeal level.

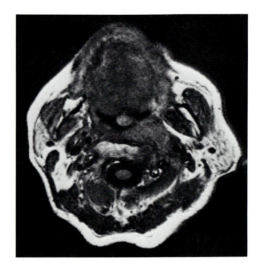

Figure 45.2 (SE 500/40). Axial scan at the oropharyngeal level.

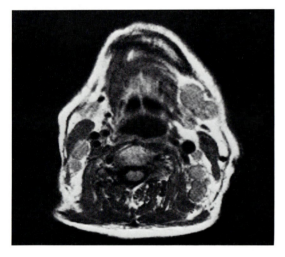

Figure 45.3 (SE 500/40). Axial scan at the hypopharyngeal level.

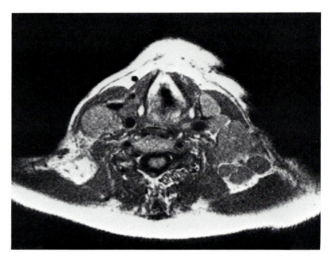

Figure 45.4 (SE 500/40). Axial scan at the supralaryngeal level.

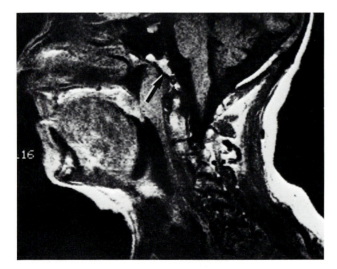

Figure 45.5. (SE 500/40). Midsagittal scan.

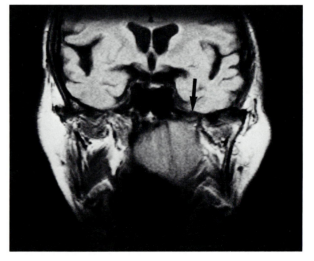

Figure 45.6 (SE 1000/30). Coronal scan through the nasopharynx.

MR TECHNIQUES

	1	2	3	4
a. Coil	Head	Head	Head	Neck
b. Centering point	Maxilla	Midline	Mid-coronal	Thyroid cartilage
c. Imaging planes	Axial	Sagittal	Coronal	Axial
d. Contrast	Moderate T1W	Moderate T1W	Mild T1W	Moderate T1W
e. Slice thickness	Thin	Routine	Routine	Thin
f. Spatial resolution	High	High	Routine	High

As discussed in the introductory section, the anatomic details and lymphadenopathy are best demonstrated with T1WIs, especially with high-resolution scanning techniques. The axial plane is our standard view in the head and neck area. The sagittal and coronal images provide better appreciation of the longitudinal extent of the tumor as well as possible skull base invasion.

MR FINDINGS

Figure 45.1. There is a soft tissue mass in the left side of the nasopharynx. On this moderate T1WI, the mass has a homogeneous intensity, slightly greater than that of the surrounding skeletal muscle. It extends laterally into the left parapharyngeal space. Although the left pharyngobasilar fascia is not seen, the lateral border of the mass (arrowheads) is relatively well defined. The left prevertebral muscle is also involved.

Figure 45.2. The mass extends inferiorly to the level of the oropharynx.

Figures 45.3 and 45.4. There is diffuse bilateral cervical lymphadenopathy, slightly more prominent on the left than the right. The enlarged nodes are predominately located in the posterior triangles. On these moderate T1WIs the lymph nodes have an intensity slightly greater than that of the skeletal muscle but lower than of the surrounding fat.

Figures 45.5 and 45.6. The mass appears to extend to the skull base (arrowheads) There is no evidence of intracranial extension.

DIFFERENTIAL DIAGNOSIS

Close to 99% of the malignancies arising in the nasopharynx are carcinomas, with 80% of these tumors being squamous cell carcinomas.[1] Approximately 50% of nasopharyngeal carcinomas present with bilateral cervical adenopathy. The next most common malignant tumor arising in the nasopharynx is non-Hodgkin's lymphoma, which also frequently causes bilateral cervical adenopathy.[1]

The location of the enlarged nodes may provide clues as to the site of the primary tumor.[2] Nasopharyngeal carcinoma is the most common head and neck tumor that metastasizes to the posterior triangle nodes. Otherwise, these nodes are likely to be lymphomatous or rarely metastatic from other sources (e.g., scalp, melanoma, primary carcinoma below the clavicles). Hence, the most likely diagnosis is either nasopharyngeal carcinoma or non-Hodgkin's lymphoma.

A possible differential finding in this case is the marked enlargement of the nodes without evidence of necrosis. This is more characteristic of lymphoma.[1]

The patient underwent transnasal biopsy of the left nasopharyngeal mass, which was found to be non-Hodgkin's lymphoma.

Final Diagnosis

Non-Hodgkin's lymphoma of the nasopharynx.

Table 45.1. Pattern of Lymph Node Involvement of Head/Neck Tumors[1-3]

Location	Frequency	Cervical Nodes (Metastatic) Side	Cervical Nodes (Metastatic) Group
Nasopharynx	85%–90%	Ipsilateral (50%) Bilateral (50%)	Internal jugular Spinal accessory
Paranasal sinus	Rare		
Tongue			
Anterior two thirds	Frequent	Ipsilateral	Submental and jugulodigastric
Posterior third	75%	Ipsilateral (70%) Bilateral (30%)	Jugulodigastric, submandibular, and spinal accessory
Oropharynx			
Tonsillar pillar	45%–75%	Ipsilateral Contralateral (5%–11%)	Jugulodigastric and submandibular
Soft palate	35%–50%	Ipsilateral Bilateral (16%)	Jugulodigastric and retropharyngeal
Larynx			
True cord	Rare		
Infraglottic	Rare	Ipsilateral	Lower deep cervical group
Supraglottic	>55%	Ipsilateral Bilateral (16%)	Jugulodigastric

Note: The majority of the tumors are squamous cell carcinomas.

Sources: Data from *Computed Tomography and Magnetic Resonance Imaging of the Head and Neck* (pp 428-497) by AA Mancuso and WN Hanafee, Williams & Wilkins Company, © 1985; *MRI of the Head and Neck* by WN Hanafee and RB Lufkin, Brian Decker, Inc, in press.

SUMMARY OF MR FINDINGS FOR NON-HODGKIN'S LYMPHOMA OF THE NASOPHARYNX

1. Soft tissue mass in the nasopharynx. The pattern of spread is similar to that of nasopharyngeal carcinoma (see Case 39).

2. Bilateral cervical adenopathy. The nodes are often in both the internal jugular and spinal accessory (posterior triangle) groups. The nodes tend to be quite large and usually do not cavitate. Table 45.1 summarizes the pattern of nodal involvement of head/neck tumors.

REFERENCES

1. Mancuso AA, Hanafee WN: Nasopharynx and parapharyngeal space, in *Computed Tomography and Magnetic Resonance Imaging of the Head and Neck*, ed 2. Baltimore, Williams & Wilkins, 1985, pp 428–497.

2. Mancuso AA, Hanafee WN: The neck, in *Computed Tomography and Magnetic Resonance Imaging of the Head and Neck*, ed 2. Baltimore, Williams & Wilkins, 1985, pp 169–240.

3. Hanafee WN, Lufkin RB: *MRI of the Head and Neck*. New York, Brian Decker Inc, in press.

5

SPINE IMAGING

TECHNIQUE

T1-weighted images of the spinal cord are most useful for depicting cord contour abnormalities, while T2-weighted images are more useful for detecting intrinsic cord abnormalities associated with edema or increased water content.[1] Evaluation of the subarachnoid space can be accomplished with either T1-weighted images (in which the long-T1 CSF is dark) or heavily T2-weighted images (in which the long-T2 CSF is bright). The relative disadvantage of heavily T1-weighted images is that they may make it difficult to distinguish dark CSF from dark ligaments and cortical bone. The relative disadvantage of heavily T2-weighted images is that they are more susceptible to CSF flow artifacts and decrease the conspicuity of intrinsic cord lesions. For these reasons, we prefer mildly to moderately T1- and T2-weighted sequences.

The sagittal plane has been shown to be most useful for the evaluation of the spinal canal and its contents. Levels of disease can be assessed directly by reference to known landmarks, such as the dens or the L5–S1 junction. Thin (5 mm or less), contiguous (either directly or by interleaving) sections are required, with a coverage spanning at least the distance from one neural foramen to the other. Positioning is facilitated by having a localizer scan from which to offset electronically. As in CT, transverse axial scans continue to be useful both to evaluate cord abnormalities and to distinguish between surgical and nonsurgical disc disease. Axial sections have proven to be more technically difficult to implement than sagittal sections, particularly in the cervical spine. This may be due to the normal curvature of the spine and the oblique course of the neural foramina with respect to the standard axial plane. The implementation of angled axial sections (similar to gantry angulation in CT) is considered a most useful feature. Additional angulation in the sagittal-coronal plane is useful for evaluation of the cervical neural foramina and their contents. Coronal sections are generally less useful than sagittal or axial sections because of the cervical and lumbar lordosis and thoracic kyphosis, and the resulting susceptibility to partial volume averaging.

The use of specialized local coils for the spine has the advantage of improving signal-to-noise near the coil, but there is generally an associated reduction in the field of view.[2] Such coils may require implementation with a localizing body coil image to assess the level of disease and associated abnormalities beyond the spine.

MYELOPATHY

Intrinsic cord pathology may be due to trauma, tumors, inflammation, demyelination, syringomyelia, infarction, and arteriovenous malformations.[3-8] Patients with acute cord trauma are often best evaluated with CT with or without intrathecal contrast material, as this examination can be performed quickly and in conjunction with evaluation of injuries to the head, torso, and extremities. Furthermore, the patient may be closely monitored during a CT procedure; if necessary, the examination may be interrupted for therapeutic interventions. Furthermore, CT allows more effective demonstration of spinal bony injuries, which probably will determine the need for decompressive or stabilizing surgical procedures. Nevertheless, MR imaging may be used in the acute setting to demonstrate cord contusion and/or transection. Delayed effects, including posttraumatic atrophy and syringomyelia, are better studied with MRI than with myelography or CT.

The most common intrinsic cord tumors are astrocytomas and ependymomas, both of which tend to produce fusiform enlargement of the cord and a focal increase in cord water content; the latter is conspicuous as a region of increased signal intensity on moderately T2-weighted images. T1-weighted sequences are effective in demonstrating abnormal cord contours associated with neoplastic involvement but are relatively insensitive to alterations in tissue composition. Other intrinsic cord tumors include intraspinal dermoids, hemangioblastomas, and cord metastases. Of these, only dermoids have a characteristic MR appearance, appearing hyperintense on both T1- and T2-weighted images, reflecting their fat content.

Intrinsic inflammatory diseases of the cord include transverse myelitis and multiple sclerosis.[9] In the acute inflammatory stage of either of these diseases, one may see focal alterations in cord signal intensity, most conspicuous as hyperintense regions on T2-weighted images. There may be focal cord swelling, simulating the appearance of a tumor. More commonly, multiple sclerosis involving the cord is characterized as a relatively subtle inhomogeneity of cord signal, usually associated with typical multifocal intracranial abnormalities. We have had occasion to observe cord abnormalities, however, in patients with suspected multiple sclerosis and no demonstrable intracranial disease.

Spinal infarcts are difficult to demonstrate unless the lesion is well localized clinically, permitting detailed examination using localized coils.[10] Similarly, demonstration of arteriovenous malformations requires a spatial resolution somewhat greater than that generally available with MRI at this time. In addition, signal loss due to normal CSF flow phenomena may mimic an intraspinal vascular abnormality.[11]

Nonneoplastic syringomyelia[7] is well evaluated by MRI, appearing as an intramedullary collection of CSF-intensity fluid. T1-weighted sagittal images best depict the longitudinal extent of the lesion and associated cord expansion or atrophy. Appropriate MR sequences also allow assessment of associated Chiari malformations, arachnoiditis, and traumatic injury. Tumor cysts often have a more irregular appearance. This fluid tends to be proteinaceous, which distinguishes these lesions from nonneoplastic cysts but also decreases lesion conspicuity. Solid tumor may be depicted as a nodularity along with margins of the cyst or, more frequently, as alteration of cord contour and signal intensity above or below the level of the cyst.

Patients with spinal dysraphism complexes may present with progressive myelopathy, although this diagnosis is usually made on the basis of physical stigmata at birth in patients who appear to be neurologically intact. MRI has proven useful in the evaluation of affected patients, as posterior element defects, (myelo)meningoceles, intraspinal/subcutaneous lipomas, and cord tethering can all be effectively demonstrated by a combination of T1-weighted sagittal and axial images. CT may be better suited to the evaluation of congenital abnormalities with subtle bony components, such as diastematomyelia.

Extrinsic myelopathy (e.g., cord compression) may be produced by primary tumors (e.g., meningiomas and neurofibromas), metastases, or—more often—degenerative disc disease. Frank disc herniation, spondylosis, and ligamentous spinal stenosis may all lead to cord impingement and long tract signs. While MRI may not be capable of differentiating ligamentous and bony causes of canal compromise, cord position and size are well evaluated without the necessity of injecting intrathecal contrast material.[12,13]

RADICULOPATHY

Evaluation of lumbar radiculopathy is facilitated by the fact that the lumbar neural foramina are displayed in cross section on parasagittal images. The low intensity nerve root is well seen as it exits the spinal canal beneath the pedicle and is surrounded by high intensity perineural and epidural fat.[13] Lesions that impinge on the nerve roots within the lateral recesses and neural foramina are usually visualized, although low intensity lesions (bone, disc fragment, or fibrosis) may be indistinguishable. The distinction of a bulging annulus fibrosis (which is generally considered a nonsurgical lesion) from herniation of the nucleus pulposus may not be possible in the sagittal projection. While this differentiation can often be made with axial sections using current technology, the occasional use of high-resolution angled axial CT may be required prior to anticipated surgery.

Evaluation of cervical radiculopathy is currently hampered by the general lack of availability of angled oblique sections that are required to visualize optimally the cervical neural foramina and cervical nerve roots.[14] While midline disc degeneration and osteophyte formation may be visualized, the degree of correlation between midline disease (which can be visualized) and uncovertebral or foraminal disease (which is difficult to visualize) has yet to be established. In our opinion, thin-slice, high-resolution CT without intrathecal contrast is more effective in evaluating bony disease, and CT with intrathecal contrast remains the most sensitive and specific method of evaluating cervical radiculopathy.

DISEASE OF THE BONY SPINE

Replacement or modification of the signal from the high-intensity marrow is the basis for visualization of abnormalities of the bony spine. Metastatic disease and less common primary tumors are associated with T1 prolongation and, therefore, with decreased signal, particularly on T1-weighted images. Discitis and osteomyelitis are well evaluated by a combination of T1- and T2-weighted images.[3] Radiation changes result in increased intensity of the involved vertebral bodies because of replacement of the hematopoietic marrow by fatty marrow. Paravertebral soft tissue abnormalities are well evaluated, as are lesions that impinge on the cord substance and nerve roots.

REFERENCES

1. Bradley WG: Fundamentals of MR image interpretation, in Bradley WG, Adey WR, Hasso AN (eds): *Magnetic Resonance Imaging of the Brain, Head, and Neck: A Text Atlas.* Rockville, Md, Aspen Publishers, 1985.

2. Edelman RR, Shoukimas GM, Stark DD, et al: High-resolution surface-coil imaging of lumbar disk disease. *AJNR* 1985;6:479–486.

3. Modic MT, Weinstein MA, Pavlicek W, et al: Nuclear magnetic resonance imaging of the spine. *Radiology* 1983;148:757–762.

4. Modic MT, Weinstein MA, Pavlicek W, et al: Magnetic resonance imaging of the cervical spine: Technical and clinical observations. *AJR* 1983;141:1129–1136.

5. Han JS, Kaufman B, El Yousef SJ, et al: NMR imaging of the spine. *AJR* 1983;141:1137–1145.

6. Norman D, Mills CM, Brant-Zawadzki M, et al: Magnetic resonance of the spinal cord and canal: Potentials and limitations. *AJR* 1983; 141:1147–1152.

7. Yeates A, Brant-Zawadzki M, Norman D, et al: Nuclear magnetic resonance imaging of syringomyelia. *AJNR* 1983;4:234–237.

8. Hawkes RC, Holland GN, Moore WS, et al: Craniovertebral junction pathology: Assessment by NMR. *AJNR* 1983;4:232–233.

9. Maravilla KR, Weinreb JC, Suss R, et al: Magnetic resonance demonstration of multiple sclerosis plaques in the cervical cord. *AJNR* 1984;5:685–689.

10. Axel L: Surface coil magnetic resonance imaging. *J Comput Assist Tomogr* 1984;8:381–384.

11. Rubin JB, Enzmann DR: Imaging spinal CSF pulsation by 2DFT MR: Significance during clinical imaging. Presented at the Annual Meeting of the ASNR, San Diego, CA, Jan 19–23, 1986.

12. Modic MT, Pavlicek W, Weinstein MA, et al: Magnetic resonance imaging of intervertebral disc disease. *Radiology* 1984;152:103–111.

13. Chafetz NI, Genant HK, Moon KL, et al: Recognition of lumbar disc herniation with NMR. *AJR* 1983;141:1153–1156.

14. Norman D, Newton TH: MRI of the spine and cord: A present perspective. Presented at the Annual Meeting of the ASNR, San Diego, CA, Jan 19–23, 1986.

CASE 46

HISTORY

An 8-month-old boy with a fatty subcutaneous lower lumbar mass.

QUESTIONS

1. What are your differential considerations?

_____

_____

2. What MR techniques would you use?

	1	2	3
a. Coil	___	___	___
b. Centering point	___	___	___
c. Imaging plane(s)	___	___	___
d. Contrast	___	___	___
e. Slice thickness	___	___	___

3. What do you expect to find?

_____

_____

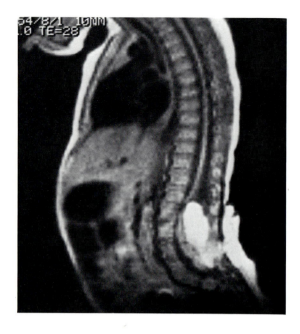

Figure 46.1 (SE 1000/28). Midsagittal section through thoracolumbar spine.

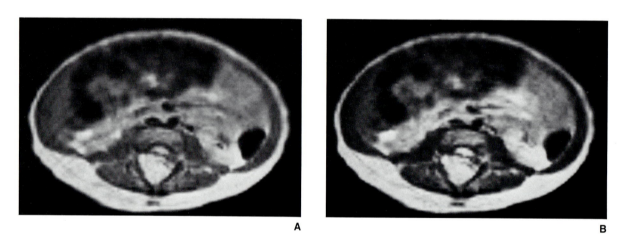

A   B

Figures 46.2A (SE 2000/28) and **46.2B** (SE 2000/56). Axial sections through midlumbar spine.

MR TECHNIQUES

		1	2
a.	Coil	Head	Head
b.	Centering point	Midabdomen	Over palpable mass
c.	Imaging planes	Sagittal	Axial
d.	Contrast	Mild T1W/mild T2W	Mild T2W/ moderate T2W
e.	Slice thickness	Thin	Thin

As discussed in Chapter 5, a mildly T1-weighted sagittal sequence provides sufficient T1 weighting to enable the evaluation of cord contour and for recognition of short T1 abnormalities, such as hemorrhage and fatty tissue. The mildly T2-weighted (second echo) images provide adequate contrast between higher intensity CSF and lower intensity cortical bone and disc material. In addition, there is sufficient T2 weighting to identify abnormalities within the cord (i.e., areas of edema and neoplastic and inflammatory changes).

The axial mild to moderate T2WI provides confirmation of changes in intensity due to T2 prolongation, and allows cross-sectional depiction of pathologic processes.

Note that a head instead of a body coil was used because of the small size of the subject. As discussed in Chapter 2, in some pediatric patients a smaller diameter coil can be used to provide better signal to noise.

MR FINDINGS

Figure 46.1. There is a well-defined, lobulated, high intensity (short T1) mass located within an expanded spinal canal and extending through a posterior element defect to the subcutaneous tissue. The spinal cord is tethered to the superior aspect of the mass, and the nerves of the cauda equina are clumped and displaced anteriorly.

Figure 46.2. The findings are confirmed on the axial images. The mass remains increased in signal intensity on the second echo image, indicating a relatively prolonged T2 relaxation time.

DIFFERENTIAL DIAGNOSIS

The differential diagnosis of a high intensity mass (a short T1 lesion) would include a fatty tumor or a hematoma. However, the combination of cord tethering, posterior element defect, and a subcutaneous fatty mass is pathognomonic of an intraspinal lipoma and a spinal dysraphic complex.

Final Diagnosis

Spinal dysraphism with an intraspinal lipoma.

SUMMARY OF MR FINDINGS FOR SPINAL DYSRAPHISM[1]

1. Intraspinal lipoma (short T1 and long T2, high intensity mass) with or without a subcutaneous lipoma.
2. Conus located below the L 2 level due to cord tethering.
3. Meningocele or meningomyelocele (i.e., nerve roots or cord substance in meningocele).
4. Posterior element defect (spina bifida).

REFERENCE

1. Kortman KE, Bradley WG, Van Dalsem W, et al: MRI of spinal dysraphism, submitted for publication.

CASE 47

HISTORY

This 40-year-old man sustained a lifting injury 1 week earlier, resulting in low back pain and bilateral sciatica.

QUESTIONS

1. What are your differential considerations?

   _____

   _____

2. What MR techniques would you use?

	1	2	3
a. Coil	_____	_____	_____
b. Centering point	_____	_____	_____
c. Imaging plane(s)	_____	_____	_____
d. Contrast	_____	_____	_____
e. Slice thickness	_____	_____	_____

3. What do you expect to find?

   _____

   _____

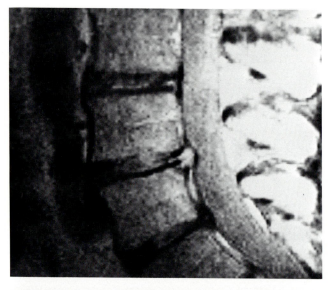

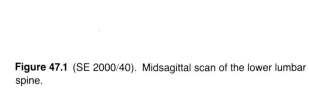

Figure 47.1 (SE 2000/40). Midsagittal scan of the lower lumbar spine.

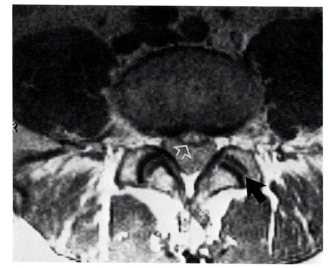

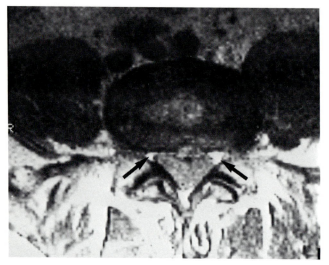

Figure 47.2 (SE 2000/40). Axial section through the L 4–L 5 neuroforamina.

Figure 47.3 (SE 2000/40). Axial section 5 mm inferior to Figure 47.2.

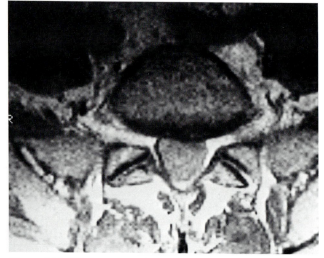

Figure 47.4 (SE 2000/40). Axial section 5 mm inferior to Figure 47.3 through the L 4–L 5 disc.

Figure 47.5 (SE 2000/40). Axial section through the posterior margin of the L 5–S 1 disc.

MR TECHNIQUES

		1	2
a.	Coil	Surface	Surface
b.	Centering point	Iliac crest	Iliac crest
c.	Imaging planes	Sagittal	Axial
d.	Contrast	Mild T2W	Mild T2W
e.	Slice thickness	Thin	Thin

As with all spinal examinations, our first sequence was performed in the sagittal plane. In this instance, a 12.5-cm-diameter, circular surface coil was used. Because of the limited field of view, care must be taken to position the coil exactly over the area of interest. This was accomplished by using a fast localizing scan with the surface coil in place and repositioning as needed. Surface coils offer two advantages.[1] First, there is increased signal to noise compared with the body coil. Second, artifact due to respiration or bowel motion is reduced since this is not "seen" by the coil because of its restricted field of view.

Since thin (5 mm) contiguous slices without an interslice gap were needed to ensure sufficient detail, a mild T2WI was obtained with a TR of 2,000 mseconds to provide sufficient coverage so that the spinal canal, the neuroforamina, and the paraspinal soft tissues were evaluated (see Chapter 2). With this TR, the CSF has an intermediate intensity. In some cases where visualization of cord contour is important, a mild to moderate T1WI may be necessary.

The second sequence was performed in the axial plane using thin slices at the level of interest. A similar contrast setting was used to provide adequate coverage over several levels. A shorter TR with reduction of the scan time could be used, especially if the amount of coverage is less (e.g., one disc level).

MR FINDINGS

Figure 47.1. On this sagittal image, there are degenerative changes involving the L 3–L 4, L 4–L 5, and L 5–S 1 discs manifested by decreased height and intensity. This decreased signal intensity is due to the loss of normal water content. Compare these discs with the normal upper lumbar discs in Figure 49.2. At the L 4–L 5 disc, a posterior protrusion of soft tissue with increased signal intensity, representing extruded nuclear material, can be seen. There is associated anterior impression of the thecal sac.

At the L 5–S 1 level, there is greater loss of disc height and desiccation. Posterior protrusion of low signal intensity with encroachment into the high intensity anterior epidural fat is seen. This represented a concentric annular bulge on the axial images (Figure 47.5).

Figures 47.2 through 47.4. The most superior image of this series (Figure 47.2) demonstrates normal appearing bilateral nerve roots surrounded by high intensity fat. The dimensions of the spinal canal are normal. More inferiorly, a focal area of increased signal (open arrow, Figure 47.3) corresponding to the findings on the sagittal view is confirmed. There is adjacent compression of the thecal sac. Note the normal facet joints (solid arrow, Figure 47.3) composed of opposing, low signal intensity, cortical bone separated by higher intensity joint cartilage.

On Figure 47.4, there is now predominately low signal intensity through the vertebral body. This corresponds to a section through the midportion of the disc. Note the preservation of the epidural fat (arrows) bilaterally.

Figure 47.5. Crescentic low signal intensity is noted along the posterior and posterolateral margin of the L 5–S 1 disc. This represents an annular bulge.

DIFFERENTIAL DIAGNOSIS

The differential should consider any cause for an epidural mass, including *herniated disc, osteophyte, metastasis, primary bone or soft tissue neoplasm, or abscess*. In this example, the focal area of epidural compression seen on both views is in direct continuity with a degenerated disc, compatible with a herniation.

Metastasis, other neoplasm, or abscess are much less likely because of the absence of osseous destruction, alteration of the marrow signal, or involvement of the adjacent soft tissues (see Case 50).

Final Diagnosis

Multilevel lumbar disc degeneration with L 4–L 5 disc herniation and L 5–S 1 annular bulge.

SUMMARY OF MR FINDINGS FOR HERNIATED DISC[1–4]

1. The involved disc generally has low intensity indicating desiccation and degeneration. Acute or traumatic disc herniation may have normal signal intensity.
2. Loss of the normal height of the disc space.
3. Focal epidural mass posterior and adjacent to a degenerated disc. In the preceding demonstration, the herniation is in the midline. Figure 47.6 is an example of a right posterolateral disc herniation in another patient.
4. Herniations may cause cord compression and edema.
5. Commonly associated with degeneration of disc(s) at other levels.

REFERENCES

1. Edelman RR, Shoukimas GM, Stark DD, et al: High-resolution surface-coil imaging of lumbar disk disease. *AJR* 1985;144:1123–1129.
2. Han JS, Kaufman B, el Yousef SJ, et al: NMR imaging of the spine. *AJR* 1983;141:1137–1145.
3. Modic MT, Weinstein MA, Pavlicek W, et al: Nuclear magnetic resonance of the spine. *Radiology* 1983;148:757–762.
4. Pech PP, Haughton VM: Lumbar intervertebral disk: Correlative MR and anatomic study. *Radiology* 1985;156:699–701.

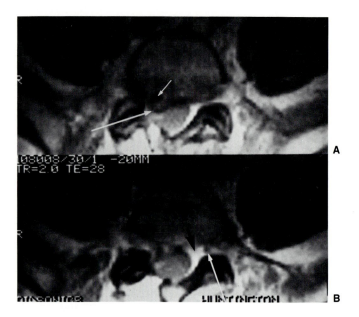

Figures 47.6A (SE 2000/28) and **47.6B** (SE 2000/28). Axial sections demonstrating a right posterolateral herniation of the L 5–S 1 disc. In Figure 47.6A, focal protrusion of intermediate-signal disc material (long arrow) and a low intensity focus representing portions of the annulus and/or calcification (short arrow) are noted. In Figure 47.6B, 5 mm superior to Figure 47.6A, the right epidural fat is obliterated and a clearly defined right L 5 nerve root cannot be identified. Compare with the normal left epidural fat (black arrow) and nerve root (long white arrow).

CASE 48

HISTORY

Five months previously, this 25-year-old man sustained a C 6 and C 7 fracture subluxation with immediate loss of bilateral lower extremity function and preservation of upper extremity function. More recently, however, there has been progressive upper extremity motor and sensory deficits and acute onset of respiratory compromise necessitating emergency surgical intervention. He is now referred for a follow-up MR examination.

QUESTIONS

1. What are your differential considerations?

   _____

   _____

2. What MR techniques would you use?

	1	2	3
a. Coil	_____	_____	_____
b. Centering point	_____	_____	_____
c. Imaging plane(s)	_____	_____	_____
d. Contrast	_____	_____	_____
e. Slice thickness	_____	_____	_____

3. What do you expect to find?

   _____

   _____

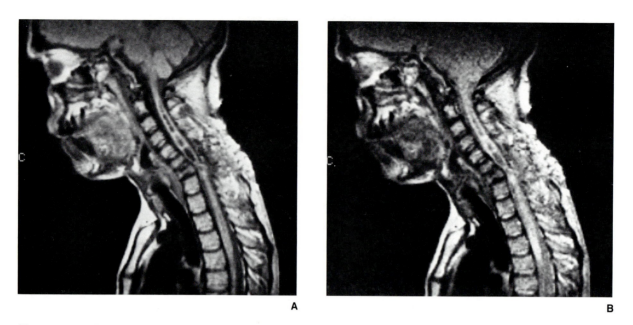

A

B

Figures 48.1A (SE 1000/40) and **48.1B** (SE 1000/80). Parasagittal section through the posterior fossa, cervical cord, and proximal thoracic cord.

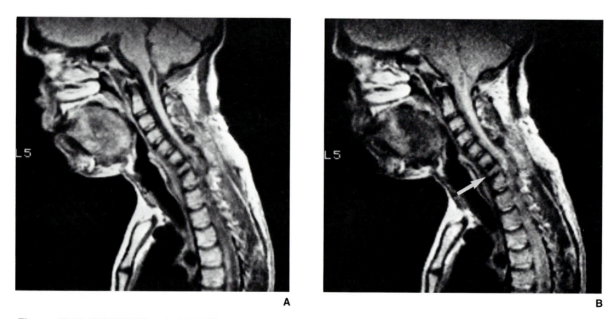

A

B

Figures 48.2A (SE 1000/40) and **48.2B** (SE 1000/80). Section 5 mm to the left of Figure 48.1.

MR TECHNIQUES

a. Coil   Body
b. Centering point   Sternal notch
c. Imaging plane   Sagittal
d. Contrast   Mild T1W
e. Slice thickness   Thin

A body coil was used, rather than a surface coil (as in Case 47), to increase the field of view. In this example, the field of view on the nonmagnified images covered from the posterior fossa to the T 9–T 10 level. This has a distinct advantage when a survey study is desired.[1] Other coils, such as a planar surface coil (Figure 47.1) and a cervical coil (Figure 20.4), have a more limited field of view. The cervical coil used in Figure 20.4 is actually a modified, double-saddle head coil with its shape altered to fit over the shoulders. In a normal size patient, the field of view with this coil extends to the T 1–T 2 level.

As discussed in Chapter 2, the phrase *field of view* should not be confused with the term *coverage*. In this example, *field of view* refers to the total area portrayed on a single image, for example, the cranial-caudal or anterior–posterior dimensions of a sagittal section. *Coverage* refers to the dimension perpendicular to the imaging plane and depends on the number of slices, each with a given thickness and interslice gap, obtained with each acquisition. With a field of view of about 30 cm, a centering point of the sternal notch was used for this survey.

We have found that the sagittal plane is the most efficient projection for screening the cord compared with either the axial or coronal projection. This is in agreement with other investigators.[2] In this example, we felt that the sagittal study yielded sufficient information, and no additional sequences were performed. As described in Case 46, mild T1-weighting was utilized.

MR FINDINGS

Figures 48.1 and 48.2. There is loss of height and decreased signal intensity of the C 6 and C 7 vertebral bodies. There is abnormal kyphosis at the C 7 level with associated focal compression of the cervical cord. The C 6–C 7 and C 7–T 1 discs are narrowed, with loss of normal signal intensity. The end plates are grossly intact except along the superior margin of the C 7 vertebral body. Note the obliteration of the posterior elements compatible with a prior decompressive laminectomy.

The most striking abnormalities are the focal areas of low signal intensity within the proximal cervical cord and extend-

ing into the caudal medulla. The cord contour is minimally expanded.

DIFFERENTIAL DIAGNOSIS

As discussed in Case 3, the differential for a cystic lesion within the cord should include the following:

a. *Hydromyelia,* or enlargement of the central canal characteristically associated with Chiari malformations. The enlarged canal may communicate with the ventricular system; however, the communication may be difficult to visualize with MR.
b. *Syrinx,* which primarily resides outside the central canal and is associated with trauma, intramedullary hematoma, or tumor. Differentiating between hydromyelia and syrinx per se is generally not possible with MRI.
c. *Cystic cord tumor.*
d. *Myelomalacia* from either postinflammatory, infectious, or posttraumatic causes.

The findings, when combined with the patient's history, most certainly represent a posttraumatic syrinx.

Final Diagnosis

Posttraumatic syrinx.

SUMMARY OF MR FINDINGS FOR SYRINX OF THE CORD[1–3]

1. Intramedullary foci of CSF intensity.
2. The cause of the syrinx may be apparent on the study—for example, focal trauma, arachnoiditis, or cord tumor.
3. Making the distinction between syrinx and hydromyelia may not be possible on MRI.
4. The segment of the cord affected by the syrinx may have either increased, normal, or decreased diameter.

REFERENCES

1. Gebarski SS, Maynard FW, Gabrielsen TO, et al: Posttraumatic progressive myelopathy. *Radiology* 1985;157:379–385.
2. Pojunas K, Williams AL, Daniels DL: Syringomyelia and hydromyelia: Magnetic resonance evaluation. *Radiology* 1984;153:679–683.
3. Lee BCP, Zimmerman RD, Manning JJ, et al: MR imaging of syringomyelia and hydromyelia. *AJNR* 1985;6:221–228.

CASE 49

HISTORY

A 41-year-old man presents with low back pain and left leg pain. A screening examination of the entire lumbar spine was requested.

QUESTIONS

1. What are your differential considerations?

_____

_____

2. What MR techniques would you use?

	1	2	3
a. Coil	___	___	___
b. Centering point	___	___	___
c. Imaging plane(s)	___	___	___
d. Contrast	___	___	___
e. Slice thickness	___	___	___

3. What do you expect to find?

_____

_____

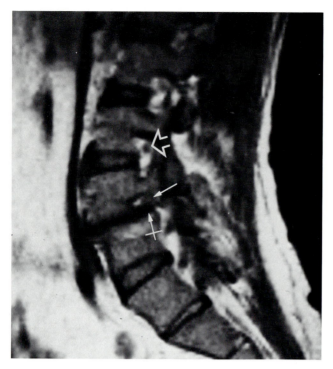

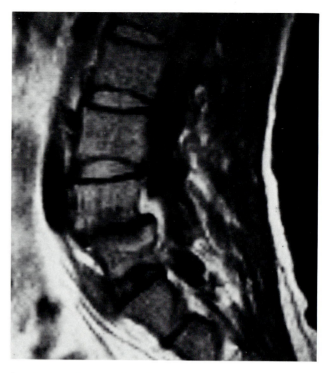

Figure 49.1 (SE 1000/28). Parasagittal scan 1.5 cm to the right of midline.

Figure 49.2 (SE 1000/28). Parasagittal scan 5 mm to the left of midline.

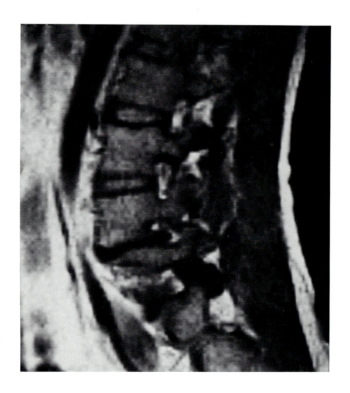

Figure 49.3 (SE 1000/28). Parasagittal scan 1.5 cm to the left of midline.

MR TECHNIQUES

		1	2
a.	Coil	Body	Body
b.	Centering point	Iliac crest	Iliac crest
c.	Imaging planes	Sagittal	Axial
d.	Contrast	Mild T1W/mild T2W	Mild T1W/mild T2W
e.	Slice thickness	Thin	Thin

The first sequence is the routine screening protocol for the entire lumbar spine. In this case, the body coil was used because of its increased field of view compared with the surface coil's limited field of view (see Case 37) available at the time of this examination. The body coil allowed adequate visualization from the midsacrum to the middle to lower thoracic spine. The entire field of view is not apparent on the preceding images because they are magnified to show the area of abnormality. With the increasing use of surface coils, more specialized shapes, including ellipses or rectangles with increased fields of view, will become available.

The second sequence, with a similar contrast and slice thickness setting, was less helpful in evaluating this disorder and is not shown.

MR FINDINGS

Figures 49.1 through 49.3. There is a grade I spondylolisthesis of L-4 on L-5, associated with loss of normal disc height and intensity indicating severe degeneration. The exiting nerve roots of L-4 (short white arrow, Figure 49.1) are impinged bilaterally by low-signal structures protruding into the neuroforamina (crossed white arrow, Figure 49.1). These low-signal structures may represent osteophytes or degenerated, possibly calcified disc material. Differentiating between these two entities is difficult owing to their similar low intensities. Intraforaminal nerve roots appear as small, round, intermediate intensity structures (short white arrow and open white arrow, Figure 49.1) surrounded by high intensity fat.

DIFFERENTIAL DIAGNOSIS

The causes of spondylolisthesis are either a congenital or acquired pars defect or severe spondylosis with ligamentous degeneration. Even though a pars defect was not seen, it cannot be excluded because MRI is relatively insensitive to bony abnormalities. In this case, since there is severe spondylosis manifested by loss of normal disc signal and height at the involved level, this is thought to be the cause of the spondylolisthesis.

Final Diagnosis

Lumbar spondylolisthesis with neural foraminal stenosis.

SUMMARY OF MR FINDINGS FOR LUMBAR SPONDYLOLISTHESIS[1]

1. Vertebral body anterolisthesis of varying severity commonly affecting the lower lumbar spine.
2. The causes of spondylolisthesis may include pars defect(s) or disc and ligamentous degeneration. The former may be difficult to diagnose with MRI.
3. MRI may have an advantage in showing neural foraminal narrowing because of its ability to image in the sagittal plane.

REFERENCE

1. Modic MT, Weinstein MA, Pavlicek W, et al: Nuclear magnetic resonance imaging of the spine. *Radiology* 1983;148:757–762.

CASE 50

HISTORY

A 50-year-old man with a history of lung carcinoma now presenting with back pain and midthoracic radiculopathy. An enhanced CT is shown in Figure 50.1.

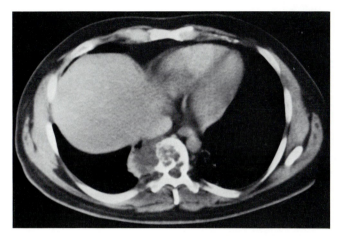

Figure 50.1. Enhanced axial CT through the T-9 vertebral body.

QUESTIONS

1. What are your differential considerations?

_____

_____

2. What MR techniques would you use?

	1	2	3
a. Coil	___	___	___
b. Centering point	___	___	___
c. Imaging plane(s)	___	___	___
d. Contrast	___	___	___
e. Slice thickness	___	___	___

3. What do you expect to find?

_____

_____

Source: Courtesy of Washington MR Center, Whittier, CA.

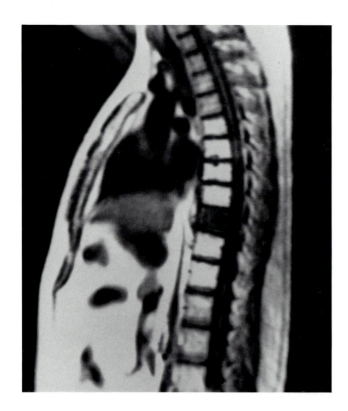

Figure 50.2 (SE 600/20). Sagittal section through the midthoracic spine.

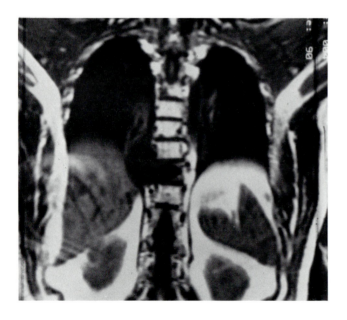

Figure 50.3 (SE 600/20). Coronal section through the region of interest.

MR TECHNIQUES

		1	2
a.	Coil	Body	Body
b.	Centering point	Midsternum	Posterior thorax
c.	Imaging planes	Sagittal	Coronal
d.	Contrast	Moderate T1W	Moderate T1W
e.	Slice thickness	Thin	Thin

Our routine screening examination of the spine is performed in the sagittal plane. Because of suspected metastatic disease and the lack of clinical localizing signs, a body coil was used to increase the field of view. In addition, T1 weighting was utilized to improve the MR sensitivity to malignant infiltration of bone marrow.[1,2] In addition, the scanning time can be reduced when compared to that for T2-weighted sequences. Thin slices were used to reduce partial volume averaging.

The second sequence in the coronal plane was used to provide additional localizing information. Such a sequence is particularly useful in evaluating paraspinal masses that may be more difficult on the sagittal view. An argument for performing an axial study could have been made, since the paraspinal mass would probably have been adequately evaluated and the degree of spinal canal narrowing may have been better appreciated on the cross-sectional view.

MR FINDINGS

Figure 50.1. The CT examination demonstrates extensive destruction of the T 9 vertebral body and a right paraspinal mass. The spinal canal appears to be grossly intact without significant encroachment by the tumor.

Figure 50.2. There is replacement of the normal vertebral body marrow signal by decreased signal intensity within the T 9 vertebral body. The endplates are intact, and the disc spaces are preserved. The thoracic cord can readily be identified and does not appear to be displaced. Note the low intensity CSF surrounding the cord. On this midsagittal view, there is no evidence of spinal stenosis by the mass. (The astute observer may notice the increased signal intensity within several of the midthoracic vertebral bodies. This is due to fatty replacement within the marrow secondary to previous radiation therapy. This is discussed further in Case 52.)

Figure 50.3. The coronal section demonstrates the right-sided paraspinal mass. The intensity of the mass on this T1-weighted image is only slightly greater than that of CSF.

DIFFERENTIAL DIAGNOSIS

The most striking finding is the replacement of the normally high vertebral body signal, indicating loss of the normal fatty component of bone marrow. This finding is nonspecific since tumor cells, fibrous tissue, or inflammatory infiltration may replace normal marrow elements. Therefore

the differential should include any disease that affects the marrow, including metastases, myeloma, osteomyelitis, or ischemic necrosis. Neoplastic disease is the most likely cause for these MR findings. Both metastases and myeloma can infiltrate the vertebral body and leave the endplate intact. Associated paraspinal masses are more characteristic of metastatic disease. In contradistinction, vertebral osteomyelitis is generally associated with loss of distinction between the disc and the adjacent vertebral body.[3] Ischemic necrosis also causes altered marrow signal (see Case 54); however, the location, the osseous destruction, and the associated paraspinal mass would be atypical.

What vertebral body signal intensity would you expect to see on a T2-weighted image with either tumor infiltration or osteomyelitis? From calculated relaxation values of both bone and soft tissue neoplasms, there is a slight tendency for tumor T2 values to be slightly prolonged compared with those of normal fat, although there can be considerable variation.[2] Therefore, the signal intensity may be greater on a T2-weighted exam (see Figure 50.4). Similar increased signal intensity may be seen with osteomyelitis (see Figure 50.5).[3]

Final Diagnosis

Spinal metastases.

SUMMARY OF MR FINDINGS FOR METASTATIC DISEASE OF THE SPINE[1,2,4–6]

1. On T1-weighted images, low intensity signal within the vertebral bodies represents replacement of the marrow with tumor cells.
2. Increased signal intensity may be seen with T2 weighting.
3. This altered signal intensity pattern may be heterogeneous.
4. Pathologic fractures may have altered signal intensity due to edema and/or hemorrhage. Cord compression may result in myelopathy (Figure 50.6).
5. Paraspinal masses may be seen.

REFERENCES

1. Daffner RH, Lupetin AR, Dash N, et al: MRI in the detection of malignant infiltration of the bone marrow. *AJR* 1986;146:353–358.
2. Aisen AM, Martel W, Braunstein EM, et al: MRI and CT evaluation of primary bone and soft-tissue tumors. *AJR* 1986;146:749–756.
3. Modic MT, Feiglin DH, Piraino DW, et al: Vertebral osteomyelitis: Assessment using MR. *Radiology* 1985;157:157–166.
4. Han JS, Kaufman B, el Yousef SJ, et al: NMR imaging of the spine. *AJR* 1983;141:1137–1145.
5. Modic MT, Weinstein MA, Pavlicek W, et al: Nuclear magnetic resonance of the spine. *Radiology* 1983;148:757–762.
6. Norman D, Mills CM, Brant-Zawadzki MB, et al: Magnetic resonance imaging of the spinal cord and canal: Potentials and limitations. *AJR* 1983;141:1147–1156.

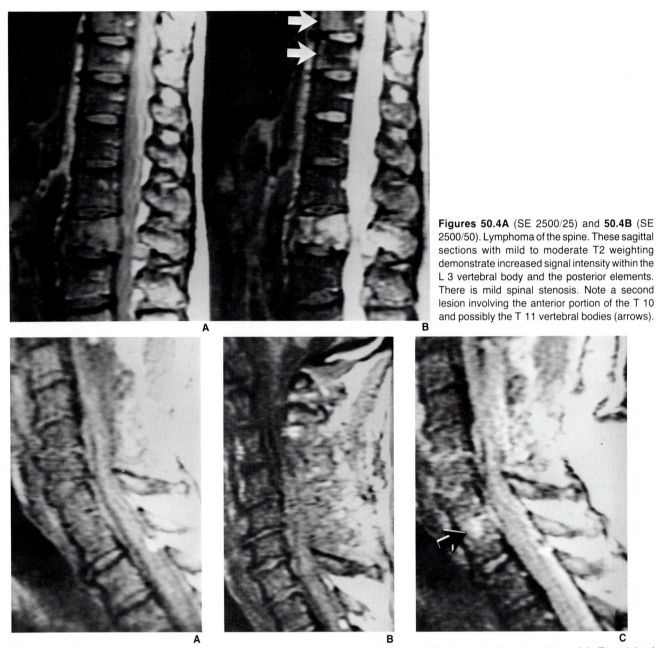

Figures 50.4A (SE 2500/25) and **50.4B** (SE 2500/50). Lymphoma of the spine. These sagittal sections with mild to moderate T2 weighting demonstrate increased signal intensity within the L 3 vertebral body and the posterior elements. There is mild spinal stenosis. Note a second lesion involving the anterior portion of the T 10 and possibly the T 11 vertebral bodies (arrows).

Figures 50.5A (SE 800/20), **50.5B** (SE 1500/25), and **50.5C** (SE 1500/50). Vertebral osteomyelitis. Figure 50.5A is a baseline, mildly T1-weighted image and shows a laminectomy defect following drainage of an anterior epidural abscess. Several weeks later (Figures 50.5B and 50.5C), there is new indistinctness between several of the vertebral endplates and adjacent disc spaces in the mid to lower cervical spine. On the second echo image (with mild T2 weighting), at least one focal area of increased signal intensity (arrow) can be identified.

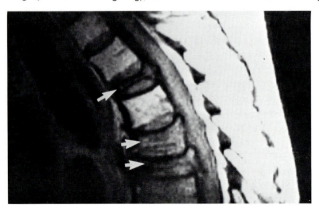

Figure 50.6 (SE 1000/40). *Vertebra plana* due to lung metastases. Multiple levels of vertebral body compression are indicated by arrows. Note the retropulsion of portions of the vertebral bodies causing spinal stenosis.

248

CASE 51

HISTORY

An 18-year-old woman with a 1-month history of spastic paraparesis.

QUESTIONS

1. What are your differential considerations?

   _____

   _____

2. What MR techniques would you use?

	1	2	3
a. Coil	___	___	___
b. Centering point	___	___	___
c. Imaging plane(s)	___	___	___
d. Contrast	___	___	___
e. Slice thickness	___	___	___

3. What do you expect to find?

   _____

   _____

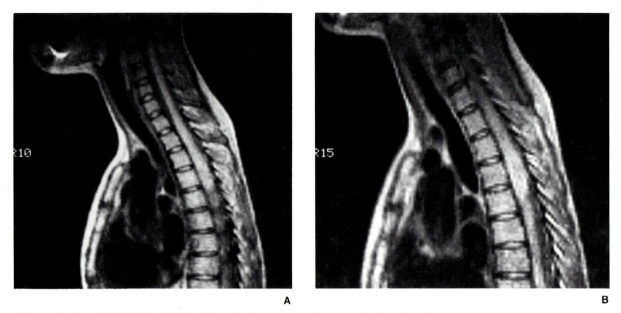

A   B

Figures 51.1A and **51.1B** (SE 1000/28). Midsagittal images through the cervicothoracic cord.

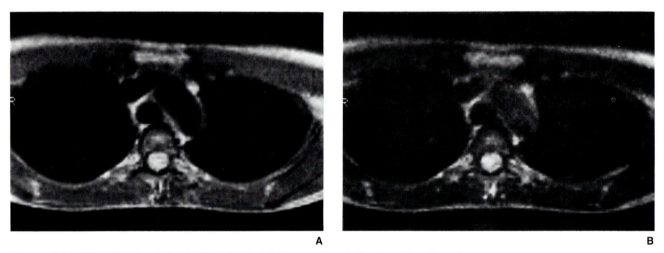

A   B

Figures 51.2A (SE 2000/28) and **51.2B** (SE 2000/56). Axial images through the upper thoracic cord.

MR TECHNIQUES

	1	2
a. Coil	Body	Body
b. Centering point	Sternal notch	Sternal notch
c. Imaging planes	Sagittal	Axial
d. Contrast	Mild T1W/mild T2W	Mild T2W/ moderate T2W
e. Slice thickness	Thin	Thin

See the discussion of techniques for evaluation of spine and cord in Chapter 5 and Case 46.

MR FINDINGS

Figure 51.1. Fusiform enlargement of the upper thoracic cord is demonstrated. The intensity of the involved portion of the cord is slightly increased, indicating increased water content and prolongation of T2.

Figure 51.2. On the axial T2WI, the enlarged cord occupies nearly all of the spinal canal. Cord signal intensity is markedly increased.

DIFFERENTIAL DIAGNOSIS

Possible causes of cord enlargement and alteration of signal intensity include *contusion, acute inflammatory disease,*[1] and *neoplasm.* In the absence of compelling history or evidence of fracture, contusion is effectively excluded. Inflammatory conditions, such as transverse myelitis or fulminant multiple sclerosis, may cause cord swelling but not usually to this degree. When MS is being considered clinically, the brain should be examined in addition to the cord, as the cord is rarely involved in isolation and MRI is more sensitive to demyelineating disease in the brain (because of the smaller head coil's greater efficiency compared with that of the larger body coil). Hence, the most likely cause for these findings is a tumor of the spinal cord.

Final Diagnosis

Anaplastic astrocytoma of the thoracic cord.

SUMMARY OF MR FINDINGS FOR CORD ASTROCYTOMA[2]

1. Cord enlargement, typically fusiform.
2. T2 prolongation.
3. Associated block may produce increased CSF intensity due to elevation of CSF protein.

REFERENCES

1. Maravilla KR, Weinreb JC, Suss R, et al: Magnetic resonance demonstration of multiple sclerosis plaques in the cervical cord. *AJR* 1985;144:381–385.
2. De Chiro G, Doppman JL, Dwyer AJ, et al: Tumors and arteriovenous malformations of the spinal cord: Assessment using MR. *Radiology* 1985;156:689–697.

CASE 52

HISTORY

A 5-year-old boy with postsurgical resection of a thoracic cord glioma. He underwent chemotherapy and spinal irradiation therapy. MRI of the spine and cord was requested.

QUESTIONS

1. What MR techniques would you use?

	1	2	3
a. Coil	_____	_____	_____
b. Centering point	_____	_____	_____
c. Imaging plane(s)	_____	_____	_____
d. Contrast	_____	_____	_____
e. Slice thickness	_____	_____	_____

2. What do you expect to find?

_____

_____

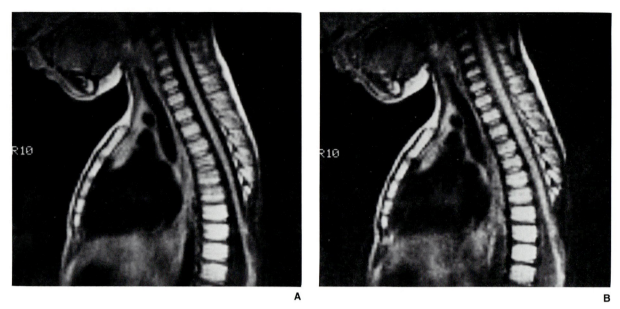

Figures 52.1A (SE 1000/28) and **52.1B** (SE 1000/56). Midsagittal scan through the thoracic spine.

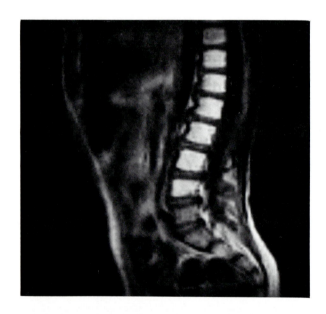

Figure 52.2 (SE 500/28). Midsagittal scan through the lumbar spine.

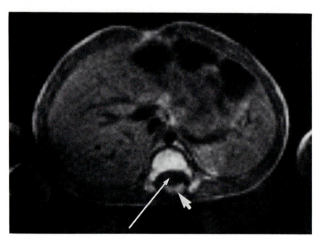

Figure 52.3 (SE 1000/28). Axial scan through the T 11 vertebral body.

MR TECHNIQUES

	1	2	3
a. Coil	Head	Head	Head
b. Centering point	Midsternum	Midabdomen	Xyphoid
c. Imaging planes	Sagittal	Sagittal	Axial
d. Contrast	Mild T1W/ mild T2W	Moderate T1W	Mild T1W/ Mild T2W
e. Slice thickness	Thin	Thin	Routine

The first pulsing sequence is the routine screening sequence for spine pathology. A second sagittal sequence with more T1 weighting was used to better illustrate changes in the marrow signal (see following discussion). The third pulsing sequence was used to provide a cross-sectional view of the contents of the spinal canal.

MR FINDINGS

Figures 52.1 and 52.2. There is homogeneous, increased intravertebral signal intensity extending from the midportion of T 7 to L 3. This increase in signal intensity is more apparent on the more heavily T1-weighted (TR of 500 msec) sequence indicating a shortened T1. The disc spaces, spinal alignment, and the shape of the vertebral bodies are normal.

The distal spinal cord is atrophic and displaced posteriorly, presumably because of adhesion at the operative site. Note the absence of the posterior elements related to the prior laminectomy procedure.

Anterior to the spinal cord is a widened subarachnoid space filled with CSF. This can be differentiated from an epidural tumor or hematoma because of the characteristic intensity changes on the two pulsing sequences. On the moderately T1-weighted image, the CSF has a low signal intensity owing to its low protein content. On the mildly T2-weighted (TR = 1,000 mseconds, TE = 56 mseconds) image, the CSF signal is increased to an intermediate intensity. With even greater T2 weighting, the CSF signal becomes more intense than that of the cord, making it difficult to evaluate intrinsic cord lesions.

Figure 52.3. The axial image confirms the posterior position of the cord (short arrow) and the enlarged, anterior subarachnoid space (long arrow).

DIFFERENTIAL DIAGNOSIS

The differential diagnosis for T1 shortening in the vertebral column includes *fatty marrow replacement* and *hemorrhage* with the formation of methemoglobin. Fatty marrow replacement may be due to *osteoporosis*[1] or *postradiation* changes.[2] In this case, the signal changes are confined to a specific segment of the vertebral column, corresponding to a radiation port. The marked T1 shortening is greater than anticipated for osteoporosis alone. A diffuse hemorrhagic process within the marrow would be extremely unlikely.

The atrophy and posterior displacement of the spinal cord are most likely due to postoperative changes, including resection, devascularization, and adhesions. On serial scans, the appearance of the cord has remained stable; therefore, tumor recurrence is not suspected.[3]

Final Diagnosis

1. Postradiation fatty replacement of bone marrow.
2. Spinal cord myelomalacia and postoperative adhesions.

SUMMARY OF MR FINDINGS

1. Postradiation Fatty Replacement of Bone Marrow[2]

a. Marked and uniform T1 shortening of the levels of the vertebral bodies limited to the radiation port.
b. These findings are probably permanent.
c. Secondary hypoplasia of the vertebral column in children may result.

2. Spinal Cord Myelomalacia[3]

a. Atrophy.
b. Altered signal intensity (i.e., prolonged T2).
c. Intramedullary cyst formation may result.

3. Adhesions

a. Abnormal location of the spinal cord. Scanning the patient in the prone position may help in verifying cord fixation.
b. Ill definition and angulation of cord contours.

REFERENCES

1. Dooms GC, Fisher MR, Hricak H, et al: Bone marrow imaging: Magnetic resonance studies related to age and sex. *Radiology* 1985; 155:429–432.
2. Ramsey RG, Zacharias CE: MR imaging of the spine after radiation therapy: Easily recognizable effects. *AJR* 1985;144:1131–1135.
3. Kucharczyk W, Brant-Zawadzki M, Sobel D, et al: Central nervous system tumors in children: Detection by magnetic resonance imaging. *Radiology* 1985;155:131–136.

6

MUSCULOSKELETAL IMAGING

Compared with other imaging modalities, magnetic resonance imaging (MRI) has several advantages in the evaluation of musculoskeletal pathology. These include multiplanar capability and increased soft tissue contrast resolution with improved tissue specificity. Motion artifacts in a cooperative patient are not a significant problem in musculoskeletal imaging, in contrast to thoracic and abdominal imaging. The diameter of extremities permits the use of efficient volume coils or surface coils. Relative disadvantages with MR imaging include technical factors, such as limited spatial resolution and insensitivity to cortical bone pathology, and nontechnical factors, such as increased costs, limited availability, and patient claustrophobia. Occasionally, metallic prostheses and/or surgical clips may cause artifactual degradation of the image, but this is less pronounced than that seen with CT.[1]

NORMAL ANATOMY

Synovial Fluid

As with other solutions, synovial fluid can be characterized by relatively long T1 and T2 relaxation values[2] compared with those of surrounding soft tissues. As a result, decreased signal can be anticipated with T1-weighted imaging and increased signal with T2-weighted images. The degree of T1 prolongation is less than that of less proteinaceous fluids, such as CSF or urine. Joint effusions have been noted to have similar intensity patterns; however, the exact nature of the joint effusion may not be discernible with MRI. For example, it has been noted that experimental hip effusions formed by intracapsular injection of either fresh blood or saline have similar signal intensity characteristics.[3] These signal characteristics of proteinaceous fluid may aid in distinguishing effusions from the adjacent joint capsule and articular cartilage. More importantly, synovial fluid within a tear can readily be distinguished from the normal meniscus.

Cartilage

There are two types of cartilage: fibrous and hyaline. Each has a characteristic MR signal. Fibrous cartilage has a short T2 relaxation time and is therefore a low intensity structure. An example is the meniscus of the knee. On the other hand, hyaline or articular cartilage is noted to have an intermediate MR signal. The signal differences between fibrous and hyaline cartilage are thought to be due to differences in collagen composition; that is, the collagen found in hyaline cartilage is slightly more hydrophilic.[4] The articular cartilage adjacent to subchondral cortex, however, may be of lower signal intensity on T2-weighted images.[5] As a result, it may be difficult to distinguish this cartilage from the low intensity cortex, resulting in apparent but artifactual cartilage thinning. A similar finding has been noted also with inversion recovery pulsing sequences.[5]

Ligaments and Tendons[6]

As with fibrous cartilage, a low signal intensity is noted with ligaments and tendons. This is thought to be due to a decreased proton density and T2 relaxation times.

Skeletal Muscle[7]

Normal skeletal muscle has a moderately long T1 and a short T2. It has a low intermediate intensity between that of fat and cortical bone. The fascial planes between muscle bundles are readily demonstrated because of high intensity fat.

Skeletal Bone

Cortical bone contains little MR-visible hydrogen and thus produces a minimal MR signal. As a result, very low intensity is noted. In contradistinction, the medullary cavity contains visible protons in two different types of marrow: hematopoietic and fatty.[8] Therefore, a relatively uniform high signal is seen within the medullary cavity. In some cases, the dense bony trabecula may reduce the signal intensity within the medullary cavity.

Vascular Structures

Flowing blood has natural contrast on MR images. The anticipated signal intensities can vary from complete absence due to flow void to increased signal, which can be noted with various phenomena, such as even-echo rephasing, flow-related enhancement, or diastolic pseudogating.[9]

MUSCULOSKELETAL TUMORS[10–13]

Compared with CT, MRI has been shown superior in demonstrating the extent of tumors within the medullary canal, the size of any extraosseous soft tissue mass, and the extent of muscle invasion. Both coronal or sagittal images may help in defining the tumor's longitudinal extent, which is of critical importance in planning the level of therapy (i.e., amputation, radiation, and/or limb salvage procedures). Vascular involvement is better seen with MR, and the use of contrast material may be avoided. In some cases, skip lesions within the marrow are better demonstrated on MRI.[10] Postoperatively, MRI may be valuable in the assessment of tumor recurrence since metallic artifacts from orthopedic plates, screws, and surgical clips are generally nonferromagnetic and cause less image degradation with MRI than CT.[14] On the other hand, CT is superior in showing cortical destruction, periosteal reaction, matrix mineralization, and pathologic fractures.

Criteria for Tumor Detection

Radiographic criteria for detecting osseous tumors include expansion, thinning, and destruction of the cortex, periosteal new bone formation, and soft tissue masses. These criteria also apply to MR imaging. In addition, several new MR criteria have been developed.[1]

1. *Alteration of the normal marrow signal within the medullary cavity.* Since the calculated relaxation times (T1 and T2) of bone and soft tissue tumors are prolonged compared with those of normal muscle and fat, one can predict how normal signal intensities may change because of neoplastic involvement. First, replacement of normal fatty marrow (short T1) by tumor (longer T1) will decrease the signal on T1-weighted images. With T2-weighted images, increased signal may occur.
2. *Cortical invasion.* When the cortex is invaded, the signal of cortex is increased and thus appears gray and mottled, this being most obvious on T2-weighted images. The cortex may lose its sharp interface with medullary bone and soft tissue.
3. *Soft tissue changes.* Changes within the soft tissue may include direct tumor extension, hemorrhage, adjacent joint effusion, and edema. The contrast differences between the primary tumor and the adjacent muscle can be accentuated on T2-weighted images.
4. *Intensity differences.* The signal intensity of intraosseous vs. extraosseous components of the tumor may be different, with the extraosseous component having a slightly higher intensity.

On the basis of the T1 and T2 characteristics alone, differentiation cannot be made between benign and malignant lesions. Established criteria should still be applied; that is, sharply delineated lesions tend to be benign. Heterogeneity of signal (excluding calcium matrix), irregular and poorly defined margins, and invasion into adjacent muscle and vascular structures suggest malignancy.

Aneurysmal Bone Cyst[15]

The MR findings noted with this entity can be striking. The internal structure within the cyst may contain fluid–fluid levels with a wide range of signal intensities, reflecting intracystic hemorrhage of varying age, as well as the presence of small, diverticulumlike projections arising in the walls of larger cysts. The margin of the cyst may be defined by a rim of low signal. The specificity of MRI may be greater than that of CT because of its ability in demonstrating these characteristics.

MUSCLE DISEASES[7]

Many muscle disorders result in the fatty replacement of normal muscle, thus allowing easy detection of affected muscle. MRI can characterize the disease in terms of size, number, and distribution of the involved muscle(s) and the pattern of fatty replacement. With an increasing degree of clinical severity and greater muscle involvement, more complete replacement by fat can be seen. Unfortunately, MRI is nonspecific and cannot be used to determine the etiology of the disorder. However, the distribution and pattern of muscle involvement may be used to distinguish radicular disease, plexopathy, and peripheral neuropathies.

The technique used to evaluate fatty replacement should include a spin echo pulsing sequence with a relatively short TR (500 to 1,000 mseconds) and a short TE (30 to 60 mseconds). This optimizes the contrast between fat, muscle, and bone. Some investigators note that there is no additional advantage in using spin density images or T2-weighted sequences. For most purposes, the transaxial plane appears adequate; coronal sections can be added when longitudinal spatial localization is desired.

TRAUMA[16]

MRI may be useful in assessing soft tissue injury. Edematous changes in the ligaments and tendons may be noted as areas of abnormally increased signal intensity on T2-weighted spin echo sequences. Subacute hemorrhage with T1 shortening may be seen on T1-weighted sequences. However, on T1-weighted images, edema within soft tissues may not be readily appreciated and low intensity synovial fluid may obscure the margin of a torn ligament. Thus, both T1- and T2-weighted sequences should be used in the evaluation of soft tissue injury.

KNEE IMAGING[17,18]

The main advantages of MRI in evaluating the knee are its noninvasiveness compared with arthroscopy or arthrography and its ability to examine an acutely injured knee. The use of a local coil (either saddle, solenoidal, or planar) is the recommended technique. The knee should be extended and externally rotated approximately 15 to 20 degrees without stress or distraction. Meniscal and ligamentous tears are effectively demonstrated on T1-weighted (e.g., TR 500 mseconds and TE 28 mseconds), high-resolution (e.g., 0.75 mm) thin slices (e.g., 4 mm). The sagittal plane has been found to be the most useful projection.

Meniscal injuries are noted as areas of increased signal intensity within the substance of the meniscus, presumably representing synovial fluid within the cleft created by the tear. Severe degeneration of the meniscus may appear as increased signal within the central portion. Early work has shown that MRI is very accurate in the diagnosis of meniscal tear, with a greater than 90% correlation with arthroscopic findings in one study.

Osteochondral fragments are noted to be of low signal intensity. Osteonecrosis is seen as a region of decreased signal intensity within the high intensity marrow (see following discussion on hip imaging). Cruciate ligament tears may be difficult to identify because of the oblique course of these ligaments. Nonorthogonal planes may be helpful in evaluation. With the knee externally rotated 15 degrees, sagittal imaging may demonstrate the normal intact, anterior cruciate ligament. The integrity of the thicker posterior cruciate ligament is more easily assessed. Patellar tendon injuries can be recognized as areas of discontinuity or irregularity.

HIP IMAGING[19]

The normal femoral head is rounded, smoothly marginated, and surrounded by a sharply defined, low intensity cortex. The medullary cavity has a high signal intensity on conventional imaging sequences because of its marrow fat content. Surrounding the cortical bone is a thin, high intensity line corresponding to the combined articular cartilage of the femoral head and acetabulum. The acetabular marrow is slightly lower and less uniform in intensity than that of the marrow of the femoral head. On coronal images, the femoral heads contain a vertically oriented, low intensity band resulting from the prominent central weight-bearing trabeculae. These weight-bearing trabeculae can also be seen as focal low intensity signals within the marrow on axial views.

AVASCULAR NECROSIS

Various patterns of abnormal signal intensity due to avascular necrosis have been described.[9] Typically, those are focal areas of either homogeneous or heterogeneous, low signal intensity. These changes may be confined to the superior portion of the femoral head adjacent to the joint or may be more extensive so that the entire head and portions of the neck are involved. Bandlike and ringlike patterns of decreased signal surrounding central higher intensity can also be seen. There is poor correlation between the type of MR involvement and the stage of the disease and the findings on either bone scan or plain radiographs. These areas of decreased signal intensity can be seen irrespective of the pulse sequence used; however, coronal images with short TR and short TE are the most efficient in detecting these abnormalities. Preliminary studies indicate a high sensitivity of MRI; these findings may be nonspecific, however, since any process that replaces fatty marrow would produce similar results.

Legg-Calve-Perthe Disease

MRI has been reported to be effective in detecting Legg-Calve-Perthe disease.[20] It has been postulated that synovitis is a possible cause of this disorder and leads to increased intracapsular pressure, which in turn decreases blood supply to the ossification center of the femoral head.[21] MRI may also be an important tool in detecting joint effusions in these patients.

SHOULDER IMAGING[22]

In evaluation of the shoulder, MRI may have a distinct advantage compared with CT because of its multiplanar capability and better soft tissue contrast. On the other hand, MRI's disadvantages in this region are due primarily to the poor differentiation between the distal rotator cuff, cortical bone, glenoid labrum, articular capsule, and the long tendon of the biceps, since they all have similar low signal intensities.

The rotator cuff includes the supraspinatus, infraspinatus, teres minor, and subscapularis muscles and is best evaluated in the coronal and sagittal planes. With the exception of a small central band, the fibrotendinous or most distal portion of the cuff has almost no signal at its insertion and cannot be differentiated from cortical bone. The long tendon of the biceps is best visualized on axial sections as a round signal void in the bicipital groove. Owing to the absence of signal within the glenoid labrum and articular capsule, these structures may merge imperceptibly with the cortical bone of the scapula and humerus. At this time, the relative effectiveness of MR imaging in determining a rotator cuff tear compared with that of arthrography has not been fully evaluated.

ARTHRITIS[23]

The potential role of MR imaging in the evaluation of arthritis is yet to be fully defined. The cartilage and soft tissue components of the joints can be seen clearly with good contrast distinction between those structures and the low signal intensity of synovial fluid on T1-weighted sequences. We have found MRI useful in evaluating atlantoaxial synovitis in rheumatoid arthritis. MRI may prove to be a useful adjunct in the evaluation of joint disease.

OSTEOMYELITIS[24]

Infectious processes within the medullary canal may cause a reduction in the normal high signal intensity, and this is best shown on T1-weighted pulse sequences. MRI is also helpful in determining the extent of adjacent soft tissue involvement. Inflammatory disease may be difficult to distinguish from neoplasm on the basis of MR imaging findings alone.

REFERENCES

1. Li DKB: Magnetic resonance imaging of the musculoskeletal system, in *Syllabus for the Categorical Course on Magnetic Resonance 1985*. Presented at the Annual Meeting of the American College of Radiology, Montreal, 1985, pp 301–317.

2. Moon KL, Genant HK, Davis PL, et al: Nuclear magnetic resonance imaging in orthopedics: Principles and applications. *J Orthop Res* 1983;1:101–114.

3. Beltran J, Noto AM, Herman LJ, et al: Joint effusions: MR imaging. *Radiology* 1986;158:133–137.

4. Li KC, Henkelman M, Poon PY, et al: MR imaging of the normal knee. *J Comput Assist Tomogr* 1984;8:1147–1154.

5. Adams ME, Li DK, Jenkin J, et al: Magnetic resonance imaging of experimental osteoarthritis. *Clin Exp Med* 1984;7:52–86.

6. Fullerton GD, Cameron IL, Ord VA: Orientation of tendons in the magnetic field and its effect on T2 relaxation times. *Radiology* 1984;155:433–435.

7. Murphy WA, Totty WG, Carroll JE: MRI of normal and pathologic skeletal muscle. *AJR* 1986;146:565–574.

8. Dooms GC, Fisher MR, Hricak H, et al: Bone marrow imaging: Magnetic resonance studies related to age and sex. *Radiology* 1985;155:429–432.

9. Bradley WG, Waluch V: Blood flow: Magnetic resonance imaging. *Radiology* 1985;154:443–450.

10. Zimmer WD, Berquist TH, McLeod RA, et al: Bone tumors: Magnetic resonance imaging versus computed tomography. *Radiology* 1985;155:709–718.

11. Moon KL, Genant HK, Helms CA, et al: Musculoskeletal applications of nuclear magnetic resonance. *Radiology* 1983;147:161–171.

12. Brady TJ, Gebhardt MC, Pykett IL, et al: NMR imaging of forearms in healthy volunteers and patients with giant cell tumor of bone. *Radiology* 1982;144:549–552.

13. Aisen AM, Martel W, Braunstein EM, et al: MRI and CT evaluation of primary bone and soft-tissue tumors. *AJR* 1986;146:749–756.

14. Berquist TH: Magnetic resonance imaging: Preliminary experience in orthopedic radiology. *Magnetic Resonance Imaging* 1984;2:41–52.

15. Beltran J, Simon DC, Levy M, et al: Aneurysmal bone cysts: MR imaging at 1.5 T. *Radiology* 1986;158:689–690.

16. Turner DA, Prodromos CC, Petasnick JP: Acute injury of the ligaments of the knee. Magnetic resonance evaluation. *Radiology* 1985;154:717–722.

17. Reicher MA, Raushning W, Gold RH, et al: High-resolution magnetic resonance imaging of the knee joint: Normal anatomy. *AJR* 1985;145:895–902.

18. Reicher MA, Bassett LW, Gold RH: High-resolution magnetic resonance imaging of the knee joint: Pathologic correlations. *AJR* 1985;145:903–909.

19. Totty WG, Murphy WA, Ganz WI, et al: Magnetic resonance imaging of the normal and ischemic femoral head. *AJR* 1984;143:1273–1280.

20. Scoles P, Yoon YS, Makley JT, et al: Nuclear magnetic resonance imaging in Legg-Calve-Perthes disease. *J Bone Joint Surg (Am)* 1984; 66A:1357–1363.

21. Resnick D: The osteochondrosis, in Resnick D, Niwayama G (eds): *Diagnosis of Bone and Joint Disease*. Philadelphia, Saunders, 1981, pp 2883–2885.

22. Huber DJ, Sauter R, Mueller E, et al: MR imaging of the normal shoulder. *Radiology* 1986;158:405–408.

23. Adams ME, Li DK, Ho KB, et al: Magnetic resonance imaging of knee arthritis: Preliminary experience. *Arthritis Rheum* 1984;27:65.

24. Fletcher BD, Scoles PV, Nelson AD: Osteomyelitis in children: Detection by magnetic resonance. *Radiology* 1984;150:57–60.

CASE 53

HISTORY

This 21-year-old man suffered a recent twisting injury to the right knee and presents with medial joint line pain.

QUESTIONS

1. What are your differential considerations?

   _____

   _____

2. What MR techniques would you use?

	1	2	3
a. Coil	____	____	____
b. Centering point	____	____	____
c. Imaging plane(s)	____	____	____
d. Contrast	____	____	____
e. Slice thickness	____	____	____

3. What do you expect to find?

   _____

   _____

Sources: Figures 53.1, 53.2, 53.3, 53.5A, and 53.5B courtesy of Irwin Grossman, MD, Beverly Hills, CA. Figures 53.5C and 53.5D courtesy of Washington MR Center, Whittier, CA.

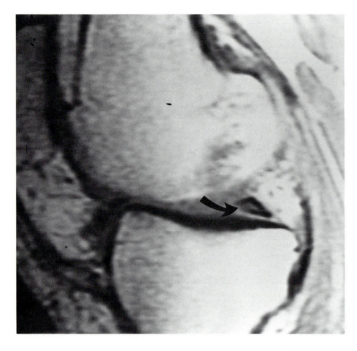

Figure 53.1 (SE 800/25). Sagittal scan through the posterior horn of the medial meniscus.

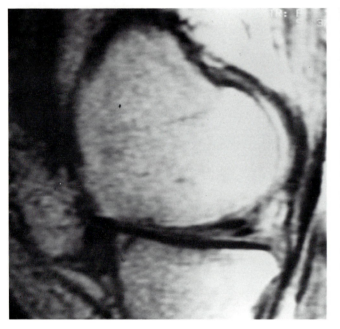

Figure 53.2 (SE 800/25). Sagittal scan 4 mm lateral to Figure 53.1.

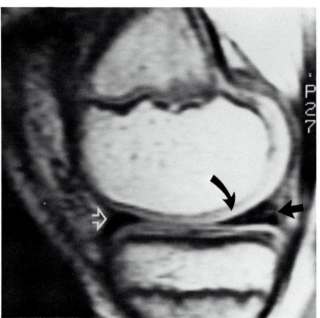

Figure 53.3 (SE 800/25). Sagittal section through the medial condyle in an asymptomatic patient for comparison.

MR TECHNIQUES

	1	2
a. Coil	Surface	Surface
b. Centering point	Joint space	Joint space
c. Imaging planes	Sagittal	Coronal
d. Contrast	Mild to moderate T1W	Mild to moderate T1W
e. Slice thickness	Thin	Thin

Internal derangements of the knee (meniscal tears and cruciate ligament injuries) are best studied in the sagittal plane.[1,2] Both anterior and posterior meniscal horns can be evaluated on the same section, and the articular cartilages are seen tangentially. With the foot externally rotated 20 degrees, both anterior and posterior cruciate ligaments can be visualized along their long axes. Coronal scans are utilized to confirm findings and to evaluate the collateral ligaments. Some investigators have also reported that the coronal plane may aid in evaluating the anterior and posterior horns of the menisci.[3] The use of T1-weighted images provides adequate contrast between the various osseous and soft tissue components of the knee while allowing for reasonable scan times. Depending on the desired slice thickness, the interslice gap, and type of coil used, several acquisitions may be necessary to cover both menisci. Alternatively, a longer TR may be necessary to increase coverage. Contiguous or nearly contiguous thin slices (5 mm or less) are mandatory.

Adequate signal-to-noise requires either a surface coil or an efficient double-saddle (quadrature) coil. For example, Figures 53.1 through 53.3 and Figure 53.4 were obtained with a flat surface coil and a quadrature coil, respectively.

MR FINDINGS

Figures 53.1 and 53.2. Within the low intensity, triangular-shaped posterior horn, there is a horizontally oriented, linear area of medium signal intensity, extending from the inferior aspect of the meniscus anteriorly (curved arrow) traversing the midportion, disrupting the normal low intensity fibrocartilaginous meniscus. This should be compared with the normal example in Figure 53.3.

Figure 53.3. This is an example of a normal meniscus. Note that there is subtle heterogeneity within the posterior horn of the meniscus (closed arrow) compared with the anterior horn (open arrow). This well-defined, horizontal band of slightly increased signal intensity does not extend to the articulating surface of the meniscus. It is frequently noted in normal individuals. This finding is of questionable significance; it probably represents a degenerative horizontal cleft and is unlikely to represent a tear. This should not be confused with the *definite tear* seen in the preceding example.

The articulating hyaline cartilage (curved arrow) has increased signal and can be identified between the low intensity cortical bone and the meniscus. Note the thinning and partial absence of this cartilage over the medial condyle adjacent to the tear on Figures 53.1 and 53.2.

DIFFERENTIAL DIAGNOSIS

The normal medial meniscus is homogeneously low in signal intensity. A linear or irregular focus of medium or increased signal intensity within the meniscus, with or without fraying or separation, is diagnostic of a tear. The cause of this increased intensity is not definitely known but is presumed to be due to synovial fluid within the tear.[3] As in arthrography, this finding may be simulated by synovial redundancy ("synovial recess") at the margin of the meniscus.

Final Diagnosis

Horizontal tear of the posterior horn of the medial meniscus.

SUMMARY OF MR FINDINGS FOR MENISCAL TEARS[1-3]

1. Linear area of medium or high signal intensity within the low intensity meniscus.
2. High intensity joint effusion due to high protein content.
3. Secondary thinning or disruption of articular cartilage.

Comments

Preliminary studies have shown that the knee can be effectively evaluated with MRI with an accuracy comparable to that of arthrography. MRI offers the advantages of tomographic display and is painless, noninvasive, and nonionizing. Arthrography, on the other hand, is less expensive and more readily available; it also has better spatial resolution. As MR imaging becomes more efficient, the cost of an examination may decrease. In some centers, MRI has already replaced arthrography as the imaging modality for evaluating knee injury.

Other current indications for MR examination of the knee include cysts (Figure 53.4), cruciate ligament injuries (Figure 53.5), avascular necrosis (Figure 54.8), infection, and neoplastic diseases.

REFERENCES

1. Reicher MA, Rauschning W, Gold RH, et al: High-resolution magnetic resonance imaging of the knee joint: Normal anatomy. *AJR* 1985; 145:895–902.
2. Reicher MA, Bassett LW, Gold RH: High-resolution magnetic resonance imaging of the knee joint: Pathologic correlation. *AJR* 1985; 145:903–910.
3. Beltran J, Noto AM, Mosure JC, et al: Meniscal tears: MR demonstration of experimentally produced injuries. *Radiology* 1986;158:691–693.

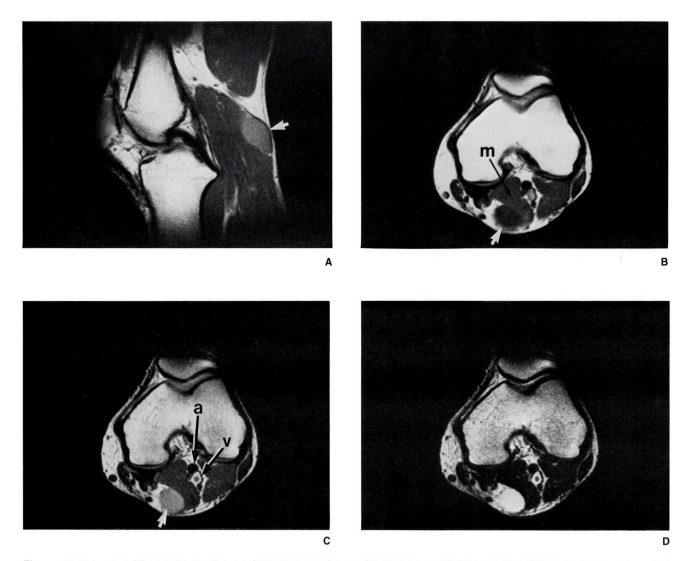

Figures 53.4A (sagittal, SE 1000/40), **53.4B** (axial, SE 500/30), **53.4C** (axial, SE 1500/40), and **53.4D** (axial, SE 1500/80). Popliteal cyst (arrow) of the knee, posterior to the medial head of the gastrocnemius muscle (m). The cyst has a long T1 (low signal on T1-weighted images) and a long T2 (high signal on T2-weighted images) characteristic of fluid. The popliteal artery (a) with flow void and the popliteal vein (v) with flow-related enhancement can readily be identified.

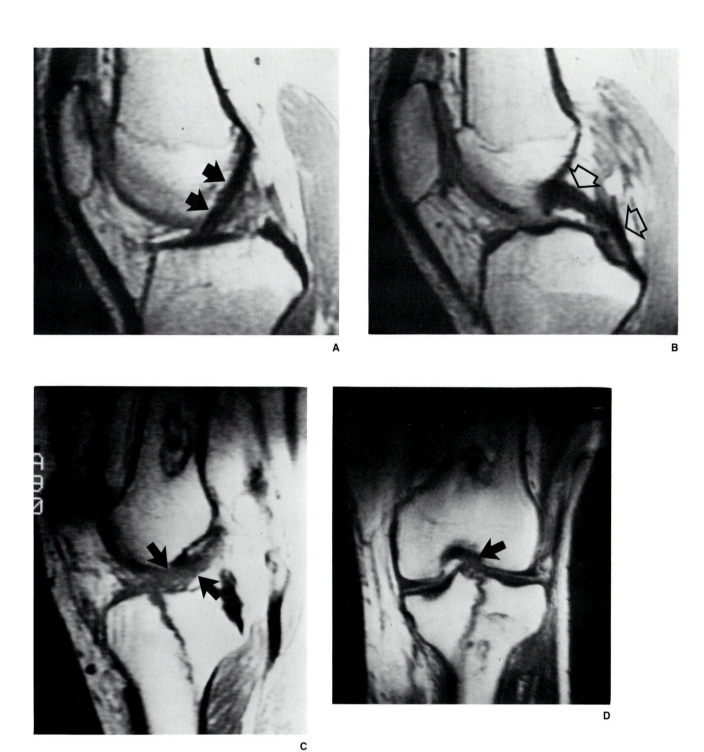

Figures 53.5A (sagittal, SE 800/25), **53.5B** (sagittal, SE 800/25), **53.5C** (sagittal, SE 800/25), and **53.5D** (coronal 800/25). Cruciate injury. Figures 53.5A and 53.5B are normal examples of the anterior (closed arrows) and posterior (open arrows) cruciates. These ligamentous structures have low proton density and, therefore, low signal intensity. With the leg extended during the scan, the posterior cruciate has a normal arcuate appearance. Figures 53.5C and 53.5D illustrate changes following trauma. There is thickening, irregularity, and increased signal intensity within the anterior cruciate (closed arrow) consistent with an incomplete tear. A fracture line is evident. (To the astute observer: Did you notice the altered signal intensity within both the distal femoral and proximal tibial metaphyses? These represent bone infarcts.)

CASE 54

HISTORY

This 46-year-old man developed the sudden onset of right hip pain after a course of prednisone therapy for sulfa allergy. A bone scan was performed (Figure 54.1).

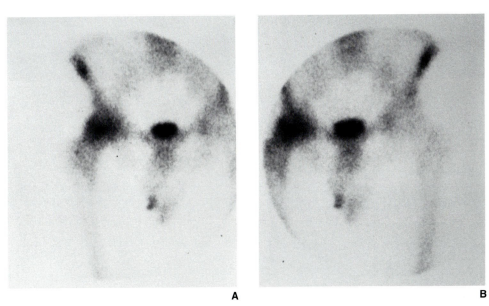

Figure 54.1. Anterior view of both hips from a radionuclide bone scan. (A) right and (B) left.

QUESTIONS

1. What are your differential considerations?

_____

_____

2. What MR techniques would you use?

	1	2	3
a. Coil	___	___	___
b. Centering point	___	___	___
c. Imaging plane(s)	___	___	___
d. Contrast	___	___	___
e. Slice thickness	___	___	___

3. What do you expect to find?

_____

_____

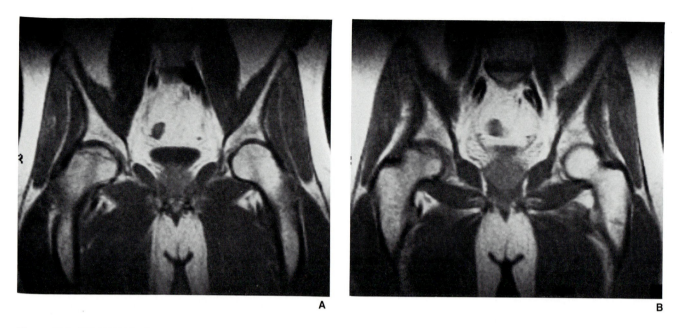

A

B

Figure 54.2 (SE 1000/28). Coronal scan through both hips. Figure 54.2B is 1 cm posterior to Figure 54.2A.

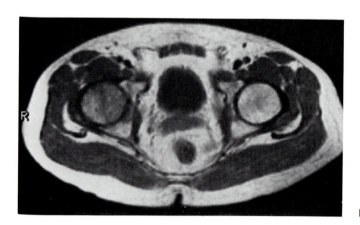

Figure 54.3 (SE 1000/28). Axial scan through the femoral heads.

Figures 54.4 and **54.5** were taken from a second study performed 6 months after the initial study (Figures 54.2 and 54.3). What has happened between the two studies?

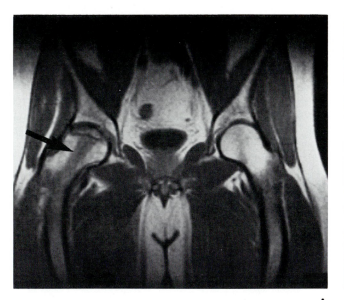

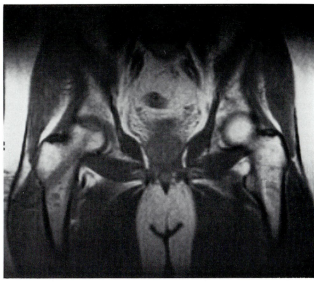

A

B

Figure 54.4 (SE 1000/28). Coronal scan of both hips. Figure 54.4B is 1 cm posterior to Figure 54.4A.

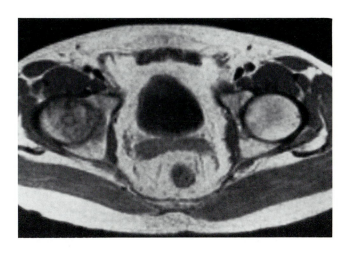

Figure 54.5 (SE 1000/28). Axial scan through the femoral heads.

MR TECHNIQUES

		1	2
a.	Coil	Body	Body
b.	Centering point	Greater trochanter	
c.	Imaging planes	Coronal	Axial
d.	Contrast	Mild T1W	Mild T1W
e.	Slice thickness	Routine	Routine

As discussed in the introductory section, T1-weighted coronal images are the most efficient in evaluating hip disorders involving the medullary space. Axial images provide another view of the femoral heads and are useful in confirming any questionable abnormalities detected on the coronal views. We favor the use of coronal and axial views because they provide direct comparison of both hips on a single image.

MR FINDINGS

Figure 54.1. There is a focal area of increased activity localized to the right femoral head.

Figure 54.2. On Figure 54.2A, a thin, irregular band (solid arrow) of low signal intensity is seen in the superior one third of the right femoral head. On Figure 54.2B, there is mild heterogeneity and decreased signal intensity in the same area. There is also slight irregularity along the superior and posterior cortical margins of the right femoral head. Note the normal appearance of the left femoral head, with uniform high signal intensity within the medullary cavity and a central, faint, low intensity vertical band resulting from the prominent central weight-bearing trabeculae (open arrow).

Figure 54.3. There is abnormal low signal intensity in the medial half of the right femoral head.

Figure 54.4. There is a new, well-defined, low intensity band traversing the right femoral neck (arrow). This represents a surgical defect caused by core biopsy and decompression. The previously seen low intensity band in the upper portion of the right femoral head appears to be slightly thicker than before.

Figure 54.5. The signal intensity of the right femoral head is now shown to be uniformly low. There are two new, low intensity rings identified in the anterior and central portions of the right femoral head. These rings represent the core biopsy sites. The inner bony cortex of the right femoral head is less well defined than that of the left femoral head.

DIFFERENTIAL DIAGNOSIS

The findings are characteristics of osteonecrosis of the femoral head. As described in the introductory section, the pattern of involvement can be variable.[1] In this example, the superior portion of the femoral head has abnormal, decreased signal with slight heterogeneity. A low intensity band is also

seen. These changes in MR intensity are thought to represent loss of both the fatty and hematopoietic marrow cells, with replacement by fibrous reactive tissue. Another pattern of altered signal intensity is shown in Figure 54.6. In this example, the avascular necrosis is bilateral, and there is diffuse involvement of the head and proximal femoral neck. Since avascular necrosis can be bilateral, MRI is a good screening test for evaluating early contralateral disease in patients with known avascular necrosis (AVN).

Core decompression is both a diagnostic and therapeutic procedure. It is usually performed on those at risk for osteonecrosis who have a painful but radiologically normal hip. This procedure is designed to decrease the intramedullary pressure within the femoral head in the hope of arresting the pathologic process indefinitely. It may also be performed for palliation on those in whom more extensive surgical procedures are contraindicated. The procedure consists of

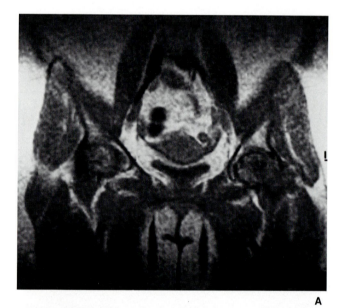

A

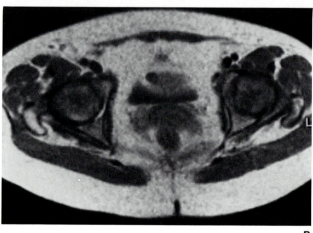

B

Figure 54.6 (SE 1000/28). Coronal (A) and axial (B) images from another patient demonstrating bilateral avascular necrosis of the hips.

removing an 8-mm to 10-mm core of bone from the antero-lateral segment of the femoral head through a lateral trochanteric approach.[2]

For those patients who have developed collapse of the femoral head, rotational osteotomy (Sugioka's procedure) may be considered.[2] The purpose is to bring the collapsing segment (usually the anteromedial surface) out of weight-bearing contact with the acetabulum. Hence, it is important to determine the integrity of the posterior and lateral surface of the femoral head that will be rotated into the weight-bearing area. This portion of the femoral head is generally difficult to examine with conventional modalities. MRI in the sagittal and coronal projections can be used to assess this area effectively.

Avascular necrosis can affect other sites. As with the hip, the MR signal intensity of the involved area is decreased. Examples involving the lunate (Figure 54.7) and femoral condyle (Figure 54.8) are shown.

Final Diagnosis

Avascular necrosis of the right hip.

SUMMARY OF MR FINDINGS FOR AVASCULAR NECROSIS OF THE HIP[1]

1. Low signal intensity within the femoral head.
2. Variable pattern of involvement.
3. The MR pattern may not correlate well with the clinical stage or findings on either plain films or radionuclide scintigraphy.

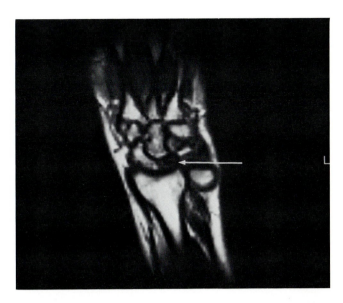

Figure 54.7 (SE 500/40). Coronal section of the right wrist. Avascular necrosis of the lunate is evident by resultant decrease in intensity (arrow). The hamate, pisiform, and triquetrum are partially outside the plane of section and are incompletely visualized.

REFERENCES

1. Totty WG, Murphy WA, Ganz WI, et al: Magnetic resonance imaging of the normal and ischemic femoral head. *AJR* 1984;143:1273–1280.
2. Hungerford DS: Treatment of ischemic necrosis of the femoral head, in Evarts CMC (ed): *Surgery of the Musculoskeletal System.* New York, Churchill Livingstone, 1983, vol 3, pp 5–29.

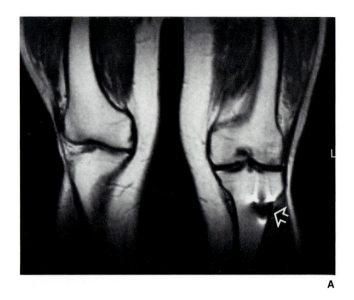

A

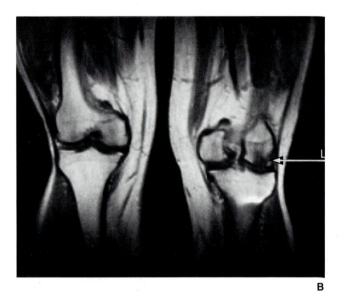

B

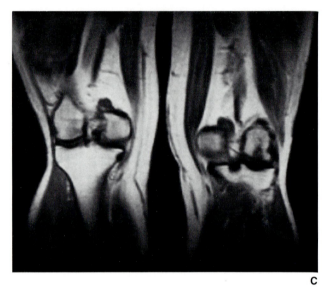

C

Figures 54.8A through **54.8C** (SE 1000/30). Coronal sections through the knees. C is the most posterior section. The closed arrow indicates a subarticular focus of decreased signal intensity in the left lateral femoral condyle, consistent with avascular necrosis. Note the surgically placed metallic artifact (open arrow), related to prior surgery.

CASE 55

HISTORY

A previously healthy 6-year-boy with a 1-week history of fever presents with a painful left hip held in a flexed position. A bone scan of the pelvis (not shown) was unremarkable. Hip aspiration was performed, but the aspirate was found to be sterile. An MR study was requested for further evaluation of the hip and pelvis.

QUESTIONS

1. What are your differential considerations?

   _____

   _____

2. What MR techniques would you use?

	1	2	3
a. Coil	___	___	___
b. Centering point	___	___	___
c. Imaging plane(s)	___	___	___
d. Contrast	___	___	___
e. Slice thickness	___	___	___

3. What do you expect to find?

   _____

   _____

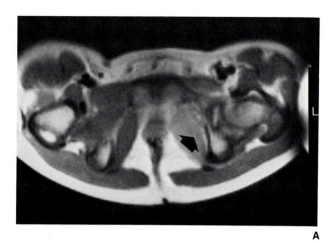
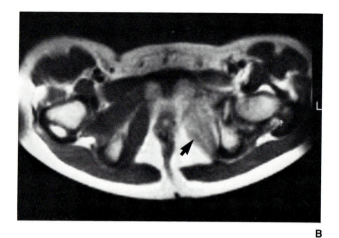

A

B

Figures 55.1A (SE 2000/28) and **55.1B** (SE 2000/60). Axial scans through the inferior hips.

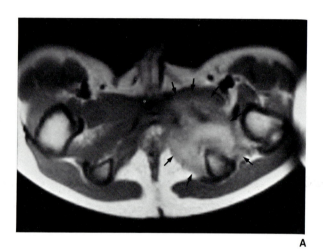
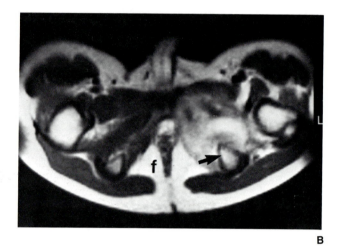

A

B

Figures 55.2A (SE 2000/28) and **55.2B** (SE2000/56). Axial scans 1 cm inferior to Figure 55.1.

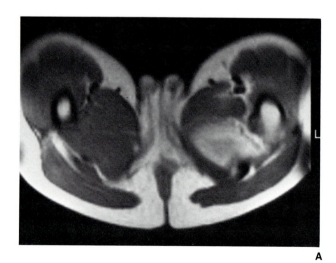
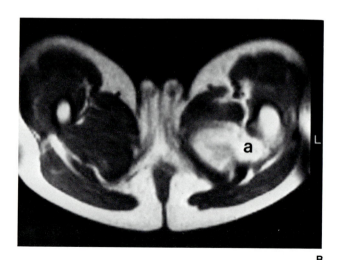

A

B

Figures 55.3A (SE 2000/28) and **55.3B** (SE 2000/56). Axial scans 2 cm inferior to Figure 55.2.

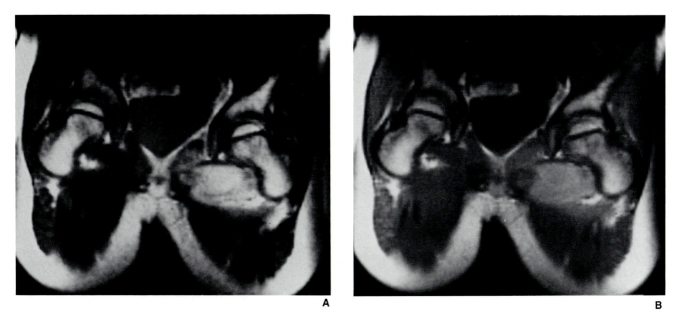

A

B

Figures 55.4A (SE 1000/28) and **55.4B** (SE 1000/56). Coronal scans through the hips.

MR TECHNIQUES

		1	2
a.	Coil	Body	Body
b.	Centering point	Greater trochanter	Greater trochanter
c.	Imaging planes	Axial	Coronal
d.	Contrast	Mild to moderate T2W	Mild T1W
e.	Slice thickness	Routine	Routine

Most pathologic processes involving the skeletal muscles increase both the T1 and T2 relaxation times. The first pulsing sequence was performed with moderate T2 weighting to provide T2 information and to accentuate the difference in intensity between abnormal and normal muscles. The coronal image was performed with a TR of 1,000 mseconds to provide additional T1 information and to define the longitudinal extent of the pathologic process.

MR FINDINGS

Figures 55.1 through 55.3. On the axial images, there is abnormal area of increased signal intensity involving the left obturator internus muscle (arrowhead, Figure 55.1A), the adductor muscle group, obturator externus/internus, and quadratus femoris muscles (arrows, Figure 55.2A). The fascial planes separating these muscles are obliterated. On the second echo images, a focal area of markedly increased signal intensity is noted ([a] Figure 55.3B), indicating pronounced prolongation of T2 as compared with normal muscle. The ramus of the ischium (arrow, Figure 55.2B) and the fat-filled ischiorectal fossa ([f] Figure 55.2B) are readily identified.

Figure 55.4. This coronal image shows a similar abnormal signal intensity within the same muscle groups. The hips appear symmetric and there is no joint effusion. The cortical margin of the left proximal femur is intact, and the medullary cavity has a normal uniform high signal intensity.

DIFFERENTIAL DIAGNOSIS

An infiltrative process is demonstrated on MRI affecting several muscle groups while sparing the adjacent cortical bone or hip joint. The differential consideration for this includes *infectious and neoplastic* causes. These entities cannot be separated on the basis of signal intensity alone, since these changes are nonspecific (see following). The pertinent negatives include the absence of enlarged vessels, large foci of calcium, or subacute hemorrhage. The latter-most would cause significant T1 shortening and high signal of the moderately T1-weighted (SE 1000/28) image.

In general, with the exception of the most aggressive and poorly differentiated tumors, soft tissue sarcomas tend to spread along one muscle group and appear as a relatively well-defined mass. Thus, involvement of multiple muscle groups is somewhat against soft tissue sarcoma. In light of this and the clinical presentation of the patient, an infectious etiology was suggested. During surgery, a large abscess was incised and drained. The culture was positive for *Staphylococcus aureus*. No source for this infection was ever discovered. In this case, the main advantage of MRI compared with other imaging modalities was its ability to show the extent of the abnormality prior to surgery.

The nonspecificity of abnormal soft tissue signal intensity is well illustrated in the following cases. Figure 55.5 is from a patient with juvenile fibromatosis, and Figure 55.6 is from another patient with a synovial sarcoma. The MR findings in these three cases are remarkably similar, and differentiating between these entities on the basis of MRI alone is not possible.

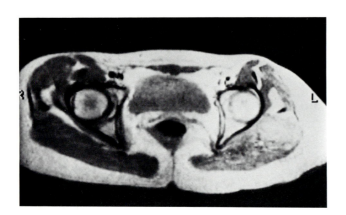

A

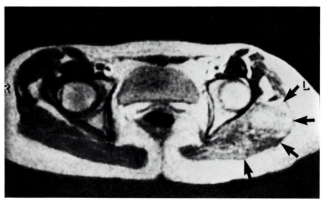

B

Figures 55.5A (SE 2000/28) and **55.5B** (SE 2000/56). Axial scans through the hips. Thickening of the left gluteal muscles with increased signal intensity is seen (arrows) in this adolescent female. Biopsy revealed juvenile fibromatosis.

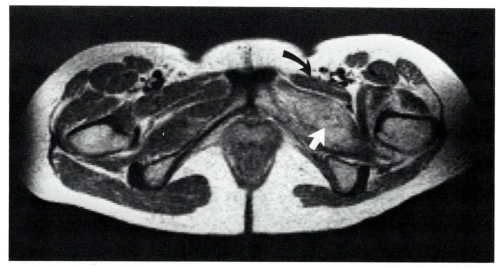

A

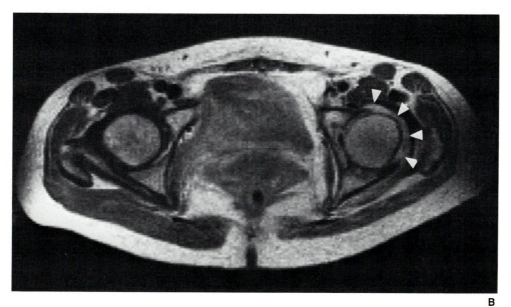

B

Figures 55.6A (SE 2000/28) and **55.6B** (SE 2000/56). Figure 55.6A is an axial scan through the lower pelvis. There is increased signal intensity in the region of the left obturator externus muscle (large arrow). The left pectineus muscle (curved arrow) is normal. On Figure 55.6B (axial section 4 cm superior to Figure 55.6A) a curvilinear high intensity signal is seen anterior and lateral to the left femoral head (arrow heads) consistent with an effusion. This 30-year-old female had a synovial sarcoma. (Courtesy of Arthur Radow, MD, Glendale, AZ.)

Final Diagnosis

Soft tissue staphylococcus abscess.

SUMMARY OF MR FINDINGS FOR SOFT TISSUE ABSCESS[1]

1. Alteration of the expected normal signal intensity with increased T2 and increased T1 relaxation times. Lesions are most conspicuously demonstrated as areas of increased signal intensity on T2-weighted images.

2. The signal intensity changes may be nonspecific and similar to that of a soft tissue neoplasm, surrounding edema, or other abnormal body fluids.[2]
3. MRI may have an important role in preoperative assessment by accurately defining the limits of the abscess.

REFERENCES

1. Wall SD, Fisher MR, Amparo EG, et al: Magnetic resonance imaging in the evaluation of abscesses. *AJR* 1985;144:1217–1221.
2. Brown JJ, vanSonnenberg E, Gerber KH, et al: Magnetic resonance relaxation times of percutaneously obtained normal and abnormal body fluids. *Radiology* 1985;154:727–731.

CASE 56

HISTORY

A 25-year-old man presented with a painful right thigh mass.

QUESTIONS

1. What are your differential considerations?

   _____

   _____

2. What MR techniques would you use?

		1	2	3
a.	Coil	_____	_____	_____
b.	Centering point	_____	_____	_____
c.	Imaging plane(s)	_____	_____	_____
d.	Contrast	_____	_____	_____
e.	Slice thickness	_____	_____	_____

3. What do you expect to find?

   _____

   _____

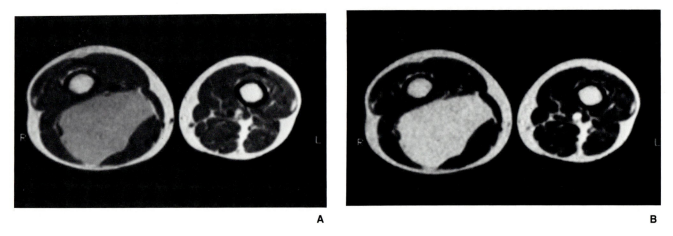

Figures 56.1A (SE 2000/28) and **56.1B** (SE 2000/56). Axial scans through the midthigh.

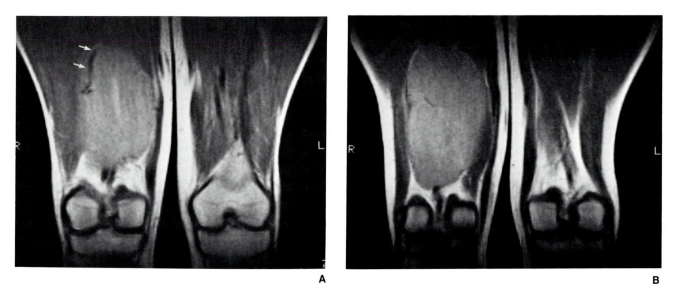

Figures 56.2A (SE 1000/28) and **56.2B** (SE 1000/28). Coronal sections through the inferior thigh; B is 1 cm posterior to A.

MR TECHNIQUES

		1	2	3
a.	Coil	Body	Body	Body
b.	Centering point	Midthigh	Midthigh	Midthigh
c.	Imaging planes	Axial	Coronal	Sagittal
d.	Contrast	Mild T1W and mild T2W	Mild T1W and mild T2W	Mild T1W and mild T2W
e.	Slice thickness	Routine	Routine	Routine

As discussed in the introductory section, T1WIs are better in demonstrating bone marrow involvement, while T2WIs are better in demonstrating soft tissue mass. The axial images are better in localizing the lesion to the different muscle compartments of an extremity. Both the axial and coronal images allow for direct comparison with the contralateral limb. The longitudinal extent of the tumor is better appreciated on coronal and sagittal images.

MR FINDINGS

Figures 56.1 and 56.2. There is a well-defined soft tissue mass in the right anterior thigh, which appears to originate in the fascial plane between the biceps femoris, semimembranosus, semitendinosus, and adductor muscle groups. The mass appears slightly heterogeneous and is intermediate in signal intensity—that is, greater than normal muscle but less than that of fat. The coronal images demonstrate dilated perforating branches of the profunda femoris artery along the superior aspect of the mass (white arrows). The sagittal images (not shown) indicated no intra-articular involvement.

DIFFERENTIAL DIAGNOSIS

Alteration of normal signal intensity within an extremity may be due to a number of etiologies, including *neoplasia,*

inflammation, trauma, or *fatty atrophy.* The lattermost can be excluded by the presence of mass effect and on the basis of clinical history. Muscular contusion or a ''pull'' injury typically results in intramuscular hemorrhage, and there is no significant T1 shortening (due to the presence of methemoglobin) to support this. Tumor and infection may be difficult to distinguish from one another, but the former is strongly favored in light of the clinical history, the marked mass effect, and the focal nature of this process.

Final Diagnosis

Liposarcoma.

SUMMARY OF MR FINDINGS FOR LIPOSARCOMA[1,2]

To date, there are limited data on the MR characteristics of soft tissue extremity tumors. In one recent report,[1] two examples of liposarcoma were described to have altered signal intensity, compared with benign lipomas or subcutaneous fat. On T1-weighted images, liposarcomas (long T1) had lower MR intensity than benign lipomas (short T1), and on T2-weighted images, these lesions had an intensity similar to that of subcutaneous fat. Note that this latter point was not demonstrated in the example shown.

The advantage of MRI in the evaluation of musculoskeletal neoplasms is its great contrast resolution. MRI is more often used to preoperatively evaluate the exact location and extent of a suspected pathologic process. While alteration in signal intensity has been seen in response to various treatment modalities, diminution of tumor bulk remains the hallmark of effective response and is readily demonstrable on serial MR exams.

REFERENCES

1. Dooms GC, Hricak H, Sollitto RA, et al: Lipomatous tumors and tumors with fatty components: MR imaging potential and comparison of MR and CT results. *Radiology* 1985;157:479–483.

2. Aisen AM, Martel W, Braunstein EM, et al: MRI and CT evaluation of primary bone and soft-tissue tumors. *AJR* 1986;146:749–756.

CASE 57

A 16-year-old man presenting with leg pain. Physical examination revealed a palpable mass in the distal half of the left thigh. Radiographs (not shown) demonstrated a predominately osteoblastic lesion involving the distal third of the left femur. Biopsy revealed osteosarcoma. MRI was requested to define the extent of the tumor.

QUESTIONS

1. What MR techniques would you use?

	1	2	3
a. Coil	———	———	———
b. Centering point	———	———	———
c. Imaging plane(s)	———	———	———
d. Contrast	———	———	———
e. Slice thickness	———	———	———

2. What do you expect to find?

_____

_____

Source: Courtesy of Lawrence Bassett, MD, UCLA.

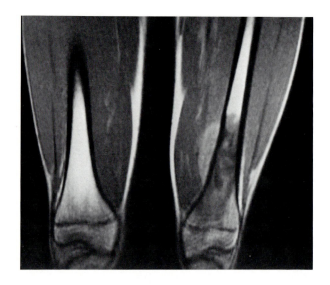

Figure 57.1 (SE 500/28). T1-weighted coronal scan through the femurs.

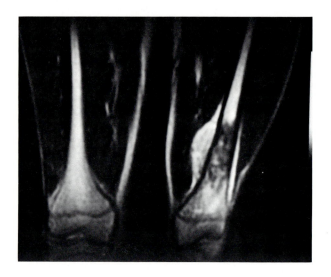

Figure 57.2 (SE 2000/84). T2-weighted coronal scans through the same area.

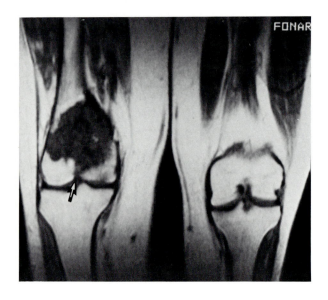

Figure 57.3. (SE 500/28). Coronal scan of the femurs of a patient with known giant cell tumor of the right distal femur.

MR TECHNIQUES

	1	2
a. Coil	Body*	Body*
b. Centering point	Middistal femur	Middistal femur
c. Imaging planes	Coronal	Coronal
d. Contrast	Moderate T1W	Heavy T2W
e. Slice thickness	Routine	Routine

*Examination performed on permanent magnet imager.

As discussed in the introductory section, T1-weighted images best demonstrate intramedullary tumor involvement, whereas T2-weighted images are better at demonstrating the soft tissue component of the tumor. Coronal imaging was performed to define longitudinal tumor extent and to compare the right and left sides.

MR FINDINGS

Figure 57.1. On this T1-weighted image, the tumor is seen as a low intensity infiltrating lesion involving the distal third of the left femur. The intensity pattern of the mass is slightly heterogeneous. The tumor crosses the epiphyseal plate to the articulating surface of the femoral condyles. The superior margin of the tumor is well demarcated by the normal high intensity fat of the medullary canal. A soft tissue mass (arrows) with intermediate intensity is seen medially between the left femur and the vastus medialis muscle. The bony cortex of the involved segment of the femur has a gray and slightly mottled appearance, indicating tumor infiltration.

Figure 57.2. On the heavily T2-weighted image, the soft tissue component of the tumor is better demonstrated because its high signal intensity contrasts against the relatively low intensity skeletal muscle. The superior intramedullary extent of the lesion is not well demonstrated. This is because both the tumor and the marrow have similar high signal intensity. The low intensity area within the involved segment of the femur represents sclerotic bone, a characteristic of osteosarcoma.

DISCUSSION

The major role of MRI in this case was to define the extent of the tumor and aid in planning the level of therapy (amputation, radiation, and/or limb salvage operation). This case illustrates the efficacy of T1-weighted images in demonstrating intramedullary tumor involvement, relating to the high contrast between the lesion and the marrow fat. The T2-weighted images would have underestimated the full extent of the tumor within the medullary canal. Conversely, the soft tissue component was better demonstrated on the T2-weighted sequence because that sequence provided greater contrast between the lesion and adjacent muscles.

It should be emphasized that the T1 and T2 relaxation times of tumors are nonspecific and cannot be used to separate benign lesions from malignant ones. A giant cell tumor of the right distal femur in a 21-year-old patient is shown in Fig. 57.3. Note that the tumor has a well-demarcated margin and extends to the subarticular surface (arrow) of the femur, a characteristic of giant cell tumor. The intensity pattern of this tumor, however, is quite similar to that of osteosarcoma.

MRI's major shortcoming in this setting is that it depicts calcification, ossification, and periosteal reaction less well than do plain radiographs or CT. Hence, the MRI findings should always be interpreted in conjunction with plain films and adequate clinical history.

Final Diagnosis

Osteosarcoma of the left femur.

SUMMARY OF MR FINDINGS FOR OSTEOSARCOMA

1. A primary bone tumor occurring in patients 10 to 25 years of age, located most frequently in the distal femur and the proximal tibia.
2. The intramedullary component of the tumor is best demonstrated on T1-weighted images and appears as an area of decreased intensity (prolonged T1) infiltrating the intramedullary canal.[1]
3. The tumor usually arises in the metaphysis of the long bone and generally does not cross the epiphyseal cartilage unless the epiphyseal plate has fused.[2]
4. Bony sclerosis is present (in more than 50% of cases).[2]
5. The cortex is frequently invaded and may have a gray or mottled appearance.
6. An adjacent soft tissue mass is a characteristic finding. There may be areas of ossification or amorphous calcification within the mass.[2]

REFERENCES

1. Aisen AM, Martel W, Braunstein EM, et al: MRI and CT evaluation of primary bone and soft-tissue tumors. *AJR* 1986;146:749–756.
2. Greenfield GB: The solitary lesion, in *Radiology of Bone Diseases,* ed 3. Philadelphia, JB Lippincott Co, 1980, pp 515–625.

CASE 58

HISTORY

An 83-year-old man with a history of prostate carcinoma presents with right hip pain. There was abnormal uptake in the right proximal femur on the bone scan (not shown). MRI was requested for further evaluation.

QUESTIONS

1. What MR techniques would you use?

	1	2	3
a. Coil	——	——	——
b. Centering point	——	——	——
c. Imaging plane(s)	——	——	——
d. Contrast	——	——	——
e. Slice thickness	——	——	——

2. What do you expect to find?

_____

_____

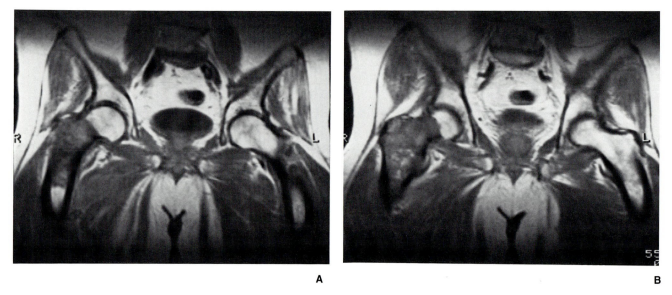

A
B

Figures 58.1A and **58.1B** (SE 1000/30). Coronal scans through the hips. Figure 58.1A is 1 cm anterior to Figure 58.1B.

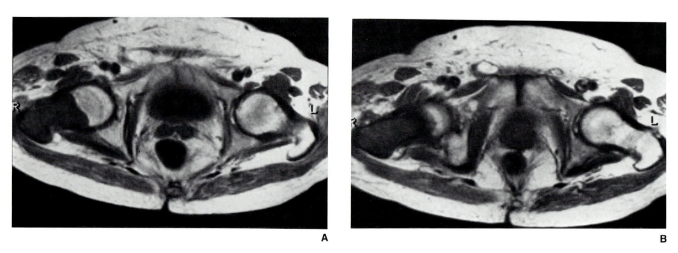

A
B

Figures 58.2A and **58.2B** (SE 500/30). Axial scans through the hips. Figure 58.2A is 1 cm superior to Figure 58.2B.

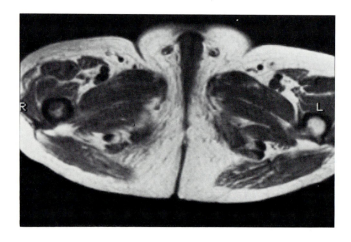

Figure 58.3 (SE 500/30). Axial scans through the proximal thighs.

MR TECHNIQUES

	1	2
a. Coil	Body	Body
b. Centering point	Greater trochanter	Greater trochanter
c. Imaging planes	Coronal	Axial
d. Contrast	Mild T1W	Moderate T1W
e. Slice thickness	Routine	Routine

As discussed in the introductory section, both pulsing sequences were performed with T1 weighting to accentuate the differences in signal intensity between the tumor and the fatty marrow of the medullary cavity. The coronal plane was chosen for the first pulsing sequence because it provides better discrimination of the superior and inferior extent of the lesion. The axial plane provides better appreciation of the cross-sectional anatomy and improves the detection of a soft tissue component associated with the bone lesion.

MR FINDINGS

Figure 58.1. This coronal study demonstrates a well-defined area of abnormally low signal intensity within the right femur, involving the neck, the intertrochanteric region, and the proximal shaft. This can readily be appreciated when compared with the contralateral side. The darker cortical margin appears relatively intact.

Figures 58.2 and 58.3. The abnormal marrow signal is conspicuously demonstrated. No associated soft tissue mass is noted.

DIFFERENTIAL DIAGNOSIS

The findings indicate an infiltrating process that is replacing the normal high signal intensity of the fatty marrow within the medullary cavity. This is a nonspecific finding and can be seen with either primary or secondary tumors of bone. In this case, the most likely diagnosis is metastatic prostate carcinoma. Avascular necrosis is another cause of altered signal intensity (see Case 54) but would be considered unlikely because of the sparing of the femoral head. The value of MRI is its ability to define the limits of the tumor, an ability that is especially helpful in planning radiation therapy.

Final Diagnosis

Metastatic prostate carcinoma to the femur.

SUMMARY OF MR FINDINGS FOR BONE METASTASIS[1]

1. Altered signal intensity within the medullary cavity. Signal changes are best seen on T1-weighted images. This signal change primarily represents replacement of the normal fatty marrow with tumor cells that have a longer T1 relaxation time.
2. There may be multiple lesions.
3. Associated soft tissue mass, which is best appreciated on T2-weighted images.
4. Pathologic fractures may be difficult to visualize because of the low signal of cortical bone.

REFERENCE

1. Aisen AM, Martel W, Braustein EM, et al: MRI and CT evaluation of primary bone and soft-tissue tumors. *AJR* 1986;146:749–756.

7

CARDIOTHORACIC IMAGING

Robert W. Henderson and Jay A. Mericle

Cardiac magnetic resonance imaging (MRI) is now in its early stages of development. Potential applications in cardiovascular disease appear virtually limitless with regard to a wide variety of pathologic processes. The ultimate role of MRI in cardiovascular diagnosis, however, will also be determined by its cost effectiveness compared with other well-established, competing modalities, such as 2D echocardiography, radionuclide dynamic and perfusion imaging, CT, and angiography.

ADVANTAGES AND DISADVANTAGES OF MRI

MRI has a number of advantages over conventional cardiac imaging modalities. Unlike CT and angiography, MRI does not require the use of iodinated material. In addition, MRI does not expose the patient to the risks of ionizing radiation.

The field of view of MRI is considerably greater than that of ultrasound and is not limited by the amount of air or bone surrounding the heart in a particular patient's chest. The absence of signal from flowing blood at normal velocities provides a natural contrast that allows exquisite visualization of endocardial and endothelial borders, considerably greater than that allowed by 2D echocardiography or blood pool scintigraphy. MRI yields soft tissue contrast many times greater than that of CT. Fat surrounding the heart provides excellent contrast with the pericardium and epicardium. In addition, imaging can be performed in any orthogonal plane without the loss of resolution associated with reformatted CT images. Finally, surgical clips, cardiac valves, sternal sutures, and other metallic intrathoracic devices produce less artifacts with MRI than with CT imaging.

The disadvantages of MRI must also be considered. Unlike echocardiography or nuclear cardiography, MRI obviously cannot be performed on critically ill patients at bedside. Further limitations are imposed by the necessity to exclude ferromagnetic equipment from the immediate proximity of the magnet. Along these same lines, MRI is contraindicated in patients who have intracranial aneurysm clips or permanent pacemakers. (The latter may not always be so in light of preliminary results from an ongoing study.)

The requirement for cardiac gating poses limitations in patients with some arrhythmias. The longer imaging times (7 to 15 minutes) pose some problems in those patients unwilling or unable to lie motionless. Here, dynamic CT (2 seconds or less) and the real-time capability of echocardiography are advantageous.

Spatial resolution is currently less than with high-resolution CT and, for some applications, this cannot be compensated by MRI's greater contrast resolution. Also, "real-time" or dynamic MR imaging is not clinically feasible at present.

TECHNIQUE

Cardiac Gating

EKG Signal

The electrocardiogram (EKG) signal is used in a way similar to its use in acquiring radionuclide studies. A three-limb lead hookup is used, monitoring lead I. The R wave serves as the triggering mechanism. The gating device has two adjustable settings—the *R-delay (RD)* and the *EKG disable.*

R-Delay (RD)

The R-Delay (RD) is the time after the R wave when data acquisition begins. It determines in which phase of the cardiac cycle the heart is imaged. At 5 mseconds, this is end-diastole (during ventricular activation, immediately prior to contraction). As systole usually occurs near the end of the T wave, the RD for end-systole is approximated by the R-T interval.

EKG Disable

The EKG disable defines a period of time after an R wave trigger during which any incoming signals within the EKG line will not be sensed. The disable serves two purposes. First, it prevents extraneous signals (gradient field shifts acting on the EKG leads as though they were antennas) from prematurely triggering the gating mechanism before the next actual R wave. Second, by increasing the EKG disable to greater than an R-R interval, gating to every second beat becomes possible.

Imaging Parameters and Multislice Acquisition

TR

The R-R interval (the patient's heart rate) determines the TR for gated acquisitions. In the usual range of heart rates (HR) of 60 to 100 beats per minute, this would correspond to a TR of 1.0 to 0.6 seconds. If a longer TR is desired, gating to every other beat can be performed. An HR of 60 would then yield a TR of 2.0 seconds; an HR of 100 would yield a TR of 1.2 seconds.

TE and Multislice Acquisition

The time required for a spin echo acquisition is much shorter than the R-R interval at normal heart rates. The time needed to obtain first and second echo acquisitions for a single slice is generally less than 20% of the cardiac cycle time. Even less time is required for a single-slice, single echo acquisition (10% of the cardiac cycle). Therefore, multiple slices, either five slices each having both first and second echo acquisitions (for example, TE = 30 and 60 mseconds) or ten slices each with only a single echo (TE = 30 mseconds), can be obtained during the R-R interval at different anatomic levels. To create an image, this process is repeated hundreds of times depending on the matrix size and the number of "averages." The routine slice thickness is 10 mm without an interspace gap. Thus if a five-slice study is performed, 5 cm will be covered with each slice at a different anatomic level through the heart. Since each slice is acquired sequentially during a unique portion of the R-R interval, each image will also depict a different part of the cardiac cycle. A ten-slice study will, of course, cover 10 cm, with each level again depicting a different portion of the cardiac cycle. In this case only a single echo will be obtained.

Anatomic Detail, Functional Parameters, and Plane of Imaging

Anatomic Detail

In the visualization of bypass grafts, proximal native coronary arteries, valvular vegetations, papillary muscles, and small mural thrombi, anatomic detail is the most important factor; therefore, contiguous thin sections (measuring 5 mm or less) should be obtained. If this is not feasible with existing software, overlapping (interleaving) of thicker sections can be performed. This is accomplished by obtaining two axial acquisitions with a table increment of 5 mm between the two studies and then interdigitating the images into a complete set. Thin sections improve resolution by reducing partial volume effect, but they do not improve spatial resolution within the plane of section.

Functional Parameters

If the goal of imaging is to assess global and regional myocardial function, the sequence can be modified accordingly. A localizing, transverse single echo 10-cm sequence can be obtained to select a midventricular level. Two additional axial acquisitions can then be performed. The first is with the table incremented to place the midventricular slice in end-diastole (RD = 5 mseconds) and the second, with the same slice imaged in end-systole (RD = RT). In this way, end-diastolic and end-systolic sections at the midventricular level can be compared. Left ventricular (LV) ejection fraction can then be calculated (overlay outline area/length method analogous to angiographic planimetry) and regional wall motion can be assessed visually.[1-3]

Rotated gating techniques give more detailed information about cyclic changes in chamber size and wall thickening at multiple levels. One method involves acquiring the five multislice double echo study described earlier and then repeating the acquisition four additional times.[4] Each time, the acquisition is "rotated" so that each slice (anatomic level) is assigned a different part of the cardiac cycle. Another method acquires five sections at the same anatomic level, each at a different part of the cycle.[5] Five levels would require correspondingly longer imaging times (30 minutes or more).

Imaging Planes

The plane of imaging can be altered to facilitate both anatomic and functional assessment of the heart. Sagittal and coronal imaging planes yield images with resolution equal to that of transverse imaging. Acquisition time, imaging parameters, and gating techniques are identical to those described for transverse imaging.

Oblique imaging can be performed by altering the patient's position within the magnet. The usual goals are to obtain long- or short-axis views of the left ventricle to facilitate evaluation of global and regional wall motion, wall thickness, and chamber size. With the patient in a 30-degree right anterior oblique (RAO) position, sagittal sections will approximate a short-axis view. Long-axis views are obtained by placing the patient supine and angled so that the right shoulder is farthest to the right of the midline of the table. Axial sections are then obtained.[6]

For some systems, gradient angles can be altered for direct acquisition of oblique sections. More precise long- and short-axis views can be obtained by selecting the angle of obliquity from an initial study in an orthogonal plane (axial or coronal).[7]

IMAGE INTERPRETATION/FLOW-RELATED PHENOMENA

Normal Anatomy

Familiarity with cross-sectional anatomy is obviously important for image interpretation. Axial sections are readily related to CT experience. Learning normal sagittal and coronal anatomy takes time and patience and is much easier when sections are related to axial images of the same patient. For the interested reader, sources describing the normal values for chamber size and wall thickness are listed in the references.[5,8–10] A series of normal images is shown in Figures 7–1A through 7–11. (Legend appears on p. 296.)

Flow-related Phenomena

The most commonly observed flow phenomenon is flow void: absence of signal results when blood protons move out of the imaging plane prior to completion of a 90-degree and 180-degree pulse cycle. Arterial flow perpendicular to the plane of section is characterized by this phenomenon.

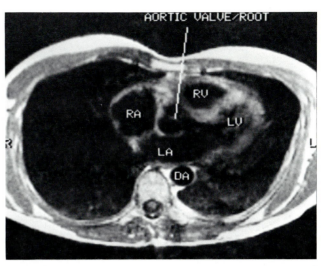

A

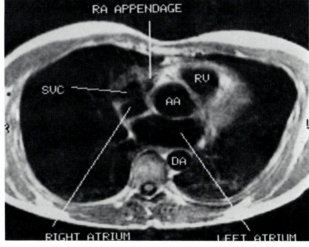

B

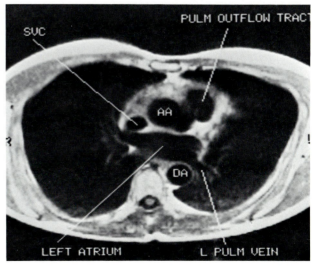

C

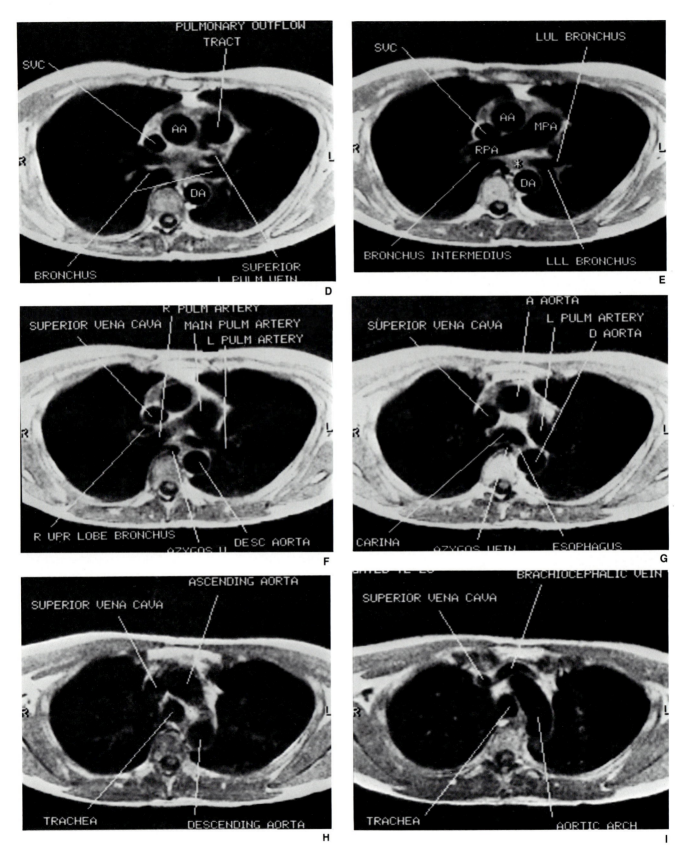

Figures 7–1A through **7–1I.** Normal study. Axial sections performed with every beat gating and TE = 28 mseconds. Ascending aorta (AA), descending aorta (DA), left atrium (LA), left ventricle (LV), main pulmonary artery (MPA), right atrium (RA), right pulmonary artery (RPA), right ventricle (RV), superior vena cava (SVC).

Flow-related enhancement may create a strong signal in structures with slow flow (generally large veins) as fully magnetized blood enters the imaging field of view.[11,12] Laminar flow can produce signal within the center of the lumen in some cases and should not be confused with thrombus.

Flow-related changes should be anticipated with *image gating* since images assembled from a specific portion of the cardiac cycle repeated over many cycles may portray the lowest velocity of the phasic flow within a specific chamber or vessel. For example, during end-systole, some atrial signal may be seen. During end-diastole, signal is commonly present in the aorta and may also be seen in the pulmonary arteries and at the apex of the ventricles. The latter phenomenon can create the false impression of subendocardial infarction or mural thrombus (see following). These flow phenomena are exaggerated in patients who have slow heart rates. Occasionally, some ventricular signal may be seen in portions of systole (making this finding less specific for low cardiac output states). Unintentional or *diastolic pseudogating* is a related phenomenon seen in nongated images and may have a similar appearance.

Even-echo rephasing[13,14] may produce strong signal in areas of slow flow on the second echo images of a double spin echo sequence. An example of this is provided in the workbook case of mural thrombus.

CLINICAL APPLICATIONS

Great Vessels

Thoracic Aorta and Major Branches

Axial sections accurately depict the external and luminal diameters of the ascending and descending aorta. An oblique sagittal image oriented parallel to the arch (about 30 degrees RAO, as determined from the transverse sections) shows the entire aorta and origins of the brachiocephalic vessels. MRI is the noninvasive method of choice for evaluating aortic coarctation, dissection, and subaortic stenosis.

Pulmonary Arteries

Axial sections best show the central pulmonary arteries. Large central arteries are readily differentiated from hilar adenopathy. Narrowing of a proximal pulmonary artery, either congenital or acquired (eg, granulomatous arteritis, or extrinsic tumor compression), is readily demonstrated.[15,16]

Central thrombotic emboli may be seen; however, distinction from hilar adenopathy can be difficult. Clots within first- and second-order branches may be directly visualized as small and relatively high intensity foci surrounded by low intensity lung parenchyma.[17,18] MRI may eventually play a role in the evaluation of pulmonary embolism. Its sensitivity and specificity are yet to be determined in this area.

With pulmonary arterial hypertension, abnormal signal in the pulmonary arteries during systole has been correlated with severity of the disease.[9,19] This phenomenon will be most intense on the second echo images. The abnormal signal tends to be uniform, proximal, and bilateral and relates to decreased arterial flow. Differentiation from chronic thrombus, an uncommon cause of pulmonary arterial hypertension, has been described.[20] The latter entity is seen equally well throughout the cardiac cycle and has relatively less signal on second echo sequences.

Pulmonary Veins

Normal central pulmonary veins are routinely seen entering the left atrium. Anomalous pulmonary vessels are difficult to see within the lung parenchyma because of poor contrast discrimination. As the vessel migrates centrally, its entry site may be more easily seen because of the surrounding soft tissues. We have imaged partial anomalous return to the inferior vena cava (IVC) below the diaphragm, above the diaphragm into the superior vena cava (SVC), and into the right atrium. Thin axial sections are helpful in evaluating the entry level.

Systemic Veins

Coronal and axial views are best for showing size, position, compression, and/or thrombosis of the SVC or IVC. Caution should be exercised in diagnosing intraluminal thrombus in light of the flow-related phenomena described earlier.

Pericardial Disease[1,21–23]

Normally the pericardium is a 2- to 3-mm-thick, curvilinear band of low intensity that is seen in contrast to the adjacent inner, epicardial fat and outer, anterior mediastinal fat. Relatively uniform thickening of the pericardium to 4 mm (suspect) or 5 mm (definite) indicates chronic disease. Nodularity of the pericardium may indicate malignancy; this can also be seen with other causes, however, such as granulomatous pericarditis.

Serous pericardial fluid tends to be low in signal intensity because of its low protein content. With increasing protein concentration, such as an exudate, increasing signal can be seen. In our experience, gross heterogeneity of signal intensity suggests a malignant cause.

Valvular Disease

Direct valvular imaging is difficult because the valves are normally thin, mobile, and obliquely oriented. These disadvantages are easily overcome by echocardiography.

Congenital Heart Disease (CHD)

Echocardiography is less expensive than MRI and is technically well suited to the examination of the infant heart. A large accumulated experience has made echocardiography the noninvasive examination of choice for CHD.

Initial experience has shown that MRI has a potential to depict certain complex malformations better, with information not obtainable from echocardiography.[24] Particularly advantageous is MRI's ability to demonstrate the size and position of the cardiac chambers and their relationship to the great vessels.

Septal defects may be accurately depicted, particularly on the long-axis views. Occasionally, normal thinning at the fossa ovalis may mimic a secundum-type atrial septal defect (ASD) in normals.[1,25]

An example of cyanotic heart disease well demonstrated by MRI is tetralogy of Fallot. The four components (ventricular septal defect, obstruction to RV outflow, overriding aorta, and right ventricular hypertrophy) can readily be depicted. There may be some advantage over sonography in certain cases, such as in distinguishing severe forms of tetralogy from truncus arteriosus. Angiography is generally needed for definitive diagnosis, however.

MRI may have an even greater role in postoperative evaluation of CHD. It can be utilized to assess patency of native vessels, grafts, and conduits and also to characterize postsurgical fluid collections. Demonstration of these and many other postoperative changes has been described and may reduce the need for repeat angiography.[26]

Coronary Artery Disease

The prevalence of coronary disease is so great relative to all forms of cardiac disease that application of MRI to only a small percentage of patients might still make it the most frequent reason for referral. Here, there are numerous highly developed, noninvasive modalities that must be compared with MRI before the expense of MRI can be justified.

Ischemic Myocardial Disease

In *acute infarction,* increased myocardial signal is seen within the first week (often within the first few days) after the event (Figure 7–2). There is prolongation of both T1 and T2 relaxation times secondary to cellular edema. Second echo images accentuate differences in T2 and yield greater contrast between normal and acutely infarcted myocardium. The increase in endocardial signal is generally equal to or greater than that of the epicardium.[1,27–29]

A potential problem is the phenomenon of even-echo rephasing of slow-flowing blood along the outer margin of the chamber lumen, which can simulate a subendocardial infarction (SEMI). Differentiating points between flow-related changes and SEMI include the former's crescentic

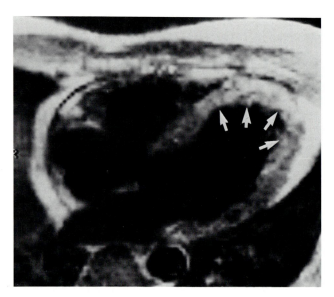

Figure 7–2. Acute MI. Axial section through the left ventricle demonstrating increased signal intensity within the myocardium of the apex and anterior septum (arrows). Every other beat gating; TE = 28 mseconds.

shape and marked signal increase on the second echo image compared with the latter's linear shape with no change to moderately increased signal on the second echo image.[1]

Acute infarction is seldom a diagnostic dilemma clinically. Evaluation of threatened (reversibly injured) myocardium, however, is an important determination. Some experimental work suggests that T1 differences between normal and ischemic myocardium might be demonstrated by using intravenous paramagnetic gadolinium-DTPA.[9]

The signal intensity of a *subacute infarct* is reported to diminish slowly over a period of 2 to 6 months, the lesion gradually appearing smaller, less homogeneous, and more subendocardial in location. The development of myocardial thinning has a more variable appearance and time course.[1]

Chronic infarction, as expected, appears as an area of thinned myocardium (Figure 7–3) with decreased signal due to fibrous replacement. Wall motion abnormalities can be visualized if a functional study is performed. LV aneurysms may be very well depicted.[1,30]

Coronary Artery Disease

Screening patients for coronary artery disease is an extremely important but difficult task. Under optimal conditions, major portions of the coronary arteries may be identified as in Figure 7–4. Currently, exercise EKG with 201-thallium tomography achieves a combined sensitivity of greater than 90% for surgically significant (more than 50%) stenosis. It is doubtful that MRI with gadolinium-DTPA will achieve this sensitivity at rest. This possibility exists, however, especially if a coronary vasodilator such as dipyridamole is used.[31]

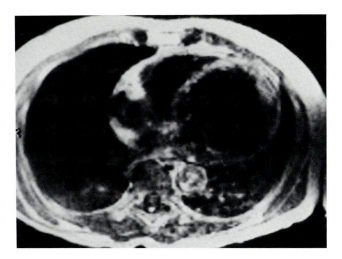

Figure 7–3. Chronic ischemia. There is diffuse thinning of the myocardium and left ventricular enlargement, consistent with ischemic cardiomyopathy. Every beat gating; TE = 28 mseconds.

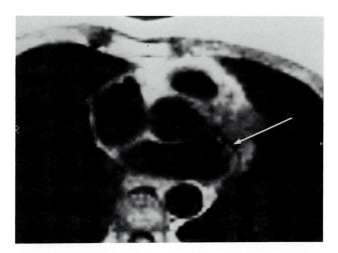

A

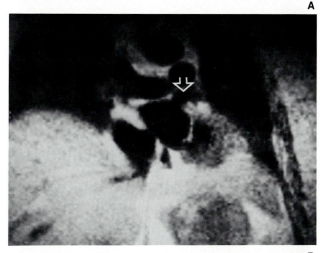

B

Coronary Bypass Grafts

Postoperative imaging after bypass graft surgery has yielded some encouraging results regarding the patency of grafts (Figure 7–5). Complications such as postcardiotomy syndrome, abscess formation, sternal infection, and mediastinal hematoma can be evaluated without the use of contrast material.

Other Cardiac Pathology

Intracavitary Thrombus

Atrial thrombus generally occurs when chronic atrial dilatation and slow atrial flow are present. Other settings include congestive cardiomyopathy and mitral stenosis. Intraventricular thrombus may be seen with severe global (e.g., congestive cardiomyopathy) or regional (e.g., ischemic cardiomyopathy) ventricular dysfunction. It is most commonly seen at the apex of the LV and can be mimicked by flow phenomena (see earlier).

Cardiac Tumors

MRI has been compared favorably with 2D echocardiography in the diagnosis and characterization of atrial myxoma.[32] We have shown intrinsic myocardial involvement with metastatic melanoma. Primary malignancies should be well delineated.

Cardiomyopathy

Congestive cardiomyopathy is characterized by four-chamber enlargement with symmetric involvement of left and right heart. Biventricular systolic wall excursion and thickening are decreased globally. *Hypertrophic car-*

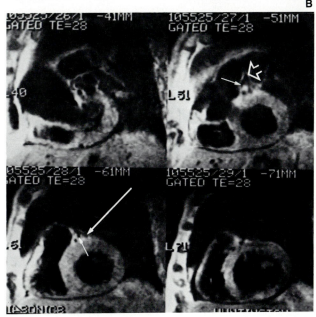

C

Figures 7–4A (axial), **7–4B** (coronal), and **7–4C** (sagittal). Normal left coronary arteries. The left main artery (open arrow), proximal circumflex (long arrow), and left anterior descending (short arrow) arteries can be identified. Every beat gating, TE = 28 mseconds.

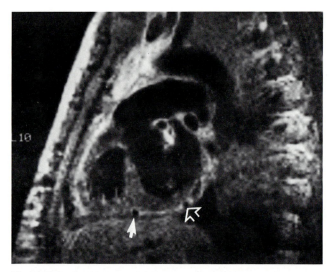

Figure 7–5. Graft patency study. Sagittal section showing flow void within posterior descending (closed arrow) and circumflex (open arrow) arterial bypass grafts. Gated every beat, TE = 28 mseconds.

diomyopathy (Figure 7–6) is readily detected and global or predominant septal involvement visualized. End-systolic images of the LV outflow tract may depict the functional severity of idiopathic hypertrophic subaortic stenosis (IHSS) at rest.

Restrictive/Infiltrating Cardiomyopathy

Pericardial thickening favors constrictive pericarditis over restrictive/infiltrating cardiomyopathy (both have similar hemodynamics).[21] Biventricular concentric wall thickening with heterogeneous signal favors infiltrating (restrictive) disease such as amyloid.[1]

Endocardial Disease

MRI may play a role in evaluating endocardial disease, such as endocardial fibroelastosis, Löffler's endocarditis, and infectious endocarditis.

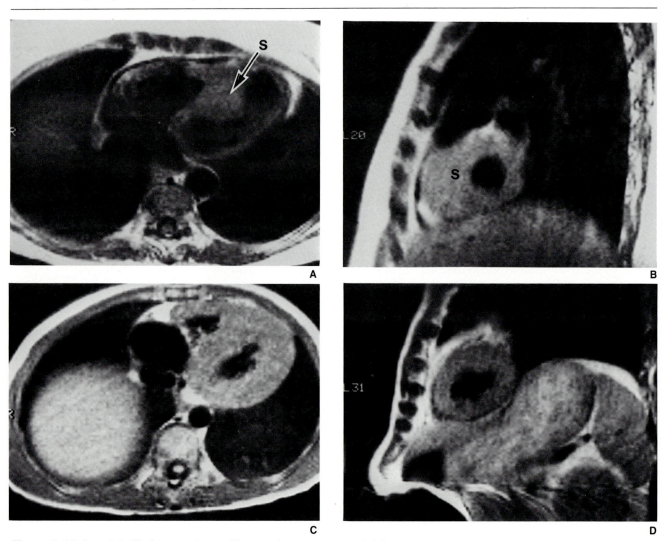

Figures 7–6A through **7–6D.** Asymmetric septal hypertrophy versus concentric left ventricular hypertrophy. Images A (axial) and B (sagittal) demonstrating asymmetric thickening of the septum(s). This is contrasted to concentric thickening in another patient on images C (axial) and D (sagittal).

Transplants

We have seen one case (referred by the Arizona Heart Institute and contributed by MRI Associates of Phoenix) that demonstrated new focal myocardial signal at the time of rejection.

MEDIASTINUM AND LUNG

As a general rule, we have found only occasional uses for MRI of the mediastinum, because it infrequently compares favorably with CT.[15,16,33–35] A distinct advantage of CT is its speed of imaging, which reduces patient (especially respiratory) artifact. Spatial resolution of CT is superior, and small nonvascular structures within the mediastinum are better delineated. For example, two smaller, contiguous, non-pathologic-size lymph nodes are less likely to be confused with a single pathologic-size node. The esophagus is less likely to be confused with subcarinal adenopathy. In addition, endobronchial lesions and bronchial wall thickening are better seen on CT. Other structures that contain little MR-visible hydrogen, such as normal lung or calcifications, can readily be seen with CT. Therefore, cancer staging and other general indications are primarily handled by CT. MRI is relegated to clarifying questions not answered by CT in preselected anatomic areas, particularly regarding patency of or tumor relation to the great vessels. It may be a reasonable alternative for tumor staging when IV contrast is contraindicated, however.

Technique

Localization

Transverse, coronal, or sagittal planes and their centering are selected after review of the chest x-ray or CT. The examination is tailored to the clinical questions raised by those studies.

Imaging Parameters

Differentiation of various mediastinal tumors from fat is best accomplished by T1-weighted sequences (e.g., TR 500 to 1,000 mseconds and TE 20 to 40 mseconds). Longer TR sequences are helpful to characterize the tumors, which generally have a prolonged T2. Longer TR images may help to avoid interpretive errors related to partial volume of blood vessels with mediastinal fat. This is because the signal of enlarged lymph nodes should increase and approach that of fat, whereas a partially volumed blood vessel should remain low in signal intensity.[15] Gating to the cardiac cycle is usually unnecessary in the examination of the superior mediastinum, since cardiac pulsations are minimal. In fact, gated images may cause spurious vascular signal intensities, as described earlier, which could conceivably be interpreted as a solid mass rather than flowing, intraluminal blood. On the other hand, adequate visualization of the lower mediastinum may require gating to improve resolution.

CONCLUSION

Cardiothoracic magnetic resonance imaging is in its formative state. The anatomic detail obtainable with MRI has already yielded occasional significant applications. More indications will become apparent with further widespread experience. Expanded use of flow-related data is to be expected as new methods of data acquisition and analysis are developed. Contrast agents may provide useful information. Ultimately, metabolic imaging may be feasible with localized phosphorus spectroscopy. If appropriate clinical questions can be answered with MR cardiothoracic imaging, there will be a significant place for this modality in the everyday management of cardiopulmonary disease.

REFERENCES

1. Miller SW, Brady TS, Dinsmore RE, et al: Cardiac magnetic resonance imaging: The Massachusetts General Hospital experience. *Radiol Clin North Am* 1985;23:745–764.

2. Dodge HT, Sandler H, Ballew DW, et al: The use of biplane angiography for the measurement of left ventricular volume in man. *Am Heart J* 1960;60:762–776.

3. Stratemeier EJ, Thompson R, Brady TJ, et al: Ejection fraction determined by magnetic resonance imaging: Comparison with left ventricular angiography. *Radiology* 1986;158:775–777.

4. Crooks LE, Barker B, Chang N, et al: Magnetic resonance imaging strategies for heart studies. *Radiology* 1984;153:459–465.

5. Fisher MR, von Schulthess GK, Higgins CB: Multiphasic cardiac magnetic resonance imaging: Normal regional left ventricular wall thickening. *AJR* 1985;145:27–30.

6. Mericle JA, Crues JV, Berman DS, et al: Optimal patient positioning and data acquisition timing in cardiac magnetic resonance imaging. *Clin Nucl Med* 1984;9(95):32.

7. Dinsmore RE, Wismer GL, Levine RA, et al: Magnetic resonance imaging of the heart: Positioning and gradient angle selection for optimal imaging planes. *AJR* 1984;143:1135–1142.

8. Bouchard A, Higgins CB, Byrd BF, et al: Magnetic resonance imaging in pulmonary arterial hypertension. *Am J Cardiol* 1985;56:938–942.

9. Tscholakoff D, Higgins CB: Gated magnetic resonance imaging for assessment of cardiac function and myocardial infarction. *Radiol Clin North Am* 1985;23:449–456.

10. Kaul S, Wismer GL, Brady TJ, et al: Measurements of normal left heart dimensions using optimally oriented MR images. *AJR* 1986;146:75–79.

11. Bradley W, Waluch V, Lai KS, et al: The appearance of rapidly flowing blood on magnetic resonance images. *AJR* 1984;143:1167–1174.

12. Mills CM, Brant-Zawadzki M, Crooks LE, et al: Nuclear magnetic resonance: Principles of blood flow imaging. *AJR* 1984;142:165–170.

13. Waluch V, Bradley WG: NMR even echo rephasing in slow laminar flow. *J Comput Assist Tomogr* 1984;8:594–598.

14. Bradley WG, Waluch V: Blood flow: Magnetic resonance imaging. *Radiology* 1985;154:443–450.

15. Aronberg DJ, Glazer HS, Sagel SS: MRI and CT of the mediastinum: Comparison, controversies, and pitfalls. *Radiol Clin North Am* 1985;23:439–448.

16. Levitt RG, Glazer HS, Roper CL, et al: Magnetic resonance imaging of mediastinal and hilar masses: Comparison with CT. *AJR* 1985;142:9–14.

17. Moore EH, Gamsu G, Webb WR, et al: Pulmonary embolus: Detection and follow-up using magnetic resonance. *Radiology* 1984;153:471–472.

18. Crues JV, Stein MG, Bradley WG, et al: The detection of pulmonary emboli by magnetic resonance imaging, abstracted in *Book of Abstracts*. Society of Magnetic Resonance in Medicine, 1985, p 1139.

19. Didier D, Higgins CB: Estimation of pulmonary vascular resistance by MRI in patients with congenital cardiovascular shunt lesions. *AJR* 1986;146:919–924.

20. Fisher MR, Higgins CB: Central thrombi in pulmonary arterial hypertension detected by MR imaging. *Radiology* 1986;158:223–226.

21. Soulen RL, Stark DD, Higgins CB: Magnetic resonance imaging of constrictive pericardial disease. *Am J Cardiol* 1985;55:480–484.

22. Stark DD, Higgins CB, Lanzer P, et al: Magnetic resonance imaging of the pericardium: Normal and pathologic findings. *Radiology* 1984;150:469–474.

23. McMurdo KK, Webb WR, von Schulthess GK, et al: Magnetic resonance imaging of the superior pericardial recesses. *AJR* 1985;145:985–988.

24. Didier D, Higgins CB, Fisher MR, et al: Congenital heart disease: Gated MR imaging in 72 patients. *Radiology* 1986;158:227–235.

25. Dinsmore RE, Wismer GL, Guyer D, et al: Axial magnetic resonance imaging of the interatrial septum and atrial septal defects. *AJR* 1985;145: 697–703.

26. Soulen RL, Donner RM: Magnetic resonance imaging of rerouted pulmonary blood flow. *Radiol Clin North Am* 1985;23:737–744.

27. Revel D, Higgins CB: Magnetic resonance of ischemic heart disease. *Radiol Clin North Am* 1985;23:719–726.

28. Higgins CB, Byrd BF III, McNamara MT, et al: Magnetic resonance imaging of the heart: A review of the initial experience in 172 subjects. *Radiology* 1985;155:671–679.

29. Brown JJ, Peck WW, Gerber KH, et al: Nuclear magnetic resonance analysis of acute and chronic myocardial infarction in dogs: Alternations in spin-lattice relaxation times. *Am Heart J* 1984;108:1292.

30. Higgins CB, Lanzer P, Stark D, et al: Imaging by nuclear magnetic resonance in patients with chronic ischemic heart disease. *Circulation* 1984;69:523–531.

31. Gould KL, Sorenson SG, Albro P, et al: Thallium-201 myocardial imaging during coronary vasodilation induced by oral dipyridamole. *J Nucl Med* 1986;27:31–36.

32. Go RT, O'Donnell JK, Underwood DA, et al: Comparison of gated cardiac MRI and 2D echocardiography of intracardiac neoplasms. *AJR* 1985;145:21–25.

33. Webb WR, Gamsu G, Crooks LE: Multisection sagittal and coronal magnetic resonance imaging of the mediastinum and hila. *Radiology* 1986;155:413–416.

34. Von Schulthess GK, McMurdo K, Tscholakoff D, et al: Mediastinal masses: MR imaging. *Radiology* 1986;158:289–296.

35. Webb WR, Moore EH: Differentiation of volume averaging and mass on magnetic resonance images of the mediastinum. *Radiology* 1985;155:413–416.

CASE 59

HISTORY

A 71-year-old man presenting with fever of unknown origin for several months, cough, and nausea. The admitting chest radiograph shows an abnormal cardiac silhouette (Figure 59.1).

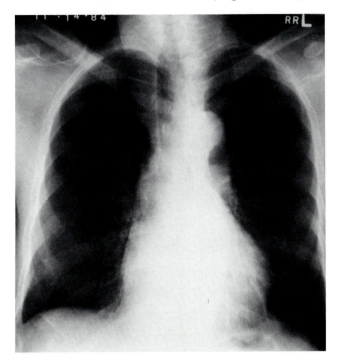

Figure 59.1. PA chest.

QUESTIONS

1. What are your differential considerations?

_____

_____

2. What MR techniques would you use?

	1	2	3
a. Coil	___	___	___
b. Centering point	___	___	___
c. Imaging plane(s)	___	___	___
d. Contrast	___	___	___
e. Slice thickness	___	___	___

3. What do you expect to find?

_____

_____

Source: Courtesy of Robert W. Henderson, MD, Pasadena, CA.

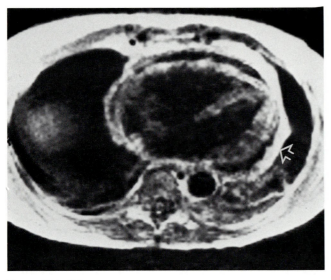

Figure 59.2 (SE gated/28). Axial scan through the midheart during early diastole.

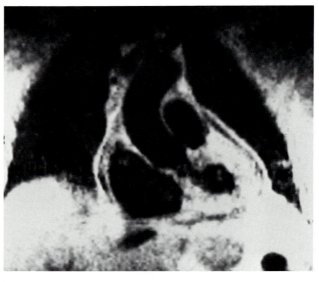

Figure 59.3 (SE gated/28). Midcoronal section.

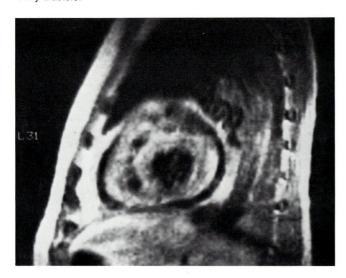

Figure 59.4 (SE gated/28). Parasagittal section through the ventricles.

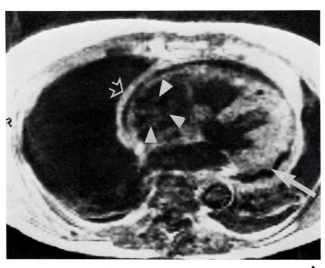

A   B

Figures 59.5A (SE gated/28) and **59.5B** (SE gated/56). Axial sections during systole, 1 cm superior to Figure 59.2.

MR TECHNIQUES

	1	2	3
a. Coil	Body	Body	Body
b. Centering point	All approximately midsternum		
c. Imaging planes	Axial	Coronal	Sagittal
d. Contrast	All gated (TR < 1000, HR > 60)		
e. Slice thickness	Routine	Routine	Routine

The TR will depend upon the heart rate (HR) and will be less than 1.0 second if the rate is greater than 60 per minute. Therefore, cardiac images will be T1 weighted at normal heart rate. T2 weighting requires every-other-beat gating (see "Technique" section in Chapter 7).

The sagittal and coronal scans were performed to provide a different imaging plane and are optional in most routine cardiac cases.

MR FINDINGS

Figure 59.1. The PA chest radiograph shows an enlarged and globular-appearing heart silhouette with a right pleural effusion and minimal pulmonary venous hypertension.

Figures 59.2 through 59.4. A band of absent signal surrounds the heart and is compatible with a pericardial effusion. (Since these are relatively T1-weighted images, fluids may have low signal, comparable to that of CSF.) A band of intermediate signal surrounds the fluid, indicating parietal pericardial thickening (open white arrow, see also Fig. 59.5A).

Figure 59.5. Irregularity adjacent to the LV (best seen along LV lateral wall, Figure 59.5A) indicates visceral pericardial thickening. Abnormal signal is present in the right atrium (arrowheads) on the first echo image (Figure 59.5A). This was confirmed as a persistent finding on additional images (not shown).

DIFFERENTIAL DIAGNOSIS

The causes of pericardial effusion/pericardial thickening are numerous and include the following: *infection* (including viral, pyogenic, and tuberculous causes), *uremia, neoplasia* (see Figure 59.6), *trauma, myxedema, irradiation, autoimmune disorders* (including collagen-vascular, and drug-induced causes), and *idiopathic disorders.* The MR appearance alone may not be specific enough to distinguish the exact etiology, although hemorrhagic (short T1) effusions should suggest neoplastic disease.

In middle-aged and elderly patients with chronic fever and cardiac enlargement due to pericardial effusion, tuberculosis is the most common cause. In this case, response to appropriate antituberculous therapy was subsequently noted.

Detecting a definite, intraluminal filling defect with MRI is difficult, as flow phenomena, such as even-echo rephasing

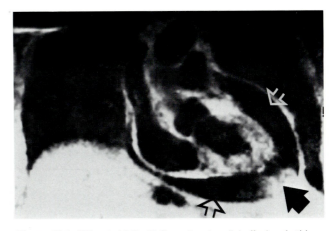

Figure 59.6 (SE gated/28). Malignant pericardial effusion. In this patient with metastatic breast cancer, a large pericardial effusion can be identified (open arrows) with an associated tumor mass (closed arrow).

on second echo images, may cause apparent filling defects. If a filling defect is seen on the first echo image of a nonentry slice, as with this case, the lesion is more likely to be real. The primary consideration should be a *mural thrombus;* however, a rare right *atrial myxoma* or primary exophytic *myocardial tumor* should be considered. This filling defect was surgically proven to be a thrombus.

Final Diagnosis

Tuberculous pericarditis and pericardial effusion with right atrial thrombus.

SUMMARY OF MR FINDINGS FOR:

1. Pericardial Effusion/Pericarditis[1,2]

    a. Separation of the pericardial layers by a crescentic fluid collection.

    b. The signal intensity may reflect its content—that is, elevated protein (long T2 and relatively short T1) or methemoglobin (marked shortening of T1).

    c. Both visceral and parietal layers may be irregularly thickened.

2. Mural Thrombus

    a. Focus of altered intraluminal signal intensity on the first echo image (nonentry slice).

    b. May be simulated by flow phenomena, such as even-echo rephasing or absence of flow, if the gated image was acquired during diastole.

REFERENCES

1. Soulen RL, Stark DD, Higgins CB: Magnetic resonance imaging of constrictive pericardial disease. *Am J Cardiol* 1985;55:480–484.

2. Stark DD, Higgins CB, Lanzer P, et al: Magnetic resonance imaging of the pericardium: Normal and pathologic findings. *Radiology* 1984;150:469–474.

CASE 60

HISTORY

A 5-month-old boy presented with a history of "failure to thrive" and two previous episodes of congestive heart failure. Physical examination revealed upper extremity hypertension. MRI was requested to rule out coarctation of the aorta.

QUESTIONS

1. What MR techniques would you use?

	1	2	3
a. Coil	____	____	____
b. Centering point	____	____	____
c. Imaging plane(s)	____	____	____
d. Contrast	____	____	____
e. Slice thickness	____	____	____

2. What do you expect to find?

_____

_____

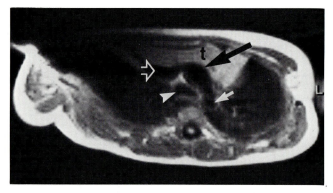

Figure 60.1 (SE gated/30). Axial scan through the aortic arch.

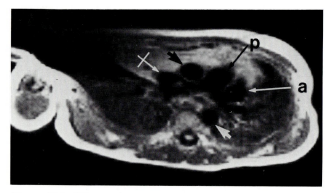

Figure 60.2 (SE gated/30). Axial scan 1 cm below Figure 60.1.

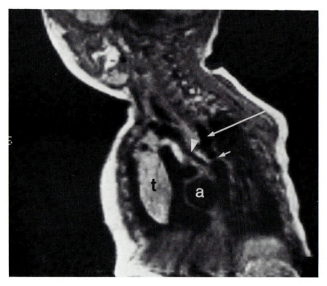

Figure 60.3 (SE gated/40). Oblique parasagittal scan through the descending aorta.

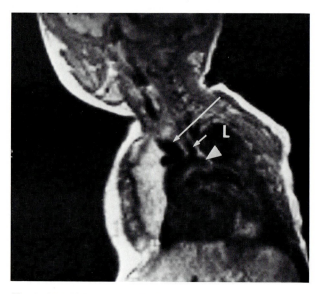

Figure 60.4 (SE gated/40). Oblique parasagittal scan through the ascending aorta 5 mm to the right of Figure 60.3.

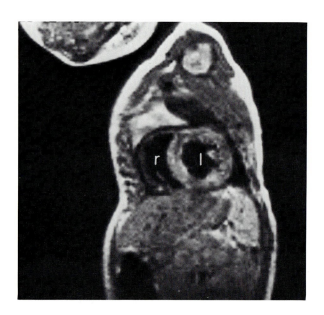

Figure 60.5 (SE gated/40). Oblique parasagittal scan through the right and left ventricles.

MR TECHNIQUES

		1	2
a.	Coil	Head	Head
b.	Centering point	Midsternum	Midchest
c.	Imaging planes	Axial	Sagittal
d.	Contrast	Gated (TR < 1000)	Gated (TR < 1000)
e.	Slice thickness	Routine	Thin

Please see introductory section on cardiac gating technique.

Because of the patient's age, sedation was required. Our standard protocol calls for chloral hydrate 50 to 75 mg/kg administered orally. A smaller diameter head coil was used instead of the regular body coil because of the patient's size. This improves the signal to noise.

Gated axial images were initially performed to examine the aortic arch, great vessels, and cardiac chambers. The obliquity of the aortic arch relative to the y axis was estimated from these axial "scout" views and was found to be approximately 15 to 20 degrees. The patient was then placed in a right anterior oblique (RAO) position, 15 to 20 degrees relative to the y axis, in order to align the plane of the aortic arch with the sagittal scanning plane. Contiguous 5-mm-thick sagittal sections were then obtained.

Nonorthogonal scanning would be ideal in this case since this would eliminate the need for repositioning the patient and thus decrease the likelihood of a positioning error. Unfortunately, this software was not available at the time of the examination.

MR FINDINGS

Figure 60.1. There is abrupt tapering of the aortic arch. The diameter of the ascending aorta (black arrow) measures approximately 13 mm, and the diameter of the descending aorta (white arrow) measures 4 mm. Note the large thymus (t) with intermediate intensity in the anterior mediastinum, the tracheal lumen (white arrowhead), and the superior vena cava (SVC) (open arrowhead). Note the image heterogeneity in the region of the right anterior thorax due to the metallic EKG lead used for gating.

Figure 60.2. The calibers of the ascending (black arrow) and descending (white arrow) aorta are similar at a level 1 cm below the aortic arch. Because of the flow void phenomenon, the mediastinal vasculature is well demonstrated. Note the pulmonary outflow tract (p), the left atrial appendage (a), and the SVC (crossed arrow).

Figure 60.3. On this parasagittal oblique view, there is a bandlike constriction (short white arrow) in the descending portion of the aortic arch distal to the origin of the left

subclavian artery (long white arrow). Note the left main stem bronchus (white arrowhead), the left atrium (a), and the large thymus (t).

Figure 60.4. On this parasagittal oblique view 5 mm to the right of Figure 60.3, the tapering of the aortic arch (arrowhead) is again demonstrated. The origin of the left common carotid artery (small white arrow), the brachiocephalic artery (long white arrow), and the medial portion of the left lung apex (L) are identified.

Figure 60.5. On this parasagittal oblique scan 3 cm to the right of Figure 60.4, a short-axis view of the heart is obtained. Both the right (r) and left (l) ventricles are noted to be slightly enlarged, and there is slight left ventricular hypertrophy (also found on echocardiography).

DIFFERENTIAL DIAGNOSIS

The findings described are characteristic of coarctation of the aorta. The distinct advantage of MRI in this case is its ability to display clearly the mediastinal vasculature noninvasively. The lack of ionizing radiation in MRI is an additional benefit in a patient of this age.

There are two types of coarctation of the aorta.[1] The most frequent is the adult or postductal type with the level of the coarctation occurring distal to the ductus arteriosus. The second type, the preductal or infantile type, is less common and more severe, presenting with a long segment of stenosis occurring proximal to the origin of the ductus arteriosus. A ventricular septal defect (VSD) and/or a patent ductus arteriosus (PDA) are often associated with the preductal type. Hemodynamically, both types may present with left ventricular overloading and hypertrophy, as seen in this case. Because of associated shunts (PDA and/or VSD), however, pulmonary hypertension with right ventricular overloading is also present in the infantile type. Clinically, the adult type usually presents in late childhood or early adulthood. Early congestive heart failure (CHF) may occur in infants with the adult type, however, particularly when it is associated with either a VSD or PDA. Patients with the infantile type usually present very early with symptoms of CHF. In addition, because of shunting of nonoxygenated blood through the PDA to the descending aorta, these patients often present with cyanosis of the lower extremities.

In this case, the segment of stenosis is noted to be very short, and the patient's clinical symptoms have been relatively mild. There was no PDA or VSD seen on the MR examination or on a cardiac angiogram.

Final Diagnosis

Postductal or adult-type coarctation of the aorta.

SUMMARY OF MR FINDINGS FOR COARCTATION OF THE AORTA[1,2]

1. Postductal (Adult) Type

a. Short segment of stenosis or narrowing of the descending aorta distal to the origin of the left subclavian artery and the ductus arteriosus.

b. May see both pre- and poststenotic dilatation of the aorta (the classic "figure-3" sign on plain film).

c. Left ventricular hypertrophy.

2. Preductal (Infantile) Type

a. Long segment of stenosis extending from the left subclavian artery to a PDA.

b. May demonstrate a PDA or VSD.

c. May demonstrate LVH and/or pulmonary arterial and venous congestion.

REFERENCES

1. Swischuk LE: Pulmonary vascular patterns, in *Plain Film Interpretation in Congenital Heart Disease*, ed. 2. Baltimore, Williams & Wilkins Co, 1979, pp 47–197.

2. Didier D, Higgins CB, Fisher MR, et al: Congenital heart disease: Gated MR imaging in 72 patients. *Radiology* 1986;158:227–235.

CASE 61

HISTORY

A 12-year-old boy with infantile hypercalcemia syndrome had undergone placement of a bypass graft from the ascending aorta to the abdominal aorta because of severe narrowing of the descending aorta. An aortogram (Figures 61.1 and 61.2) was performed to check for patency of the graft. MRI was requested as a baseline study.

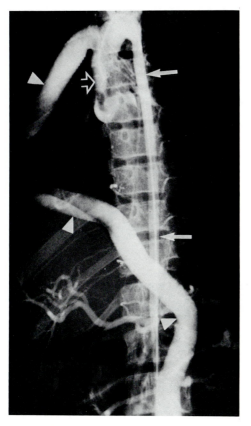

Figure 61.1. AP thoracic aortogram.

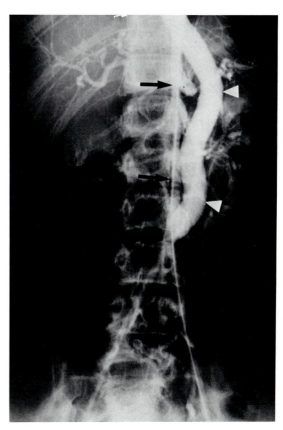

Figure 61.2. AP abdominal aortogram.

QUESTIONS

1. What is infantile hypercalcemia (or William's) syndrome?

_____

_____

2. What MR techniques would you use?

	1	2	3
a. Coil	_____	_____	_____
b. Centering point	_____	_____	_____
c. Imaging plane(s)	_____	_____	_____
d. Contrast	_____	_____	_____
e. Slice thickness	_____	_____	_____

3. What do you expect to find?

_____

_____

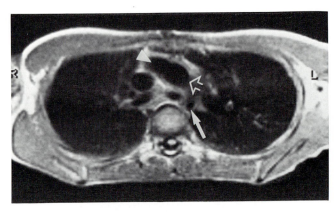

Figure 61.3 (SE gated/30). Axial scan of the aortic arch level.

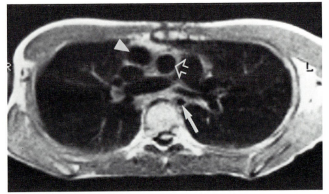

Figure 61.4 (SE gated/30). Axial scan 1 cm below Figure 61.3.

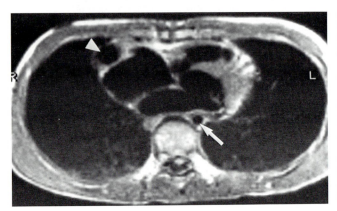

Figure 61.5 (SE gated/30). Axial scan at the level of the right atrium.

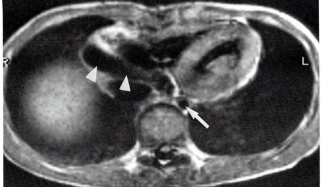

Figure 61.6 (SE gated/30). Axial scan at the level of the hepatic veins.

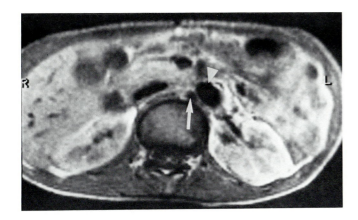

Figure 61.7 (SE gated/30). Axial scan at the level of the left renal artery.

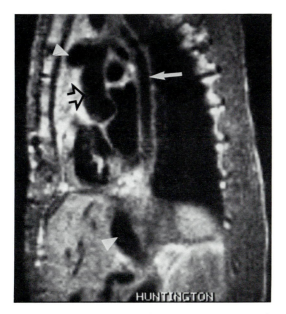

Figure 61.8 (SE gated/30). Oblique parasagittal scan through the descending aorta.

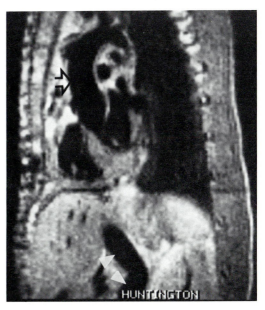

Figure 61.9 (SE gated/30). Oblique parasagittal scan through the ascending aorta 5 mm to the right of Figure 61.8.

MR TECHNIQUES

	1	2
a. Coil	Body	Body
b. Centering point	Midchest	Midchest
c. Imaging planes	Axial	Sagittal
d. Contrast	Gated	Gated
e. Slice thickness	Routine	Thin

Please see MR technique in Case 60 pertaining to examination of the aorta.

MR FINDINGS

Figures 61.1 and 61.2. The descending aorta (arrows) is shown to be very small and is about one fourth the caliber of the ascending aorta (open arrow). The Dacron graft (arrowheads) originates from the ascending aorta, deviates initially to the right, curves medially at the level of the diaphragm, and then descends to the left of the abdominal aorta. It ends at the aortic bifurcation. The angiographic catheter is seen within the lumen of the ascending and descending aorta.

Figures 61.3 through 61.7. The graft (arrowheads) is well demonstrated on these axial scans. Within the thorax, it is shown to be located anterior and lateral to the right atrium (Figure 61.5). The graft then curves around the undersurface of the heart (Figure 61.6) and penetrates the diaphragm near the midline. The native descending aorta (arrows) is again shown to be very small in caliber compared with the ascending aorta (open arrow).

Figures 61.8 and 61.9. The abrupt narrowing of the descending aorta (arrow) is better appreciated on these oblique parasagittal views (open arrow—ascending aorta; arrowheads—graft).

DISCUSSION

Infantile hypercalcemia (or William's) syndrome is rare. It consists of supravalvular aortic stenosis, other systemic and pulmonary vessel stenosis, mental retardation, and a peculiar but distinctive facial appearance. These characteristics are thought to be the sequelae of, or at least to be associated with, hypercalcemia, which may be only transient. Not all of these features need always be present. The supravalvular aortic stenosis may involve either a short or long segment of the aorta.[1]

With the exception of pulmonary vessel stenosis, this patient had all the preceding features. The supravalvular aortic stenosis involved the entire descending aorta as well as the iliac vessels. MRI is especially useful in this case because it can demonstrate the entire pathway of the graft without the use of contrast material. It is an ideal modality in following this patient because it is noninvasive and may be repeated without any known deleterious effect on the patient.

Final Diagnosis

Infantile hypercalcemia (or William's) syndrome.

SUMMARY OF MR FINDINGS FOR INFANTILE HYPERCALCEMIA SYNDROME

1. Supravalvular aortic stenosis. The involvement may be a short or long segment of the aorta.
2. Stenosis of the pulmonary or other systemic vessels may be demonstrated.

REFERENCE

1. Swischuk LE: Pulmonary vascular patterns, in *Plain Film Interpretation in Congenital Heart Disease*, ed 2. Baltimore, Williams & Wilkins Co, 1979, pp 47–197.

CASE 62

HISTORY

A 62-year-old hypertensive man presents with chest pain and abnormal chest radiograph (Figure 62.1).

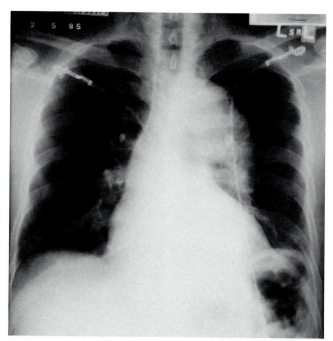

Figure 62.1. PA chest.

QUESTIONS

1. What are your differential considerations?

_____

_____

2. What MR techniques would you use?

	1	2	3
a. Coil	___	___	___
b. Centering point	___	___	___
c. Imaging plane(s)	___	___	___
d. Contrast	___	___	___
e. Slice thickness	___	___	___

3. What do you expect to find?

_____

_____

Note: This case was prepared by Robert W. Henderson and Jay A. Mericle.

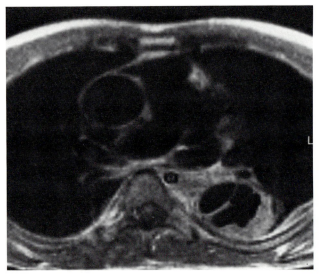

Figure 62.2 (SE gated/28). Axial scan at the level of the main pulmonary artery.

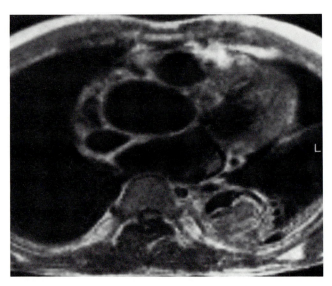

Figure 62.3 (SE gated/28). Axial scan at the level of the left atrium.

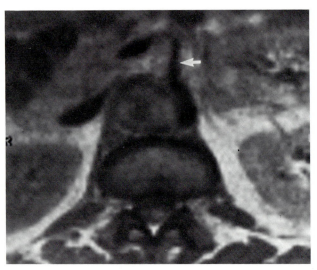

Figure 62.4 (SE gated/28). Axial scan at the level of the celiac axis.

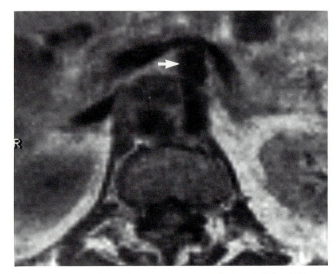

Figure 62.5 (SE gated/28). Axial scan at the level of the SMA.

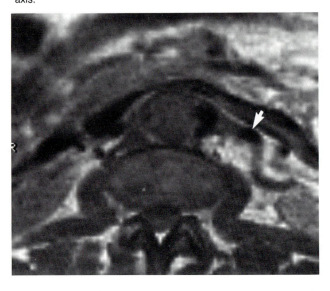

Figure 62.6 (SE gated/28). Axial scan at the level of the left renal artery.

MR TECHNIQUES

	1	2
a. Coil	Body	Body
b. Centering point	Midsternum	Subxyphoid
c. Imaging planes	Axial	Axial
d. Contrast	Gated (TR < 1000)	Mild T1W and mild T2W
e. Slice thickness	Routine	Thin

This protocol is designed for workup of aortic dissection:

1. Cardiac gating significantly improves detail in the thorax, especially for the aortic root and heart, by reducing cardiac motion. Since different portions of the aorta may be in different phases of the cardiac cycle during image acquisition, various levels of the aorta may be seen in either systole (decreased signal due to flow void or high-velocity signal loss) or diastole (increased signal due to slow flow).

2. In aortic dissection, blood flow in either the true or false lumen is best demonstrated on images acquired during systole.

3. Slow flow seen during diastole may artifactually mimic a thrombus or an occluded vessel.[1] To eliminate this diastolic artifact, one must obtain systolic gated images through the area of interest.

4. Thin slices may be required to identify the major branches of the aorta (e.g., celiac, SMA, and renal arteries).

5. The preferred scanning plane in the workup of aortic dissection is axial; the oblique sagittal plane, however, may provide additional information on the aortic arch.

MR FINDINGS

Figure 62.1. There is widening of the mediastinum.

Figure 62.2. Intimal flaps are seen in the descending aorta separating the aorta into three lumens; all have high-velocity signal loss.[1] The descending aortic wall is thickened.

Figure 62.3. At a slightly more inferior level to Figure 62.2, there is high intensity thrombus in either the true or false lumen of the descending aorta. Lack of even-echo rephasing on the second echo image confirms the impression that this is thrombus and not slow flow.[1]

Figures 62.4, 62.5, and 62.6. The celiac artery (Figure 62.4), SMA (Figure 62.5), and left renal artery (Figure 62.6) with high-velocity signal loss are indicated by arrows and are shown to originate from the same lumen of the aorta. The right renal artery was also noted to be patent (not shown).

DIFFERENTIAL DIAGNOSIS

The preceding findings are characteristic for type III aortic dissection. The primary objective of the MR study is to define the extent and patency of the various visceral arteries.

Final Diagnosis

Chronic type III aortic dissection.

SUMMARY OF MR FINDINGS FOR AORTIC DISSECTION[2–4]

1. Division of aortic lumen by a linear band representing the intimal flap.
2. Faster flow (less signal) may be seen in either the true or false lumen.
3. High signal may be attributed to thrombus, slow flow, or normal diastole. These may be distinguished in most cases.[1]
4. Absence of involvement of the root of the aorta is the key to diagnosing type III dissection.

REFERENCES

1. Bradley WG, Waluch V: Blood flow: Magnetic resonance imaging. *Radiology* 1985;154:443–450.
2. Amparo EG, Higgins CB, Hricak H, et al: Aortic dissection: Magnetic resonance imaging. *Radiology* 1985;155:399–406.
3. Geisinger MA, Risius B, O'Donnell JA, et al: Thoracic aortic dissections: Magnetic resonance imaging. *Radiology* 1985;155:407–412.
4. Amparo EG, Hoddick WK, Hricak H, et al: Comparison of magnetic resonance imaging and ultrasonography in the evaluation of abdominal aortic aneurysms. *Radiology* 1985;154:451–456.

CASE 63

HISTORY

A 44-year-old black man was found to have prominence of the hili on a routine chest radiograph (not shown). The patient was otherwise healthy. There was a history of contrast reaction during an excretory urogram performed several years earlier. MRI was requested to examine the hili.

QUESTIONS

1. What are your differential considerations?

_____

_____

2. What MR techniques would you use?

	1	2	3
a. Coil	_____	_____	_____
b. Centering point	_____	_____	_____
c. Imaging plane(s)	_____	_____	_____
d. Contrast	_____	_____	_____
e. Slice thickness	_____	_____	_____

3. What do you expect to find?

_____

_____

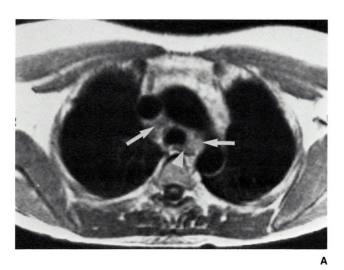
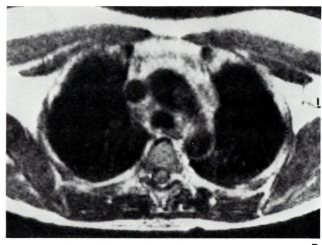

A

B

Figures 63.1A (SE 1000/30) and **63.1B** (SE 1000/60). Axial scan through the level of the aortopulmonary window.

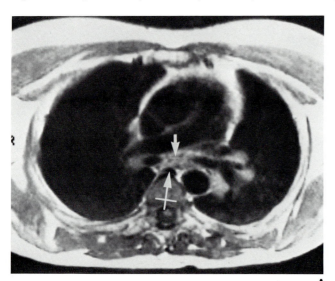
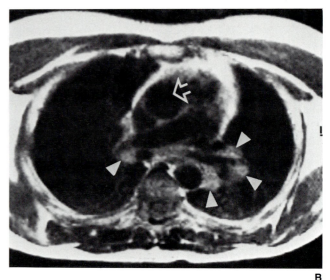

A

B

Figures 63.2A (SE 1000/30) and **63.2B** (SE 1000/60). Axial scan 1 cm below the carina.

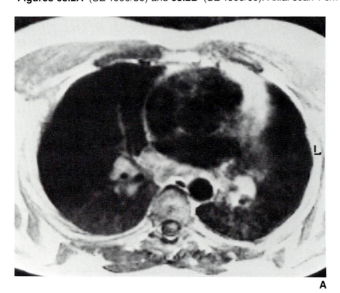
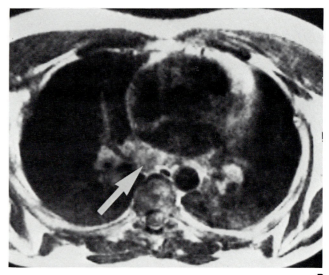

A

B

Figures 63.3A (SE 1000/30) and **63.3B** (SE 1000/60). Axial scan 2 cm inferior to Figure 63.2.

MR TECHNIQUES

	1	2
a. Coil	Body	Body
b. Centering point	Sternal notch	9.5 cm inferior to sternal notch
c. Imaging planes	Axial	Axial
d. Contrast	Mild T1W	Mild T1W
e. Slice thickness	Routine	Routine

A mildly T1-weighted pulsing sequence is used to examine the chest because it provides good contrast resolution while preserving adequate signal to noise. Two separate sequences are usually obtained, each covering 10 cm. The upper chest is scanned, centering directly over the sternal notch. The patient is then repositioned, centering 9.5 cm inferior to the sternal notch to examine the lower portion of the chest.

MR FINDINGS

Figure 63.1. There are intermediate intensity, enlarged nodes (arrows) in the right paratracheal region and in the aortopulmonary (AP) window. These nodes are easily differentiated from the mediastinal fat, which normally has a homogeneous high intensity. Note the collapsed esophagus (arrowhead) seen as an oval-shaped, intermediate intensity structure behind the trachea. This should not be mistaken for a node.

Figure 63.2. On this section, subcarinal nodes (arrow) are demonstrated. In addition, there is symmetric hilar lymphadenopathy (arrowheads) (open arrow—ascending aorta; crossed arrow—azygous vein).

Figure 63.3. The enlarged hilar nodes are again seen. In addition, there are enlarged nodes in the azygoesophageal recess (arrow). Note the image degradation due to cardiac motion.

DIFFERENTIAL DIAGNOSIS

The differential diagnosis of hilar and mediastinal adenopathy is extensive and includes numerous infectious (granulomatous and nongranulomatous) and neoplastic (e.g., lymphomatous and metastatic) etiologies.[1] The most likely cause of the bilateral hilar and mediastinal adenopathy in an otherwise healthy black male, however, would be sarcoidosis. This is a multisystem granulomatous disorder in which mediastinal and hilar adenopathy and pulmonary involvement are frequent. As in this case, the hilar adenopathy is almost always symmetric. The patient underwent mediastinoscopy with biopsy of the right paratracheal node. Pathologic examination revealed noncaseating epithelioid cell tubercles confirming the diagnosis of sarcoidosis.

Comment

This case demonstrates how well hilar and mediastinal adenopathy can be seen with MRI. The distinct advantage of MRI compared with CT in the chest is its ability to demonstrate mediastinal mass and lymphadenopathy without the use of intravenous contrast material. The natural MR contrast between high intensity mediastinal fat and the low-intensity cardiac and vascular structures allows the easy detection of intermediate intensity nodes and soft tissue masses.[2,3] Disadvantages of MRI include its longer scanning time and degradation by respiratory and cardiac motion artifacts. The latter may be partially offset by application of respiratory and cardiac gating, as discussed in the introductory section.

Final Diagnosis

Sarcoidosis.

SUMMARY OF MR FINDINGS FOR SARCOIDOSIS

1. Symmetric bilateral hilar adenopathy.
2. Mediastinal adenopathy, with the right paratracheal group of nodes most commonly involved.
3. The nodes are seen as lobulated masses with intermediate intensity. The signal intensity pattern of these nodes is nonspecific; benign and malignant lymphadenopathy cannot be differentiated on MRI.[4]
4. One may also see parenchymal abnormalities within the lung parenchyma, although MRI is relatively insensitive to these changes.

REFERENCES

1. Gamsu G: Computed tomography of the pulmonary hila, in Moss AA, Gamsu G, Genant HK (eds): *Computed Tomography of the Body.* Philadelphia, WB Saunders Co, 1983, pp 271–319.

2. Cohen AM, Creviston S, LiPuma JP, et al: NMR evaluation of hilar and mediastinal lymphadenopathy. *Radiology* 1983;148:739–742.

3. Webb WR, Gamsu G, Stark DD, et al: Magnetic resonance imaging of the normal and abnormal hila. *Radiology* 1984;152:89–94.

4. Dooms GC, Hricak H, Moseley ME, et al: Characterization of lymphadenopathy by magnetic resonance relaxation times: Preliminary results. *Radiology* 1985;155:691–697.

CASE 64

HISTORY

A 65-year-old woman smoker presenting with pain in the right axilla and right arm swelling. Chest x-ray showed a nodule in the periphery of the right apex and a right paratracheal mass. MRI was requested to evaluate the mediastinum further.

QUESTIONS

1. What are your differential considerations?

_____

_____

2. What MR techniques would you use?

	1	2	3
a. Coil	___	___	___
b. Centering point	___	___	___
c. Imaging plane(s)	___	___	___
d. Contrast	___	___	___
e. Slice thickness	___	___	___

3. Should you use cardiac gating?

_____

_____

4. What do you expect to find?

_____

_____

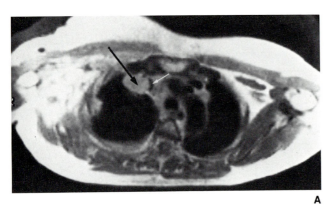
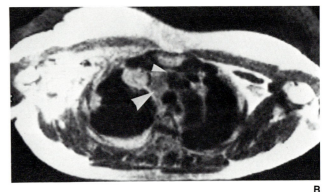

A

B

Figures 64.1A (SE 2000/28) and **64.1B** (SE 2000/56). Axial scan through the top of the aortic arch.

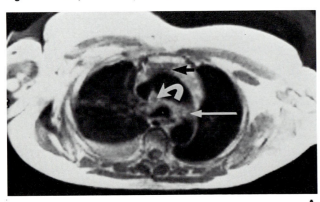
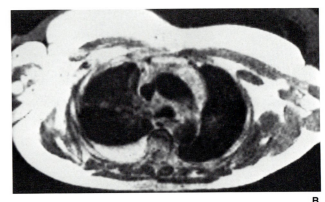

A

B

Figures 64.2A (SE 2000/28) and **64.2B** (SE 2000/56). Axial scan 1 cm inferior to Figure 64.1.

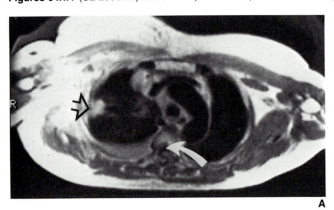
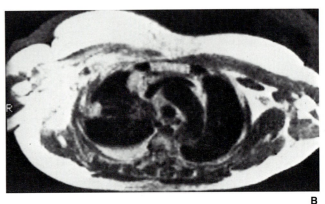

A

B

Figures 64.3A (SE 2000/28) and **64.3B** (SE 2000/56). Axial scan through the aorticopulmonary window.

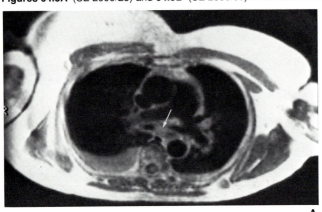
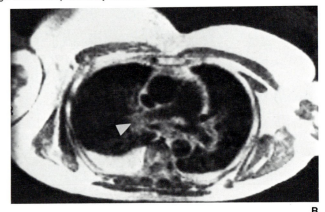

A

B

Figures 64.4A (SE 2000/28) and **64.4B** (SE 2000/56). Axial scan through the hili.

MR TECHNIQUES

a. Coil	Body
b. Centering point	Midsternum
c. Imaging plane	Axial
d. Contrast	Mild to moderate T2W
e. Slice thickness	Routine

The axial projection is the plane of choice in evaluating the chest and mediastinum. T2 weighting was used since it has been reported to increase sensitivity in detecting pulmonary nodules.[1,2] The coverage with the longer TR allows for screening most of the chest with a single acquisition. Without respiratory gating, however, MRI would be expected to provide less information about the pulmonary parenchyma when compared with either CT or plain x-rays. Alternatively, using a mild T1WI may help in evaluation of the mediastinum by accentuating the contrast differences among adenopathy, vasculature, and fat.

In this case, gating was not used since the superior mediastinum was the region of interest. When evaluating the region between the cardiac base and the diaphragm, however, we routinely utilize gating to reduce motion artifact (see Case 65).

MR FINDINGS

Figures 64.1 and 64.2. There is a mass (long black arrow) measuring 3 × 2.5 cm located just posterior to the right first costochondral junction. The mass is compressing the more medial, right innominate vein (short white arrow). The intensity of the mass is slightly heterogeneous and is intermediate between that of fat and skeletal muscle; the intensity also increases on the second echo image, indicating a prolonged T2. The mediastinal fat in the prevascular space (small arrowhead) and in the paratracheal area (large arrowhead) has an abnormally low intensity, suggesting the presence of adenopathy. There is a 2-cm, pleural-based nodule (open arrow) in the right upper lung along the midaxillary line. This nodule also has a slightly heterogeneous intensity pattern, which becomes more intense on the second echo image. There are multiple fine linear streaks extending from the nodule to the right hilus. The crescentic area of increased intensity in the dependent aspect of the right lung represents a large, right pleural effusion. The intensity of the pleural fluid is greater than that of intraspinal CSF (curved arrow) on the first echo image, indicating a shorter T1 and a higher protein content.

Figure 64.3. The enlarged nodes in the prevascular space (black arrow), pretracheal area (curved arrow), and AP window (long white arrow) are slightly better demonstrated on this image. Also note the linear streaks in the right lung and the right pleural effusion.

Figure 64.4. There are medium intensity lesions in the right hilus (arrowhead) and in the subcarinal area (short arrow), suggesting adenopathy in those regions.

DIFFERENTIAL DIAGNOSIS

The most likely diagnosis in this case is bronchogenic carcinoma, with the primary tumor being the pleural-based nodule in the right upper lung. The mass adjacent to the right innominate vein is most likely a metastatic lymph node. The compression of the right innominate vein probably caused the right arm swelling. The involvement of the mediastinal lymph nodes, clearly depicted on MRI, makes this tumor nonresectable. The patient underwent a percutaneous needle biopsy of the right upper lobe lesion, and histologic examination of the specimen revealed squamous cell carcinoma.

Comment

The most important factor in determining tumor resectability is the presence or absence of mediastinal lymph node metastases. MR imaging has been shown to be comparable to CT in the detection of mediastinal adenopathy.[2] The major advantage of MRI over CT is its ability to show adenopathy without the use of intravenous contrast material. In the detection of hilar nodes, MRI is superior to enhanced CT because of the ease with which hilar vessels and soft tissue masses can be distinguished on MR images.[2,3] It should be noted that although the presence of the *hilar* adenopathy changes the stage of the tumor, the patient's prognosis and the surgical approach, it does not render the tumor nonresectable.

CT remains the modality of choice for the detection of the primary tumor and pulmonary nodules.[1] The sensitivity of CT in nodule detection is greater than that of MRI because of respiratory artifacts encountered with the latter modality. MRI may be slightly better than CT in detecting small hilar nodules adjacent to blood vessels, however, because of its superior contrast resolution.

Chest wall involvement is a contraindication for resection.[4] CT is probably better than MRI in demonstrating chest wall invasion and rib erosion because of its greater spatial resolution and its clearer depiction of bony changes. It should be emphasized that the absence of a fascial plane between tumor and chest wall on MRI or CT does not necessarily indicate tumor invasion.

As illustrated in this case, MRI can be extremely useful in providing information about the presence, cause, and precise level of mediastinal and thoracic inlet venous obstruction.[5] This is of clinical importance because it obviates the need for a venogram to establish this diagnosis.

Final Diagnosis

Squamous cell carcinoma of the lung with involvement of the right hilar and mediastinal nodes (possible right chest wall involvement).

SUMMARY OF MR FINDINGS FOR BRONCHOGENIC CARCINOMA

1. A nodule or a mass may be seen in the lung parenchyma. Cavitation may be demonstrated.
2. The primary tumor may be better demonstrated on a T2-weighted image, appearing as a high signal intensity lesion because of the prolongation of T2. The limiting factor regardless of TR, however, is respiratory artifact.
3. Ipsilateral hilar and mediastinal nodes may be seen. In general, nodes are better demonstrated on a T1-weighted image because of the difference in T1 values between nodes and surrounding mediastinal tissue.

With a longer TR, the intensity of nodes increases relative to that of fat. Contrast decreases, and the nodes may not be detected.

4. Chest wall invasion and venous obstruction may be demonstrated.
5. Pleural effusion may be present.

REFERENCES

1. Muller NL, Gamsu G, Webb WR: Pulmonary nodules: Detection using magnetic resonance and computed tomography. *Radiology* 1985; 155:687–690.
2. Webb WR, Jensen BF, Sollitto R, et al: Bronchogenic carcinoma: Staging with MR compared with staging with CT and surgery. *Radiology* 1985;156:117–124.
3. Webb WR, Gamsu G, Stark DD, et al: Magnetic resonance imaging of the normal and abnormal pulmonary hila. *Radiology* 1984;152:89–94.
4. Armstrong JD, Bragg DG: Thoracic neoplasms: Imaging requirements for diagnosis and staging, in Bragg DG, Rubin P, Youker JE (eds): *Oncologic Imaging.* New York, Pergamon Press, 1985, pp 145–172.
5. Weinreb JC, Mootz A, Cohen JM: MRI evaluation of mediastinal and thoracic inlet venous obstruction. *AJR* 1986;146:679–684.

CASE 65

HISTORY

A 60-year-old woman presented with left scapula pain of 4 months' duration. Chest x-ray showed a large mass in the medial aspect of the apex of the left lung. Bronchoscopy and transbronchial biopsy revealed epidermoid carcinoma. Enhanced CT of the lung (Figure 65.1) showed destruction of the T-3 vertebral body. MRI was requested to rule out extension of the tumor into the spinal canal prior to radiotherapy.

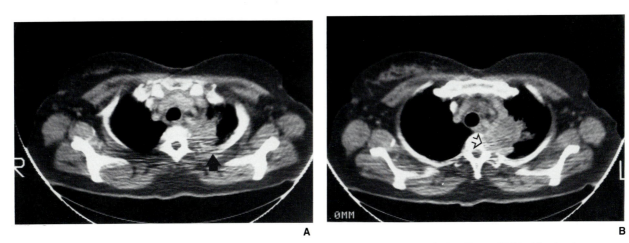

Figure 65.1A Enhanced CT at the level of the sternal notch. **B** Enhanced CT 1 cm below Figure 65.1A at the level of the T-3 vertebral body.

QUESTIONS

1. What MR techniques would you use?

	1	2	3
a. Coil	___	___	___
b. Centering point	___	___	___
c. Imaging plane(s)	___	___	___
d. Contrast	___	___	___
e. Slice thickness	___	___	___

2. What do you expect to find?

_____

_____

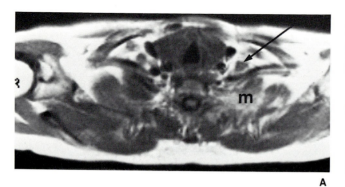

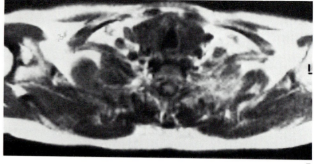

Figures 65.2A (SE 1000/30) and **65.2B** (SE 1000/60). Axial scan of the lower neck at the C 7 level.

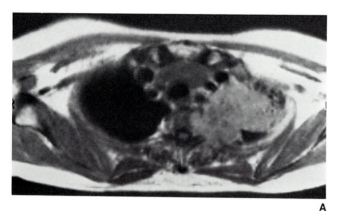

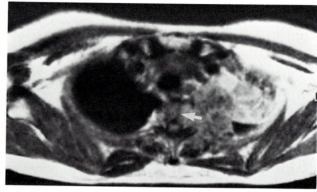

Figures 65.3A (SE 1000/30) and **65.3B** (SE 1000/60). Axial scan at the same level as Figure 65.1B.

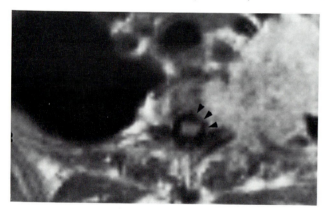

Figure 65.4 (SE 1000/30). Magnified view of Figure 65.3A.

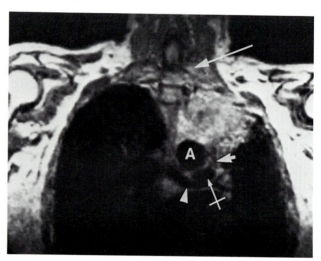

Figure 65.5 (SE 1000/40). Midcoronal scan of the upper chest.

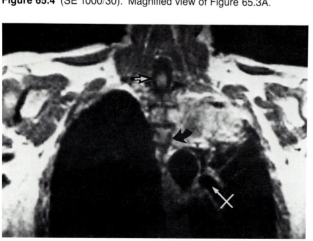

Figure 65.6 (SE 1000/40). Coronal scan 1 cm posterior to Figure 65.5.

MR TECHNIQUES

		1	2
a.	Coil	Body	Body
b.	Centering point	Sternal notch	Midcoronal plane
c.	Imaging planes	Axial	Coronal
d.	Contrast	Mild T1W and mild T2W	Mild T1W and mild T2W
e.	Slice thickness	Routine	Thin

Mild T1 weighting is used in both sequences to optimize anatomic definition and scanning time and to increase intensity differences between fat, tumor, and muscles. To define best the extent of the tumor, the chest should be scanned in at least two different imaging planes. The axial plane is the standard imaging plane for the body, so that the findings can be compared directly with those of CT. The coronal plane is chosen because it helps define both the medial-lateral and longitudinal extent of the tumor. The sagittal plane was least helpful in this case since it did not allow direct comparison of right–left symmetry on a single image, which makes the degree of spinal involvement difficult to evaluate. Because of the curvature of the spine, small lesions can easily be missed—especially in the coronal plane; hence, a thinner slice thickness was chosen for the second sequence.

MR FINDINGS

Figure 65.1. There is a large, soft tissue mass located in the medial aspect of the left upper lung. The mass has an heterogeneous density and is adherent to the mediastinum. There is destruction of the left third rib (closed arrow) at the costovertebral junction. The left side of the T-3 vertebral body (open arrow) has also been eroded by tumor. On the lung window setting (not shown), the mass appears larger, encompassing much of the left apex.

Figure 65.2. Asymmetric signal intensity is seen in the left thoracic inlet in the region of the serratus anterior muscle (m), indicating tumor infiltration. Note the low-signal tubular structures representing the subclavian vein and artery just anterior to this muscle. Although not visualized, the brachial plexus is in this region. The arrow indicates the left scalenus anterior muscle.

Figures 65.3 and 65.4. On this moderately T1-weighted image, the mass has a heterogeneous, intermediate intensity pattern, and it has a higher signal intensity on the second echo image, indicating prolongation of T2. The tumor encases most of the left upper lung. The erosion of the left side of the T-3 vertebral body (arrow) is again identified. On the magnified view of the spine (Figure 65.4), the left side of the dural sac is slightly deformed, as indicated by the asymmetry of the CSF (arrowheads), suggesting encroachment of the tumor on the spinal canal. This was not appreciated on the CT scan.

Figure 65.5. The longitudinal extent of this tumor is well demonstrated on this coronal image through the middle mediastinum. The mass spreads inframedially to involve the aortopulmonary window (short arrow). The cephalic spread of the tumor to invade the lower cervical muscles (long arrow) is again demonstrated (A—aortic arch; arrowhead—left main stem bronchus; crossed arrow—left pulmonary artery).

Figure 65.6. On this coronal scan 1 cm posterior to Figure 65.5, the involvement of the T-3 vertebral body is again demonstrated. In addition, the left side of the T-4 vertebral body (curved arrow) is also involved (arrow—spinal cord; crossed arrow—left pulmonary artery).

DISCUSSION

The preceding findings are typical of the Pancoast or superior sulcus tumor, which arises in the thoracic apex. Squamous cell carcinoma is the most common cell type; however, any cell type may be observed with Pancoast's tumor. These tumors frequently invade the ribs and the vertebrae, producing local pain. They may also involve the brachial plexus, producing sensory and motor disturbances in the upper extremity. Involvement of the sympathetic nerve chain produces an ipsilateral Horner syndrome.

In this case, the tumor was well demonstrated on both MRI and CT. Although the bony changes were better demonstrated on CT, the muscle involvement and the intraspinal spread of the tumor were much better seen on MRI because of its superior soft tissue resolution. The longitudinal extent of the lesion was also better appreciated on MRI than on CT because of MRI's multiplanar capability.

Final Diagnosis

Pancoast tumor of the left apex.

SUMMARY OF MR FINDINGS FOR PANCOAST TUMOR[1]

1. Mass in the thoracic apex.
2. The T2 of the tumor is prolonged compared with that of muscles and lung; hence, the mass has high signal intensity on a T2-weighted image. The intensity pattern is inhomogeneous, possibly representing tumor, necrotic tissue, and retained mucus due to obstructed bronchi.
3. The involved muscles also have a higher signal intensity due to prolongation of T2, probably a combination of tumor infiltration and edema.

4. Invasion of the ribs (varying involvement of the first three) and vertebrae may be demonstrated. The tumor may also invade the spinal canal, as seen in this case.
5. Invasion of the mediastinal structures may be seen.

REFERENCE

1. Armstrong JD, Bragg DG: Thoracic neoplasms: Imaging requirements for diagnosis and staging, in Bragg DG, Rubin P, Youker JE (eds): *Oncologic Imaging*. New York, Pergamon Press, 1985, pp 145–172.

CASE 66

HISTORY

A 62-year-old woman presented with pressurelike discomfort localized to the right anterior chest. A chest radiograph (not shown) demonstrated widening of the mediastinum. CT of the chest (Figure 66.1) was performed, and MRI was requested to correlate with CT findings.

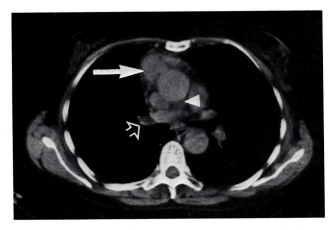

Figure 66.1. Unenhanced axial CT scan of the chest 1 cm below the carina.

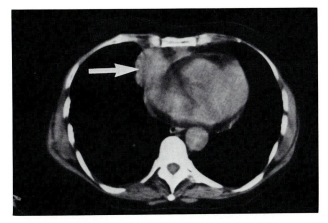

Figure 66.2 Unenhanced axial CT scan of the chest through the upper portion of the heart.

QUESTIONS

1. What are your differential considerations?

_____

_____

2. What MR techniques would you use?

	1	2	3
a. Coil	——	——	——
b. Centering point	——	——	——
c. Imaging plane(s)	——	——	——
d. Contrast	——	——	——
e. Slice thickness	——	——	——

3. What do you expect to find?

_____

_____

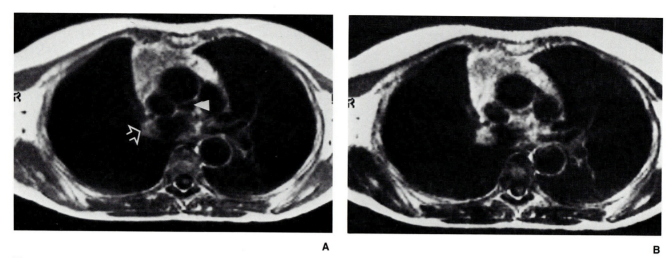

Figures 66.3A (SE 1000/30) and **66.3B** (SE 1000/60). Axial scan through same level as Figure 66.1.

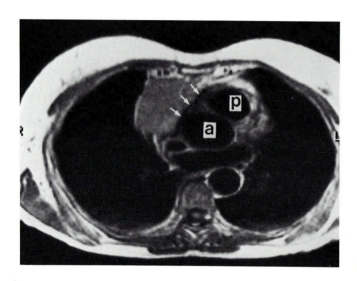

Figure 66.4 (SE gated/30). Axial scan 2 cm above the aortic valve.

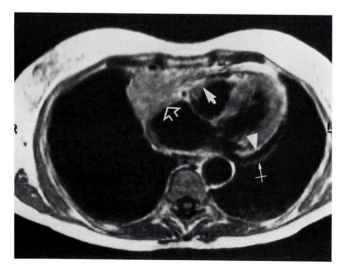

Figure 66.5 (SE gated/30). Axial scan 3 cm below Figure 66.4.

CASE 66

HISTORY

A 62-year-old woman presented with pressurelike discomfort localized to the right anterior chest. A chest radiograph (not shown) demonstrated widening of the mediastinum. CT of the chest (Figure 66.1) was performed, and MRI was requested to correlate with CT findings.

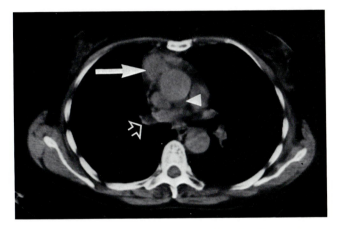

Figure 66.1. Unenhanced axial CT scan of the chest 1 cm below the carina.

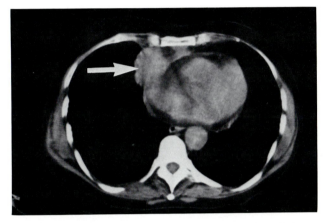

Figure 66.2 Unenhanced axial CT scan of the chest through the upper portion of the heart.

QUESTIONS

1. What are your differential considerations?

_____

_____

2. What MR techniques would you use?

	1	2	3
a. Coil	___	___	___
b. Centering point	___	___	___
c. Imaging plane(s)	___	___	___
d. Contrast	___	___	___
e. Slice thickness	___	___	___

3. What do you expect to find?

_____

_____

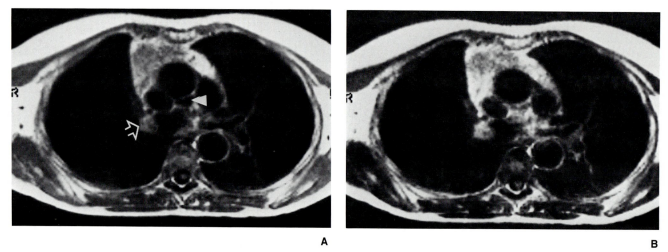

A

B

Figures 66.3A (SE 1000/30) and **66.3B** (SE 1000/60). Axial scan through same level as Figure 66.1.

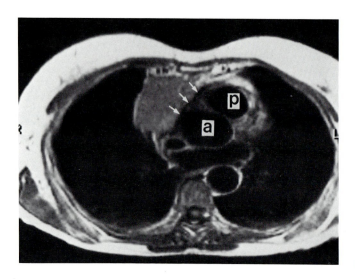

Figure 66.4 (SE gated/30). Axial scan 2 cm above the aortic valve.

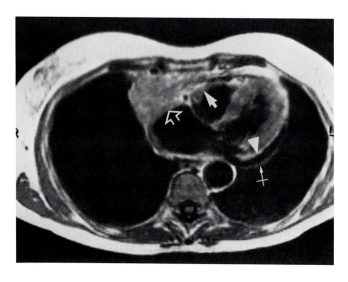

Figure 66.5 (SE gated/30). Axial scan 3 cm below Figure 66.4.

CASE 66

HISTORY

A 62-year-old woman presented with pressurelike discomfort localized to the right anterior chest. A chest radiograph (not shown) demonstrated widening of the mediastinum. CT of the chest (Figure 66.1) was performed, and MRI was requested to correlate with CT findings.

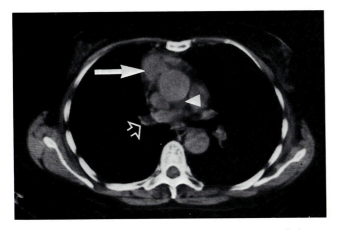

Figure 66.1. Unenhanced axial CT scan of the chest 1 cm below the carina.

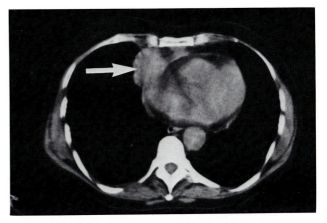

Figure 66.2 Unenhanced axial CT scan of the chest through the upper portion of the heart.

QUESTIONS

1. What are your differential considerations?

_____

_____

2. What MR techniques would you use?

	1	2	3
a. Coil			
b. Centering point			
c. Imaging plane(s)			
d. Contrast			
e. Slice thickness			

3. What do you expect to find?

_____

_____

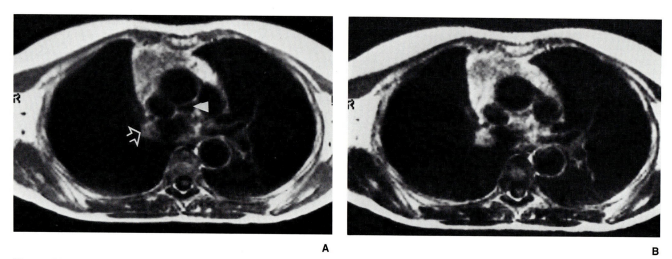

A

B

Figures 66.3A (SE 1000/30) and **66.3B** (SE 1000/60). Axial scan through same level as Figure 66.1.

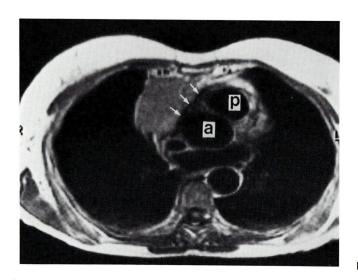

Figure 66.4 (SE gated/30). Axial scan 2 cm above the aortic valve.

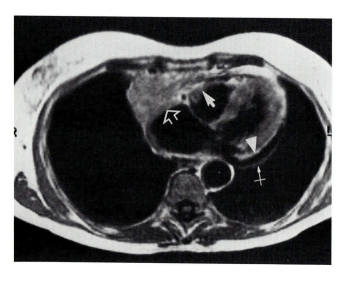

Figure 66.5 (SE gated/30). Axial scan 3 cm below Figure 66.4.

MR TECHNIQUES

	1	2
a. Coil	Body	Body
b. Centering point	Sternal notch	8 cm below sternal notch
c. Imaging planes	Axial	Axial
d. Contrast	Mild T1W and mild T2W	Gated
e. Slice thickness	Routine	Routine

Our current protocol for mediastinal lesions is to scan the chest with two separate pulsing sequences. The upper chest is examined with a mildly T1-weighted sequence, which provides good contrast resolution while preserving adequate signal to noise. A gated pulsing sequence is used to examine the lower chest to reduce the effect of cardiac motion. The axial plane is the standard imaging plane for the chest.

MR FINDINGS

Figures 66.1 and 66.2. There is a large mass (arrows) in the anterior mediastinum extending from the level of the aortic arch down to the diaphragm. The mass has a relatively homogeneous density and is adherent to the pericardium. It is predominantly located to the right of midline. The right hilus (open arrow) appears to be normal on this unenhanced scan. There is a small, semilunar-shaped soft tissue density (arrowhead) located between the ascending aorta and the right pulmonary artery.

Figure 66.3. The large, anterior mediastinal mass is well demonstrated on this mild T1WI. The mass has a relatively homogeneous intensity that is slightly greater than that of skeletal muscle but less than that of mediastinal fat. There is an intermediate intensity mass (open arrow) in the superior right hilus indicating right hilar adenopathy. This was not appreciated on the unenhanced CT scan. The semilunar-shaped structure (arrowhead) seen on CT is shown to have a low intensity on the first echo image but a higher intensity on the second echo image, indicating a prolonged T2. This structure represents the transverse sinus recess of the pericardium filled with pericardial fluid.[1] This should not be confused with adenopathy.

Figure 66.4. With cardiac gating, the margins of the mass and the mediastinal structures are better defined. The pericardium (arrows) is seen as a thin, low intensity, curvilinear structure separating the mass from the ascending aorta (a) and the pulmonary outflow tract (p).

Figure 66.5. The mass is shown to be adherent to the anterior wall of the right ventricle (closed arrow) and right atrium (open arrow). There is a small pericardial effusion seen as a low intensity curved structure separating the epicardium/visceral pericardium (arrowhead) from the parietal pericardium (crossed arrow).

DIFFERENTIAL DIAGNOSIS

The differential diagnosis of a large, solid, anterior mediastinal mass would include thymoma, teratoma, retrosternal goiter, lymphoma, and metastases. Of these, a retrosternal goiter can be excluded because its density on the CT scan should be higher than that of surrounding soft tissue.[2] A teratoma would be unusual in a patient of this age. A malignant thymoma generally is locally invasive and may spread along the pleura and pericardium.[2] It does not usually cause hilar adenopathy without lung invasion. The presence of right hilar adenopathy is more suggestive of a lymphoma and metastases.

The patient underwent percutaneous needle biopsy of the mass under CT guidance. Histologic examination revealed a poorly differentiated adenocarcinoma, probably originated from the lung. No primary lung tumor was found on CT or MRI, however.

Comment

The advantage of MRI compared with CT in this case is its ability to demonstrate clearly the mass and the presence of right hilar adenopathy without using contrast material. This is due to the good soft-tissue-to-vessel contrast resulting in easy identification of and distinction between solid and vascular lesions. MRI shows the pericardium and pericardial sinuses well, which helps in defining the cleavage lines between masses and the heart.[3] The presence of pericardial fluid was better demonstrated on MRI than CT in this case.

The disadvantages of MRI are its inferior spatial resolution compared with that of CT and its relative insensitivity to calcification, which may be helpful in determining the possible etiology of the lesion. In addition, MRI cannot guide needle biopsy, which helped establish the diagnosis in this case.

Final Diagnosis

Poorly differentiated adenocarcinoma metastasized to the anterior mediastinum and the right hilus.

SUMMARY OF MR FINDINGS FOR MEDIASTINAL MASS

1. Soft tissue mass(es) located in the mediastinum

   a. Benign neoplastic lesions tend to be unifocal.
   b. Malignant and inflammatory lesions are more often multifocal.

2. T1 and T2 relaxation times[3]

   a. Carcinoma of the lung has high T1 and T2 values.
   b. Chronic inflammatory processes have lower mean T1 and T2 values than neoplasms.

c. Other neoplasms have relaxation times in between those of bronchogenic carcinoma and chronic inflammatory processes.

3. There may be encroachment on the tracheobronchial tree and mediastinal vessels.
4. Chronic inflammatory masses (e.g., sarcoidosis) generally have a heterogeneous intensity pattern, whereas neoplasms appear inhomogeneous.[3]

REFERENCES

1. Levy-Ravetch M, Auh YH, Rubenstein WA, et al: CT of the pericardial recesses. *AJR* 1985;144:707–714.

2. Gamsu G: Computed tomography of the mediastinum, in Moss AA, Gamsu G, Genant HK (eds): *Computed Tomography of the Body*. Philadelphia, WB Saunders Co, 1983, pp 195–269.

3. Von Schulthess GK, McMurdo K, Tscholakoff D, et al: Mediastinal masses: MR imaging. *Radiology* 1986;158:289–296.

8

ABDOMINAL IMAGING

The efficacy of MRI in evaluation of the central nervous system (CNS), head and neck, and musculoskeletal system has been firmly established. Its distinct advantages include multiplanar imaging, lack of ionizing radiation, and superb contrast resolution. In contrast, MRI of the abdomen and pelvis is still at a relatively early developmental stage. Because of its greater susceptibility to motion artifact and decreased spatial resolution, as compared with CT, clinical applications for abdominal MR imaging have been limited.

The major causes of motion artifact are respiration, cardiac pulsations, and peristalsis.[1] Respiratory motion is neither periodic nor constant in amplitude, making respiratory gating difficult. Respiratory gating requires a mechanical linkage to convert chest motion into electrical impulses in order to synchronize data acquisition. In most instances, this synchronization is imperfect. Imaging time is also significantly prolonged because it is proportional to the fractional time of the respiratory cycle, which is included by the gating process. Although minimal, cardiac pulsations transmitted to the upper abdomen can be reduced by cardiac gating (see introductory section on cardiothoracic imaging). In this instance, the TR is determined by the heart rate. Peristaltic motion of the bowel during image acquisition greatly reduces definition of bowel loops as discrete structures. This is very difficult to control, even with the use of glucagon or compression belts.

An additional difficulty in imaging the abdomen is the current lack of a reliable small-bowel contrast agent. Nonopacified loops of small bowel create significant difficulties in interpretation since they may obscure adjacent abdominal organs or mimic a solid tumor mass. Additionally, MRI is insensitive to calcification, which in the abdomen may be important in detecting, as well as diagnosing, pathology.

To minimize motion artifacts, Stark and Ferrucci have developed a protocol using a heavily T1-weighted spin echo sequence with a very short TR and TE.[1] This technique averages a large number of excitations without significantly prolonging the imaging time. For example, with a TR of 260 mseconds and a TE of 15 mseconds, 16 averages are performed to produce adequate signal to noise. (See Figure 8–1.) The motion artifacts are reduced by the multiple signal averages. The disadvantage of this technique is the restriction of image contrast to tissue T1 differences.

LIVER IMAGING

Our usual protocol in examining the liver is a combination of both T1- and T2-weighted images. We initially scan the

335

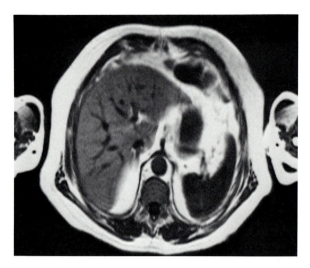

Figure 8–1 (SE 260/15, 16 acquisitions). Heavily T1-weighted image of a normal liver. The caudate lobe, intrahepatic inferior vena cava, right adrenal gland, and branching intrahepatic vessels are clearly identified. The fluid-filled stomach and colon demonstrate low signal intensity and absence of motion artifact (Courtesy of David D. Stark MD, Boston, MA).

liver with a TR of 2,000 mseconds, with echo delay times of 30 and 60 mseconds, in the transverse plane. A total of 20 sections, each covering 1 cm, are obtained. This is followed by a second sequence that utilizes a TR 500 mseconds and a single echo delay time of 30 msceconds, yielding ten sections, each covering 1 cm. Two T1-weighted acquisitions are performed to image the entire liver. As discussed earlier, the T2-weighted sequence requires a relatively long period of time and is susceptible to motion artifacts. This sequence is sensitive in the detection of pathological lesions, however, since most lesions have prolonged T2 relaxation times. The T1-weighted images have the disadvantage of less signal to noise. On the other hand, imaging time is decreased, and the vascular anatomy is better demonstrated.

LIVER MASSES

The major pathologic entities that may be encountered include primary and metastatic malignancies, cysts, and hemangiomas. Moss et al. have shown that T1 is increased by an average of 40% and T2 is increased by an average of 21% in hepatomas and metastases, as compared with normal liver parenchyma.[2] Hence, *metastases* and *primary tumors* of the liver are generally found to have a low signal intensity relative to normal liver parenchyma on a T1-weighted image and a high signal intensity relative to normal liver parenchyma on T2-weighted images. Heterogeneity is noted when there is tumor necrosis or hemorrhage. Since the tumor–liver T1 differences are significantly greater than the T2 differences, tumor–liver contrast may be better demonstrated on a T1-weighted image. In fact, using a very short

TR, short TE, heavily T1-weighted sequence, the sensitivity of MRI in the detection of metastases is equal to, if not greater than, that of CT.[1] Alternatively, if T2-weighted sequences are used, phase-contrast MR imaging may improve sensitivity in detecting hepatic tumors. The interested reader should see Reference 3.

Simple *liver cysts* are very common and, on the basis of smooth margination and homogeneous signal, are easily distinguished from solid tumors and hemangiomas both on ultrasound and on CT. Because of somewhat similar T1 and T2 values, however, they are difficult to separate from the other lesions on the basis of the MR relaxation times alone. Typically, cysts are seen as well-circumscribed lesions with low intensity on T1-weighted images and high intensity on T2-weighted images. This is because of the fluid inside these cysts, which tends to have a longer T1 and T2 than normal liver parenchyma.[4]

Hemangiomas are usually incidentally discovered lesions. They are composed of lakes of slowly flowing blood and have relatively long T2 relaxation times.[5,6] Hence, on T2-weighted images, they have significantly greater signal intensity than most solid neoplasms of the liver. They are either hypointense or isointense with liver parenchyma on moderately T1-weighted images (e.g., TR 0.5, TE 30). Mass effect may be seen if they are of sufficient size. Because of the significantly prolonged T2 relaxation times, MRI has been shown to be more sensitive in the detection of hemangiomas than either CT, ultrasound, radionuclide scanning, or selective hepatic arteriography. On the other hand, the MR appearance of hemangiomas is not totally specific, since other focal hepatic lesions (e.g., metastases and hepatomas) may have similar intensity changes.

FATTY INFILTRATION

Diffuse fatty infiltration of the liver is a common problem encountered in patients with alcoholism or obesity and in those being treated with chemotherapy. This is easily detected on CT examination and can be relatively well demonstrated by ultrasound. Fatty changes of the liver are poorly depicted on MRI, however. For reasons that are not entirely clear, fat deposited diffusely throughout the liver may not significantly alter hepatic T1 and T2 relaxation times. As might be expected, focal fatty changes may be better demonstrated than diffuse infiltration.[4] Chemical shift imaging has recently been shown to be capable of demonstrating fatty infiltration.[7]

HEPATIC IRON OVERLOAD

Hepatic iron overload can be related to various causes, including transfusions, excessive dietary intake, and idiopathic hemochromatosis. In all instances, the total hepatic iron is increased and is represented by different components, including soluble low-molecular-weight iron, hemosiderin, ferritin, and hemoproteins. When spin echo images are obtained, the intensity of iron-laden liver parenchyma is decreased predominantly because of shortening of T2. While T1 may also be decreased, this effect is overshadowed by the effect of T2 shortening. Hepatocellular water (cytosol) is the primary liver component producing a detectable MR signal. It is thought that alteration of this compartment by an increase in soluble low-molecular-weight iron may influence the relaxation times. Indeed, it has been shown *in vitro* that the relaxation rates (1/T1 and 1/T2) increase linearly with an increasing concentration of low-molecular-weight iron.[8] Ferritin deposition in the form of hemosiderin may cause selective T2 shortening because of its paramagnetic magnetic susceptibility effect and resulting locally induced, magnetic field nonuniformity. A loss of spin coherence occurs and results in a shorter T2. Therefore, iron deposition within the liver may produce a striking low intensity on clinical images. It may be possible to quantitate the degree of iron deposition by determining the relaxation rates. To a lesser extent, a similar effect is produced by iron deposition in muscle, bone marrow, and pancreas.

GALLBLADDER

Most gallbladder pathology, including cholelithiasis, cholecystitis, obstructive disease, and neoplasm, is best evaluated with ultrasound. Ultrasound of the gallbladder is both economical and accurate. A further advantage of the modality is its ability to image the gallbladder along its long axis. It may define some causes of biliary obstruction. Ultrasound can only provide anatomical information, however. Functional information may be inferred by real-time ultrasound examination of a fasting patient before, during, and after ingestion of a fatty meal.

MRI is unlikely to replace ultrasound in the evaluation of the gallbladder because of its greater cost and relatively long imaging time. There have been several studies, however, examining the use of MRI in the assessment of gallbladder function. The normal gallbladder wall is able to absorb 90% of the water content of the bile within four hours after the gallbladder is filled. This gives rise to a shortened T1, presumably due to the elevated concentrations of bile, acid, and protein. Proton spectroscopy demonstrates no MR-visible lipid in gallbladder bile.[9] On a spin echo sequence with either T1- or T2-weighted images, bile in a normal fasting subject has a high signal intensity compared with adjacent liver tissue.[10] In patients with cholecystitis, the same pulsing sequence yields relatively lower signal intensities. This is attributed to the fact that the inflamed gallbladder fails to absorb water and may actually secrete fluid into its lumen, causing T1 prolongation and a lower signal intensity. Patients with chronic cholecystitis tend to have more concentrated bile than those with acute cholecystitis;[11] there is no

significant difference between the mean T1 and T2 values in these two groups, however.

PANCREAS

At present, CT is still considered the imaging modality of choice in the examination of the pancreas. This reflects the high spatial resolution of late generation scanners. Prolonged MR scanning times result in respiratory and peristaltic motion artifacts that cause difficulty in distinguishing pancreatic parenchyma from surrounding bowel, both of which have similar intermediate MR intensities.[12] It is generally very difficult to visualize the entire gland. As in ultrasound, the posterior portion of the pancreas is outlined by the splenic vein in MRI. The anterior border and pancreatic head are frequently obscured by overlying bowel. Oral contrast (e.g., Geritol or Feosol) is recommended for duodenal opacification.

Most pathologic processes involving the pancreas increase both the T1 and T2 relaxation times. It is therefore difficult to distinguish an inflammatory mass from a neoplasm. A pseudocyst may be demonstrated on MRI as a hyperintense mass on T2-weighted images. Pseudocyst margins are poorly defined by MRI, and these lesions are generally better demonstrated on CT. The CT hallmark of chronic pancreatitis, parenchymal calcification, is poorly demonstrated on MRI. A dilated pancreatic duct is also difficult to detect. Neoplastic changes of the pancreas produce a wide range of intensities, and tumors may be isointense with normal parenchyma. There has not been any study that has correlated the intensity of the lesion with the histologic type of the tumor. The presence of contour abnormalities or invasion of surrounding structures may be helpful. In the future, a shorter TR/TE sequence may help to improve the resolution of MR in evaluating pancreatic anatomy and pathology.

ADRENALS

The adrenal glands are, similarly to the pancreas, best evaluated with CT. Currently, there is experimental work being done with surface coils that improve the spatial resolution of retroperitoneal structures as well as reduce motion artifacts by limiting the field of view to the adrenal fossa.[1] Recently, adrenal mass characterization based on signal intensity has been described.[13,14] In comparing the signal intensity of the mass to that of the liver, nonfunctioning adenomas had lower relative signal intensity ratios on both the T1- and T2-weighted images. On the other hand, nonadenomas (e.g., metastases, carcinomas, and pheochromocytomas) had higher signal characteristics.

KIDNEYS[15]

There are several imaging modalities that are very competitive in the evaluation of the kidneys. Excretory urography in many cases remains the modality of choice, because it provides functional information and anatomic detail, especially of the collecting system. Excretory urography is somewhat insensitive and nonspecific in diagnosing renal masses, however, especially those that do not indent the caliceal system or produce contour abnormalities. Ultrasound is the best imaging modality in the evaluation of renal cysts. CT is the currently accepted imaging modality of choice in the evaluation of solid tumors. MRI may play a role in evaluation of the kidneys, but this has not yet been defined.

The anatomic definition of the kidney is best demonstrated on T1-weighted images since they provide the best contrast discrimination between renal parenchyma and perinephric fat, and between renal cortex and medulla. The renal cortex has a slightly higher intensity than that of the renal medulla.[16] Gerota's fascia is not consistently seen with MRI. The renal vasculature may be differentiated from the pelvicaliceal system by the presence of flow void, and the renal arteries or veins may be traced back to their proximal origins from the aorta or inferior vena cava. As expected, parenchymal calcifications and urinary calculi may remain totally undetected on MRI.

RENAL CYSTS[16]

Simple renal cysts are generally best demonstrated on T1-weighted images, and they appear as low intensity masses. The cyst wall may be poorly defined because of its thinness. There is a smooth interface with normal parenchyma, and the cyst contents should have a homogeneous appearance. Hemorrhagic cysts may appear as high intensity lesions on both T1- and T2-weighted images, depending on the amount of protein and methemoglobin inside the cyst cavity. In this case, differentiation from an inflammatory cyst or even a solid tumor may be difficult.

RENAL CELL CARCINOMA

Specificity in differentiating between the various types of solid renal neoplasms is poor. Renal cell carcinoma generally has a prolonged T1 but not as long as that of a cyst. The intensity of the tumor may vary from hypo- to hyperintense compared with that of renal parenchyma. Characteristically, the intensity patterns of these tumors are heterogeneous secondary to focal areas of necrosis and hemorrhage. The tumors may have irregular margins and evidence of either local invasion or distant metastases. Staging of the tumor is the most important potential role of MRI, and it may have an advantage over CT in the evaluation of perinephric fat or vascular invasion.[16]

CORTICOMEDULLARY JUNCTION

Various disease processes may affect the corticomedullary junction. MRI has been shown to demonstrate best this area on T1-weighted images. In the normal kidney the cortex has a shorter T1 than the medulla and therefore has a higher signal. The hydration state of a patient influences this differentiation between the cortex and medulla, and this becomes less distinct with dehydration. In renal transplant rejection, there is also loss of definition of the corticomedullary junction on T1-weighted images. Renal artery thrombosis may have a similar appearance. Conversely, acute tubular necrosis (ATN) has been noted to increase intensity differences between the cortex and the medulla; therefore, this may serve to distinguish ATN from renal transplant rejection.[16]

A tissue-specific diagnosis using MRI may also be possible in patients with paroxysmal nocturnal hemoglobinuria.[17] This disorder is characterized by complement-mediated erythrocyte lysis leading to hemosiderin deposition within the cortex. As seen with hepatic iron deposition disease, there is a decrease in the T2 relaxation time, resulting in a decrease of the cortical signal as compared with that of the medulla.

RETROPERITONEUM

Because MRI is excellent in defining the vasculature of the abdomen, it may play a significant role in distinguishing lymphadenopathy from vessels. This is a frequently encountered problem with CT studies performed for tumor staging, particularly if contrast enhancement is limited or not used. Initial work in demonstrating retroperitoneal fibrosis has also been described.[18]

REFERENCES

1. Stark DD, Ferrucci JT: Technical and clinical progress in MRI of the abdomen. *Diagn Imaging*, 1985;7:118–127.

2. Moss AA, Goldberg HI, Stark DD, et al: Hepatic tumors: Magnetic resonance and CT appearance. *Radiology* 1984;150:141–147.

3. Stark DD, Wittenberg J, Middleton MS, et al: Liver metastases: Detection by phase-contrast imaging. *Radiology* 1986;158:327–332.

4. Haaga JR: Magnetic resonance imaging of the liver. *Radiol Clin North Am* 1984;22:879–890.

5. Stark DD, Felder RC, Wittenberg J, et al: Magnetic resonance imaging of cavernous hemangioma of the liver: Tissue-specific characterization. *AJR* 1985;145:213–222.

6. Glazer GM, Aisen AM, Francis IR, et al: Hepatic cavernous hemangioma: Magnetic resonance imaging: Work in progress. *Radiology* 1985;155:417–420.

7. Lee JKT, Dixon WT, Ling D, et al: Fatty infiltration of the liver: Demonstration by proton spectroscopic imaging. *Radiology* 1984; 153:195–201.

8. Stark DD, Moseley ME, Bacon BR, et al: Magnetic resonance imaging and spectroscopy of hepatic iron overload. *Radiology* 1985; 154:137–142.

9. Demas BE, Hricak H, Mosley M, et al: Gallbladder bile: An experimental study in dogs using MR imaging and proton MR spectroscopy. *Radiology* 1985;157:453–455.

10. McCarthy S, Hricak H, Cohen M, et al: Cholecystitis: Detection with MR imaging. *Radiology* 1986;158:333–336.

11. Loflin TG, Simeone JF, Mueller PR, et al: Gallbladder bile in cholecystitis: In vitro MR evaluation. *Radiology* 1985;157:457–459.

12. Haaga JR: Magnetic resonance imaging of the pancreas. *Radiol Clin North Am* 1984;22:869–877.

13. Glazer GM, Woolsey EJ, Borrello J, et al: Adrenal tissue characterization using MR imaging. *Radiology* 1986;158:73–79.

14. Reinig JW, Doppman JL, Dwyer AJ, et al: Adrenal mass differentiated by MR. *Radiology* 1986;158:81–84.

15. Hricak H, Crooks L, Sheldon P, et al: Nuclear magnetic resonance imaging of the kidney. *Radiology* 1983;146:425–432.

16. LiPuma JP, Bryan PJ: Magnetic resonance imaging of the genitourinary tract, in Kressel HY (ed): *Magnetic Resonance Annual 1985*. New York, Raven Press, 1985, pp 149–196.

17. Mulopulos GP, Turner DA, Schwartz MM, et al: MRI of the kidneys in paroxysmal nocturnal hemoglobinuria. *AJR* 1986;146:51–52.

18. Degesys GE, Dunnick NR, Silverman PM, et al: Retroperitoneal fibrosis: Use of CT in distinguishing among possible causes. *AJR* 1986;146:57–60.

CASE 67

HISTORY

A 36-year-old man presents with abnormal liver function tests, hepatomegaly, diabetes mellitus, and bronze-colored skin.

QUESTIONS

1. What are your differential considerations?

   _____

   _____

2. What MR techniques would you use?

	1	2	3
a. Coil	____	____	____
b. Centering point	____	____	____
c. Imaging plane(s)	____	____	____
d. Contrast	____	____	____
e. Slice thickness	____	____	____

3. What do you expect to find?

   _____

   _____

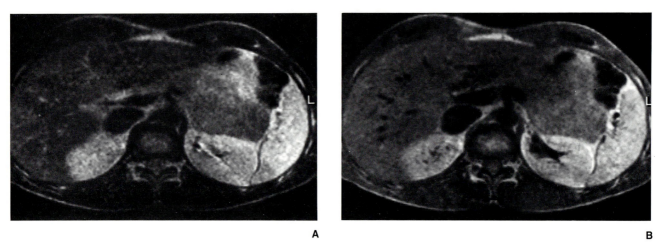

A   B

Figures 67.1A (SE 2000/28) and **67.1B** (SE 2000/56). Axial scans through the upper abdomen.

MR TECHNIQUES

	1	2
a. Coil	Body	Body
b. Centering point	Xyphoid	Xyphoid
c. Imaging planes	Axial	Axial
d. Contrast	Mild and moderate T2W	Moderate T1W
e. Slice thickness	Routine	Routine

These two sequences are our routine protocol for hepatic imaging.

MR FINDINGS

Figure 67.1. The liver is normal in size and shape and homogeneous in intensity. There is, however, a significant decrease in signal intensity of the liver on the second echo image compared with the first echo image. This indicates abnormal T2 shortening. Similar decreases in intensity are also seen in the marrow of the vertebral bodies and the paraspinal muscles.

DIFFERENTIAL DIAGNOSIS

The uniform shortening of both T1 and T2 of multiple organs is indicative of iron deposition disease, or hemochromatosis.[1,2] As discussed in the introductory section on hepatic iron overload, the relaxation rates of the liver (1/T1 and 1/T2) are influenced by the presence of low-molecular-weight iron and ferritin. The overall effect is to decrease the signal intensity of the liver parenchyma.

The causes of hemochromatosis include idiopathic sources, familial disorders of erythropoiesis, multiple transfusions, and excessive intake of iron.

The clinical findings reflect the systemic, multiorgan involvement from iron deposition and include bronze discoloration of the skin, diabetes mellitus, arthritis, and hepatic failure.

Final Diagnosis

Hemochromatosis.

SUMMARY OF MR FINDINGS FOR HEMOCHROMATOSIS

1. Multiorgan involvement
2. Liver
   a. Hepatomegaly
   b. Uniform low signal intensity due to T2 shortening effect.
3. Muscle, pancreas, and bone marrow may have changes similar to those seen in the liver, depending on the amount of iron deposited.

REFERENCES

1. Brasch RC, Wesbey GE, Gooding CA, et al: Magnetic resonance imaging of transfusional hemosiderosis complicating thalassemia major. *Radiology* 1984;150:767–771.
2. Leung AWL, Steiner RE, Young IR: NMR imaging of the liver in two cases of iron overload. *JCAT* 1984;8:446–449.

CASE 68

HISTORY

This 57-year-old woman had undergone a right mastectomy for breast cancer 15 years earlier. She was found to have a solitary enhancing lesion on a recent CT scan of the liver (Figure 68.1).

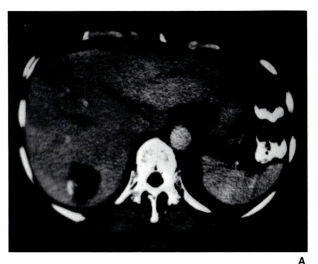
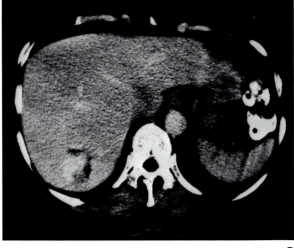

A   B

Figures 68.1A (early) and **68.1B** (late). Two axial images from a dynamic CT scan of the liver following a bolus injection of contrast material.

QUESTIONS

1. What are your differential considerations?

_____

_____

2. What MR techniques would you use?

	1	2	3
a. Coil	___	___	___
b. Centering point	___	___	___
c. Imaging plane(s)	___	___	___
d. Contrast	___	___	___
e. Slice thickness	___	___	___

3. What do you expect to find?

_____

_____

Source: Courtesy of Alan Wagman, MD, Canoga Park, CA.

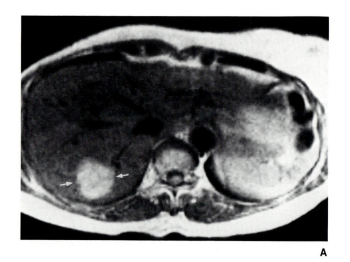 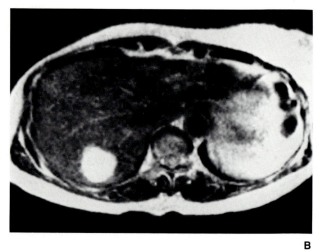

A   B

Figures 68.2A (SE 2000/28) and **68.2B** (SE 2000/56). Axial scans through the right lobe of the liver.

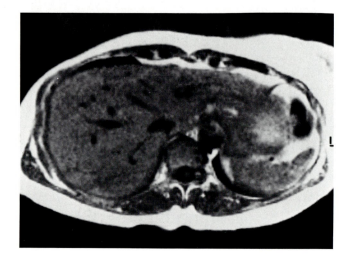

Figure 68.3 (SE 500/28). Axial scan at the same level as in Figure 68.2.

MR TECHNIQUES

	1	2
a. Coil	Body	Body
b. Centering point	Xyphoid	Xyphoid
c. Imaging planes	Axial	Axial
d. Contrast	Mild and moderate T2W	Moderate T1W
e. Slice thickness	Routine	Routine

These two pulsing sequences are our routine protocol for screening liver disease. The first sequence with T2 weighting is designed to detect lesions with a prolonged T2. The second sequence with T1 weighting is to provide additional anatomic definition and to enhance lesions with long or short T1.

MR FINDINGS

Figure 68.1. There is a well-defined, low-density lesion in the posterior segment of the right lobe of the liver. In Figure 68.1A, which is the first image from a dynamic CT scan, there is slight enhancement along the posterolateral wall of the mass. In Figure 68.1B, which is the eighth image, most of the mass is enhanced by contrast. This is the typical appearance of a liver hemangioma on dynamic CT.[1]

Figure 68.2. On MR examination, the mass (small white arrows) appears well circumscribed, homogeneous, and high in signal intensity. The mass becomes significantly brighter on the more T2-weighted second echo image, indicating a prolonged T2.

Figure 68.3. On this T1-weighted image, the mass is slightly hypointense compared with liver parenchyma, indicating a minimally prolonged T1.

DIFFERENTIAL DIAGNOSIS

The findings described are quite characteristic of a cavernous hemangioma. The marked T2 prolongation, well-defined borders, and homogeneity of the intensity have been reported as features distinguishing hemangiomas from primary and metastatic tumors of the liver.[2–4] These signs are not 100% specific, however. T2 values of hemangiomas and malignant tumors may overlap, and textures are occasionally similar. Compared with other modalities, MRI may be more sensitive in the detection of hemangioma, with a reported sensitivity as high as 100%;[2] it should be noted, however, that this study was retrospective and the MRI was performed after the diagnosis of hemangioma had been made by other modalities.

Final Diagnosis

Cavernous hemangioma of the liver.

SUMMARY OF MR FINDINGS FOR HEPATIC CAVERNOUS HEMANGIOMA

1. A well-defined, homogeneous, long-T2 mass within the liver parenchyma on a T2WI. The size of the lesion varies, and mass effect may occasionally be demonstrated (Figure 68.4).

2. The mass may be hypointense or isointense with the liver parenchyma on a T1WI, indicating slight prolongation of T1.

3. There may be multiple lesions, simulating liver metastases. Distinguishing points may be the absence of a known primary tumor, the longer T2, and the homogeneity of the intensity pattern. For comparison, Figure 68.5 demonstrates the MR findings that can be seen with liver metastases.

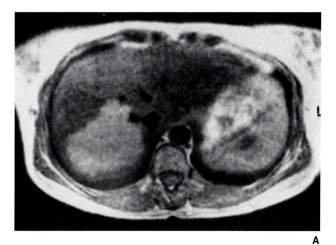

A

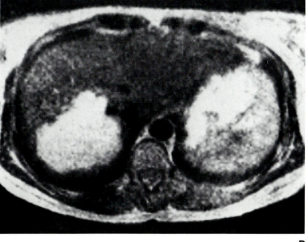

B

Figures 68.4A (SE 2000/28) and **68.4B** (SE 2000/56). Axial scan of the liver from another patient, demonstrating a large, irregularly marginated, high intensity, homogeneous mass involving most of the right lobe of the liver. There is slight mass effect, as shown by the distortion of the portal and hepatic venous structures. This was a proven hemangioma.

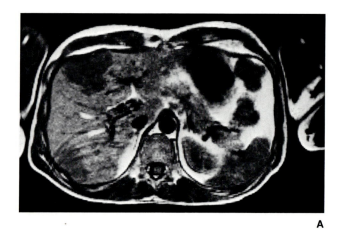

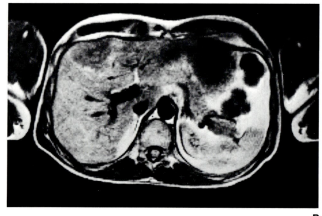

A

B

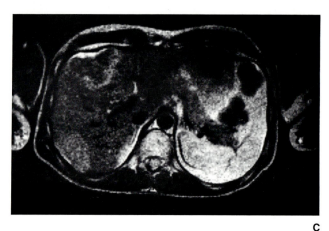

Figures 68.5A (SE 300/30), **68.5B** (SE 2000/35), and **68.5C** (SE 2000/90). Liver metastases from adenocarcinoma of the colon. In comparison with hemangiomas, the lesion is more heterogeneous and not as intense on the moderate (second echo) T2WI (Courtesy of Lee Radford, MD, Dallas, TX).

C

REFERENCES

1. Johnson CM, Sheedy PF II, Stanson AW, et al: Computed tomography and angiography of cavernous hemangioma of the liver. *Radiology* 1981;138:115.

2. Stark DD, Felder RC, Wittenberg J, et al: Magnetic resonance imaging of cavernous hemangioma of the liver. Tissue-specific characterization. *AJR* 1985;145:213–222.

3. Glazer GM, Aisen AM, Francis IR, et al: Hepatic cavernous hemangioma: Magnetic resonance imaging: work in progress. *Radiology* 1985;155:417–420.

4. Ohtomo K, Itai Y, Furui S, et al: Hepatic tumors: Differentiation by transverse relaxation time (T2) of magnetic resonance imaging. *Radiology* 1985;155:421–423.

CASE 69

HISTORY

A 70-year-old woman with a history of breast carcinoma. Hepatic imaging was performed to exclude metastases. An enhanced CT of the liver is shown in Figure 69.1.

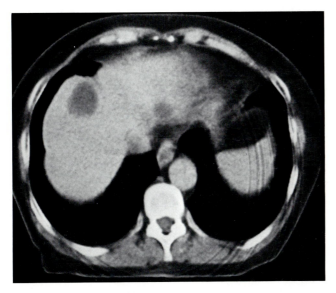

Figure 69.1. Axial enhanced CT through the dome of the liver. The mean intensity of the lesion is 4.7 HU.

QUESTIONS

1. What are your differential considerations?

_____

_____

2. What MR techniques would you use?

	1	2	3
a. Coil	_____	_____	_____
b. Centering point	_____	_____	_____
c. Imaging plane(s)	_____	_____	_____
d. Contrast	_____	_____	_____
e. Slice thickness	_____	_____	_____

3. What do you expect to find?

_____

_____

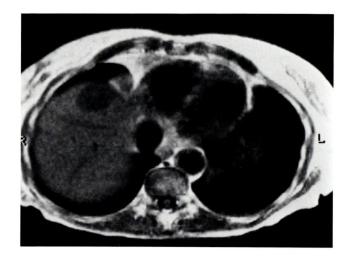

Figures 69.2 (SE 1000/28). Mildly T1-weighted axial scan through the dome of the liver.

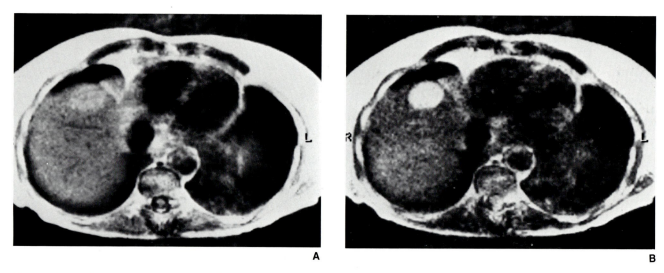

A   B

Figures 69.3A (SE 2000/28) and **69.3B** (SE 2000/56). Mildly and moderately T2-weighted axial scans at the same level as Figure 69.2.

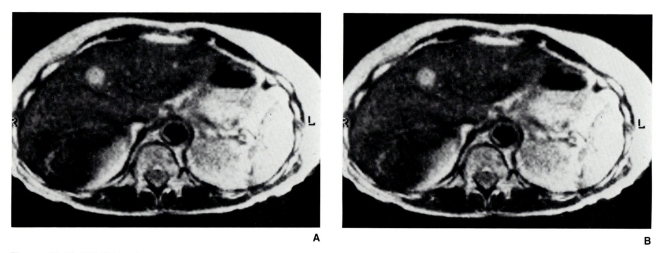

A   B

Figures 69.4A (SE 2000/28) and **69.4B** (SE 2000/56). Axial scans 4 cm inferior to Figure 69.3.

350

MR TECHNIQUES

	1	2
a. Coil	Body	Body
b. Centering point	Xyphoid	Xyphoid
c. Imaging planes	Axial	Axial
d. Contrast	Mild T1W and mild T2W	Mild and moderate T2W
e. Slice thickness	Routine	Routine

A mildly T1-weighted sequence was used initially to examine both the lower mediastinum and the upper abdomen. Such a sequence provides the greatest contrast between fat and organ parenchyma and can be utilized effectively to define organ size and contour. This sequence is moderately sensitive in the detection of focal intrahepatic lesions. The second pulsing sequence was performed with mild and moderate T2 weighting to characterize hepatic pathology further.

MR FINDINGS

Figure 69.1. The axial CT demonstrates a 3-cm, rounded, sharply circumscribed, homogeneous, low-density lesion without enhancement in the medial segment of the left lobe of the liver. The attenuation value of 4 HU suggests the lesion is cystic.

Figure 69.2. On this moderate T1WI, the lesion is homogeneously low in signal intensity, indicating a prolonged T1.

Figure 69.3. On the mild and moderate T2WI, the lesion is high in signal intensity compared with liver parenchyma, indicating prolongation of T2.

Figure 69.4. The more caudal scan demonstrates a smaller lesion with similar characteristics in the same segment of the liver.

DIFFERENTIAL DIAGNOSIS

The most likely cause of multiple lesions in the liver is metastatic disease, particularly in a patient with a history of breast carcinoma. Multiple cavernous hemangiomas and liver cysts should also be considered, however. The MR signal intensity pattern is nonspecific and can be seen with any one of the three entities. The cystic nature of these lesions shown on CT, however, would be unusual for either breast metastases or cavernous hemangiomas. A follow-up sonogram (not shown) confirmed that the lesions were simple cysts.

The case illustrates the relative lack of specificity of MRI compared with CT and ultrasound. One advantage of MRI compared with CT is its greater contrast resolution, resulting in increased sensitivity in detecting liver lesions.

Final Diagnosis

Multiple hepatic cysts.

SUMMARY OF MR FINDINGS FOR HEPATIC CYSTS[1]

1. Rounded and well-circumscribed lesions with smooth borders.
2. The internal signal intensity of the lesions is homogeneous.

   a. Prolonged T1 produces low signal intensity on T1WI.
   b. Prolonged T2 produces high signal intensity on T2WI. The intensity of hepatic cysts on T2WI, however, may not be as great as that of cavernous hemangiomas (see Case 68) because of the latter lesions' shorter T1.

3. If of sufficient size, mass effect may be demonstrated. A patient's large hepatic cyst that exhibits these features is shown on Figure 69.5. The cyst, with mass effect, demonstrates prolonged T1 (Figure 69.5A) and T2 relaxation times (Figures 69.5B and 69.5C) compared with liver parenchyma.
4. Multiple cysts are frequently seen, especially in association with polycystic kidney disease.
5. Cysts may be difficult to differentiate from metastases and cavernous hemangiomas on the basis of MR findings alone.

REFERENCE

1. Haaga JR: Magnetic resonance imaging of the liver. *Radiol Clin North Am* 1984;22:879–890.

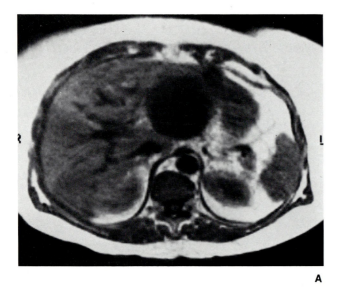

A

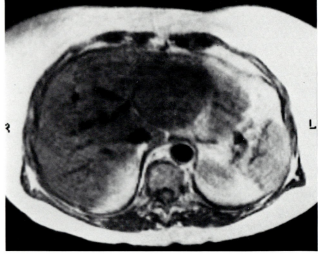

B

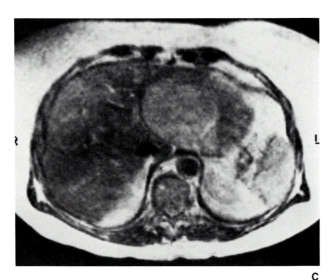

C

Figures 69.5A (SE 500/30), **69.5B** (2000/30), and **69.5C** (SE 2000/60). Axial scan of the liver demonstrating a large cyst in the lateral segment of the left lobe of the liver. The signal intensity pattern is not exactly the same as that of the reference case. This is probably due to slight variations in the protein content.

CASE 70

HISTORY

A 78-year-old woman presenting with enlarging, tender, right upper quadrant mass. There was no history of liver disease. A liver/spleen scan is shown in Figure 70.1.

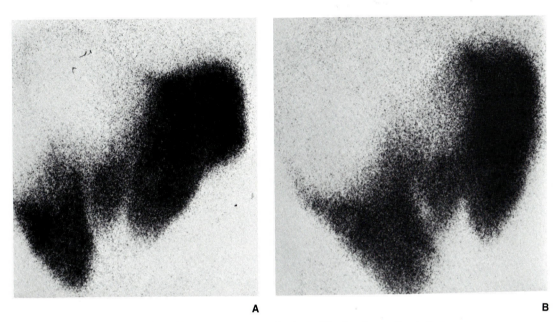

Figure 70.1. (A) Anterior and (B) right anterior oblique projections of the liver from a liver/spleen scan.

QUESTIONS

1. What are your differential considerations?

2. What MR techniques would you use?

	1	2	3
a. Coil	——	——	——
b. Centering point	——	——	——
c. Imaging plane(s)	——	——	——
d. Contrast	——	——	——
e. Slice thickness	——	——	——

3. What do you expect to find?

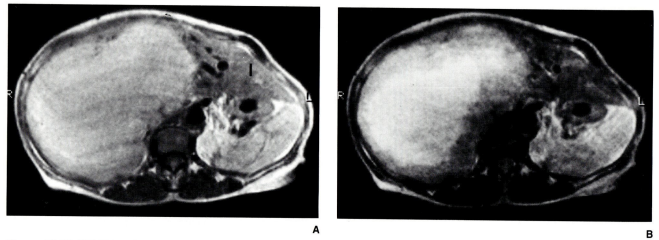

A

B

Figures 70.2A (SE 2000/30) and **70.2B** (SE 2000/60). Axial scans through the midportion of the liver.

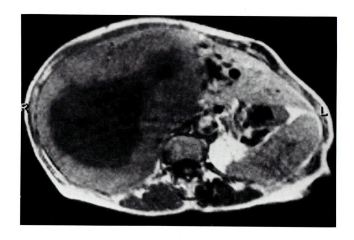

Figure 70.3 (SE 500/30). T1-weighted axial scan through the same level as Figure 70.2.

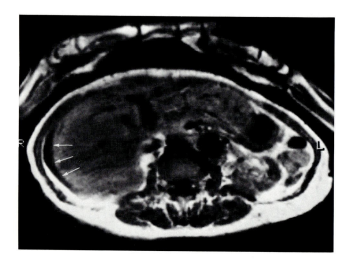

Figure 70.4 (SE 500/30). Axial image through the inferior portion of the right lobe of the liver.

MR TECHNIQUES

	1	2
a. Coil	Body	Body
b. Centering point	8 cm below xyphoid process	
c. Imaging planes	Axial	Axial
d. Contrast	Mild to moderate T2W	Moderate T1W
e. Slice thickness	Routine	Routine

The above pulsing sequences represent our standard screening protocol for the liver, as described in the introductory section.

MR FINDINGS

Figure 70.1. There is a large photopenic mass replacing most of the right lobe of the liver. The spleen is normal.

Figure 70.2. A large, well-circumscribed, heterogeneous mass is seen replacing most of the right lobe as well as the medial segment of the left lobe of the liver. The signal intensity of the tumor is greater than that of the normal lateral segment of the left lobe. On the second echo image, the central portion of the tumor becomes significantly higher in intensity, indicating prolongation of T2, presumably secondary to tumor necrosis. Note the lack of the normal signal void in the expected position of the intrahepatic portion of the inferior vena cava, suggesting compression and/or obstruction of this vessel.

Figure 70.3. On this T1WI, the central area of necrosis is low in intensity, indicating prolongation of T1 due to the increase in water content. The signal intensity of the wall of the tumor is noted to be lower than that of the normal portion of the left lobe.

Figure 70.4. A curvilinear low intensity band is seen along the lateral aspect of the tumor (arrows), representing ascites in the right subphrenic space.

DIFFERENTIAL DIAGNOSIS

The signal intensity pattern of MRI is nonspecific for hepatic tumors; however, this solitary, large hepatic mass most likely represents a hepatoma. Metastases tend to be smaller and multicentric. Rarely, metastases from infiltrating tumors, such as carcinoid and aggressive lymphoma, may have a similar appearance.

Final Diagnosis

Hepatoma.

SUMMARY OF MR FINDINGS FOR HEPATOMA

1. There are four types of hepatomas:[1]

   a. Sixty percent present as multiple nodules.
   b. Five percent present as diffusely infiltrating tumors. This type is invariably seen in patients with cirrhosis.
   c. Thirty percent present as a large mass with multiple satellite lesions.
   d. The remaining few percent present as an encapsulated mass, as in this case.

2. Signal intensity patterns:[2]

   a. Prolongation of T1 produces low signal intensity on T1WIs.
   b. Prolongation of T2 produces high signal intensity on T2WIs.

3. In tumors of sufficient size, central necrosis is frequently seen. Characteristically, the necrotic portion is heterogeneous and has longer T1 and T2 relaxation times than the surrounding tumor tissue.

4. Displacement and/or invasion of the hepatic vasculature may be demonstrated.[1]

REFERENCES

1. Lawson TL, Berland LL, Foley WD: Pancreas, liver and biliary tract, in Bragg DG, Rubin P, Youker JE (eds): *Oncologic Imaging*. New York, Pergamon Press, 1985, pp 287–342.
2. Moss AA, Goldberg HI, Stark DD, et al: Hepatic tumors: Magnetic resonance and CT appearance. *Radiology* 1984;150:141–147.

CASE 71

HISTORY

A 55-year-old woman presenting with a 4-month history of right-sided abdominal pain and hematuria. Physical examination revealed a large right flank mass. An enhanced CT is shown in Figure 71.1. A sonogram was also performed and appears in Figure 71.2.

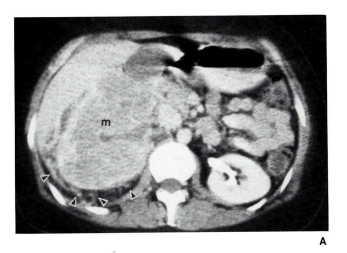
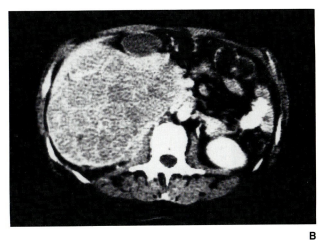

Figures 71.1A and **71.1B.** (A) Axial enhanced CT scan through the renal hili. (B) Axial CT 2 cm inferior to Figure 71.1A and with a narrower window setting.

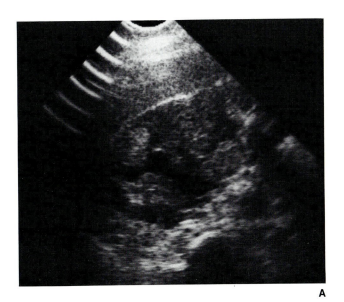
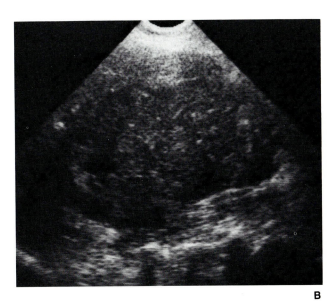

Figure 71.2. (A) Transverse and (B) longitudinal sonograms through the mass.

QUESTIONS

1. What are your differential considerations?

   _____

   _____

2. What MR techniques would you use?

	1	2	3
a. Coil	___	___	___
b. Centering point	___	___	___
c. Imaging plane(s)	___	___	___
d. Contrast	___	___	___
e. Slice thickness	___	___	___

3. What do you expect to find?

   _____

   _____

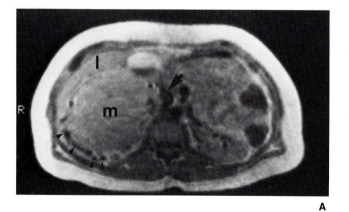
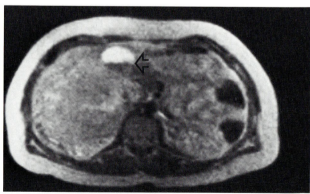

A **B**

Figures 71.3A (SE 2000/28) and **71.3B** (SE 2000/56). Axial scans through the same level as Figure 71.1.

MR TECHNIQUES

	1	2 (not shown)
a. Coil	Body	Body
b. Centering point	8 cm below the xyphoid process	
c. Imaging planes	Axial	Axial
d. Contrast	Mild and moderate T2W	Mild T1W and mild T2W
e. Slice thickness	Routine	Routine

A pulsing sequence with mild T2 weighting was chosen in an attempt to distinguish between tumor, which has a prolonged T2, and normal renal parenchyma. An additional advantage of a relatively long TR is that it makes it possible for a greater area of the abdomen to be examined with a single acquisition. The axial plane is standard for abdominal imaging. The T1-weighted sequence was used to better separate tumor from perinephric fat and to demonstrate nodal metastases.

MR FINDINGS

Figure 71.1. In Figure 71.1A, there is a large, heterogeneous right renal mass (m), with relatively lower density than the normal left kidney. The margin of the mass is slightly irregular owing to the presence of numerous curvilinear densities (arrowheads) within the perinephric space. The inferior vena cava is displaced anteromedially by the mass. In Figure 71.1B, there are numerous linear densities identified within the mass, suggesting septation in a multiloculated cyst.

Figure 71.2. The abdominal sonogram demonstrates that the mass is solid.

Figure 71.3. On this moderate T2WI, the mass (m) has a relatively well-defined border and is isointense with the liver (l) and the left kidney. There are numerous small, circular, low intensity foci (arrowheads) surrounding the mass, corresponding to the curvilinear densities seen on CT. Based on the MR findings alone, these low intensity foci could represent air, calcium, or rapidly flowing blood. Since neither air nor calcification was seen on the CT scan, these foci most likely represent parasitized capsular renal arteries. Note the markedly compressed IVC (closed arrow) being displaced anteromedially. The right renal vein cannot be adequately visualized. An incidental finding is the low- and high intensity fluid–fluid layer (open arrow) within the gallbladder. As discussed in the introductory chapter, this finding indicates an abnormally functioning gallbladder.

DIFFERENTIAL DIAGNOSIS

The findings are compatible with a hypervascular solid mass within the right kidney. Statistically, this most likely represents a renal cell carcinoma. As discussed in the introductory section, the value of MRI is not in determining the cell type of the tumor but rather in preoperative staging. Tumor extension into the renal vein and/or inferior vena cava is readily demonstrated, as is local tumor invasion into the liver or abdominal wall. In the reference case, the renal vein was poorly seen; however, a patent renal vein and IVC are well demonstrated on a coronal view (Figure 71.4B) from another patient with renal cell carcinoma. In Figure 71.4A, the axial view clearly demonstrated invasion of the adjacent abdominal musculature (arrow).

It should be emphasized that the loss of fascial planes between tumor and adjacent organs does not necessarily

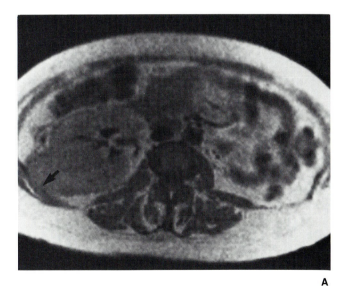

A

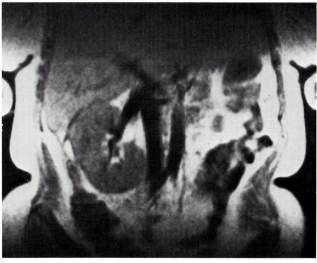

B

Figures 71.4A and 71.4B. MR scans from another patient with clear cell carcinoma of the right kidney. (A: SE 1000/28). Axial scan through the midportion of the right kidney. (B: SE 500/28). Coronal scan through the right kidney and right renal vein.

indicate direct tumor invasion. The fascia and/or renal capsule may be stretched so thin that it may not be seen on either MRI or CT. In Figures 71.1A and 71.3, there was poor separation of the tumor and the adjacent liver, suggesting possible hepatic invasion. The liver, however, was found not to be involved at surgery.

Final Diagnosis

Renal cell carcinoma.

SUMMARY OF MR FINDINGS FOR RENAL CELL CARCINOMA

1. Renal masses of varying size. Small lesions (less than 2 cm) are difficult to detect with CT, ultrasound, or MRI.[1]
2. Depending on the size of the tumor, there may be contour abnormalities, mass effect, and displacement and/or compression of the vascular structures.
3. Compared with renal parenchyma, tumor intensity may vary from hypo- to hyperintense, depending on the pulsing sequence used. The intensity pattern is usually inhomogeneous secondary to focal areas of necrosis and hemorrhage.[2]

4. One may see parasitized vessels (Figure 71.3). This finding has been found to have a poor prognostic significance, with a 5-year survival rate of only 33%.[3]
5. Central tumoral calcification may be demonstrated on CT but is difficult to appreciate on MRI.
6. Robson's staging of renal cell carcinoma[4]

   Stage I: Tumor confined to kidney
   Stage II: Tumor spread to perinephric fat but within Gerota's fascia
   Stage IIIA: Tumor spread to renal vein
   Stage IIIB: Tumor spread to local lymph nodes
   Stage IIIC: Tumor spread to local vessels and lymph nodes
   Stage IVA: Tumor spread to adjacent organ
   Stage IVB: Distant metastasis

REFERENCES

1. McClennan BL, Baife DM: Kidney and ureter, in Bragg DG, Rubin P, Youker JE (eds): *Oncologic Imaging*. New York, Pergamon Press, 1985; pp 363–387.
2. LiPuma JP, Bryan PJ: Magnetic resonance imaging of the genitourinary tract, in Kressel HY (ed): *Magnetic Resonance Annual 1985*. New York, Raven Press, 1985, pp 149–196.
3. Wong WS, Cochran ST, Boxer RJ: Radiographic grading system for renal cell carcinoma with clinical and pathological correlation. *Radiology* 1982;144:61–65.
4. Robson CJ, Churchill RM, Anderson W: The results of radical nephrectomy for renal cell carcinoma. *J Urol* 1969;101:297–301.

CASE 72

HISTORY

A 5-year-old girl presenting with a large right upper abdominal mass. A chest x-ray (Figure 72.1) and an excretory urogram (Figure 72.2) were performed. A contrast-enhanced CT (Figures 72.3 and 72.4) was also obtained. MRI was requested for further evaluation.

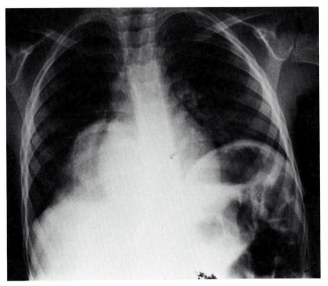

Figure 72.1. PA chest x-ray.

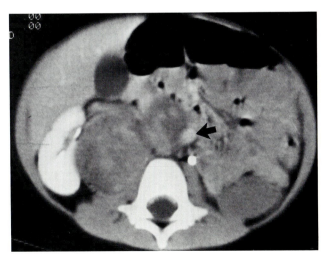

Figure 72.2. Excretory urogram.

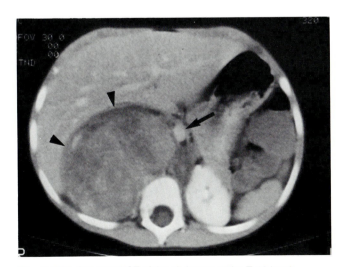

Figure 72.3. Enhanced CT of the abdomen at the T-12 level.

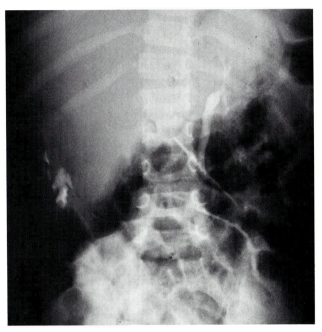

Figure 72.4. Enhanced CT of the abdomen at the L-3 level.

QUESTIONS

1. What are your differential considerations?

   _____

   _____

2. What MR techniques would you use?

	1	2	3
a. Coil	___	___	___
b. Centering point	___	___	___
c. Imaging plane(s)	___	___	___
d. Contrast	___	___	___
e. Slice thickness	___	___	___

3. What do you expect to find?

   _____

   _____

Note: Figures 72.1 to 72.4 Courtesy of Philip Stanley, MD, Los Angeles, CA.

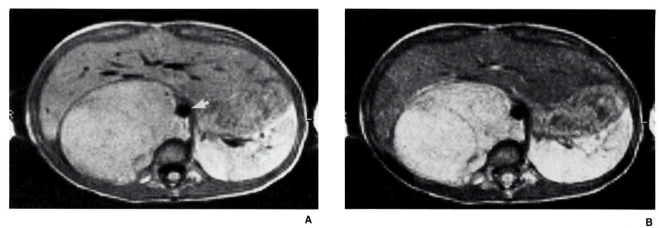

A B

Figures 72.5A (SE 1000/28) and **72.5B** (SE 1000/56). Axial scan of the upper abdomen at the T-11 level.

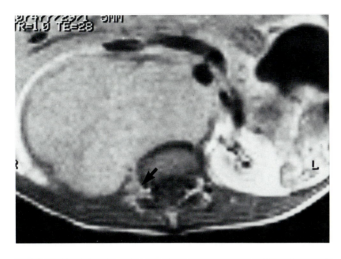

Figure 72.6 (SE 1000/28). Magnified axial view of the spine at the L-1 level.

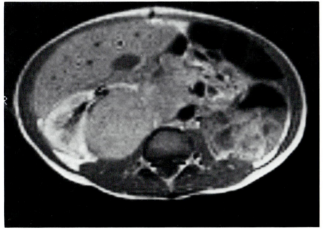

A

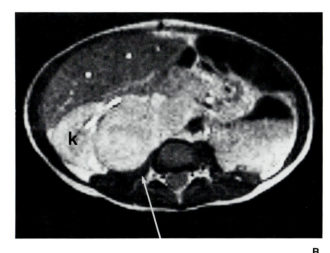

B

Figures 72.7A (SE 1000/28) and **72.7B** (SE 1000/56). Axial scans at the L-3 level.

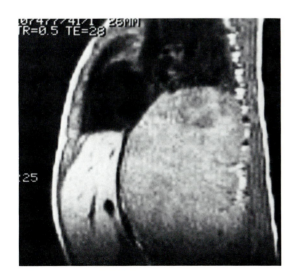

Figure 72.8 (SE 500/28). Parasagittal scan 2 cm to the right of midline.

MR TECHNIQUES

		1	2
a.	Coil	Head	Head
b.	Centering point	L-1 level	Midline
c.	Imaging planes	Axial	Sagittal
d.	Contrast	Mild T1W/ mild T2W	Moderate T1W
e.	Slice thickness	Thin	Thin

For improved signal-to-noise in this pediatric patient, a head coil was used rather than the standard adult body coil. The pulsing sequences were performed with T1 weighting to optimize anatomic definition and to limit scanning time. The first pulsing sequence was performed in the axial plane with a TR of 1,000 mseconds providing coverage of 10 cm. This is sufficient to examine the upper abdomen of a child. Thin slices were chosen to evaluate more accurately possible intraspinal tumor extension. The second sequence was performed in the sagittal plane to assess the longitudinal extent of the tumor better.

MR FINDINGS

Figure 72.1. The PA chest x-ray demonstrates a large, soft tissue mass in the right lower lung superimposed on the right cardiac border.

Figure 72.2. On the excretory urogram, the mass extends into the right upper abdomen with inferior and lateral displacement of the right kidney.

Figures 72.3 and 72.4. On this contrast-enhanced CT scan, the mass is shown to have a well-defined border and an heterogeneous density pattern. It extends superiorly through the right subcrural space (arrowheads) into the thorax. It extends medially across the midline, displacing the aorta (arrow) anteriorly and to the left. The right kidney is displaced inferiorly and laterally. There is no evidence of tumor extension into the spinal canal on CT. No calcification is identified within the mass.

Figure 72.5. The mass is homogeneous and hyperintense on the first echo image. The mass remains hyperintense on the second echo image but becomes slightly heterogeneous. There is a well-defined, low intensity rim surrounding the mass, which may represent a capsule and/or the right crus of the diaphragm (arrow—abdominal aorta).

Figure 72.6. On this magnified view of the spine at the L-1 level, the tumor appears to extend into a slightly widened, right neural foramen (arrow). This was not appreciated on the CT scan.

Figure 72.7. More inferiorly, the displaced right kidney (k) is again demonstrated. The mass is shown to abut the right psoas muscle (arrow), which has a normal intensity, indicating that the muscle has not been invaded by tumor.

Figure 72.8. The intrathoracic extension of the tumor is better demonstrated on this parasagittal scan. The mass has a more heterogeneous texture on this more heavily T1WI.

DIFFERENTIAL DIAGNOSIS

In a young child presenting with a large abdominal mass, the major consideration is a Wilm's tumor or a neuroblastoma. The mass is shown by excretory urogram, CT, and MRI to be extrinsic to the right kidney; hence, a Wilm's tumor is unlikely. The suprarenal, paraspinal location of this mass is consistent with a neuroblastoma. The intrathoracic and intraspinal extension of the tumor are also compatible with this diagnosis. On CT, however, neuroblastomas characteristically have an irregular shape, a mixed low-density center, and focal calcification. None of these features were seen in this case. In addition, the tumor capsule seen on MRI is atypical for neuroblastoma.[1] The presence of a capsule suggests that the tumor grows slowly or is benign.

The benign counterpart or mature form of a neuroblastoma is a ganglioneuroma. Like neuroblastomas, these tumors arise from the sympathetic ganglia and the adrenal medulla. Unlike neuroblastomas, ganglioneuromas are more common in females. These tumors generally cause symptoms by local expansion.[2] All the preceding MR and CT findings are consistent with this diagnosis.

At surgery, a large ganglioneuroma with intraspinal extension at the L-1 level was discovered, confirming the MR findings.

Final Diagnosis

Ganglioneuroma.

SUMMARY OF MR FINDINGS FOR GANGLIONEUROMA

1. Abdominal mass located in the suprarenal and paraspinal area in children.
2. Posterior mediastinal mass in adults.[3]
3. Homogeneous intensity pattern with prolonged T2.
4. Low intensity tumor capsule.
5. Occasional intraspinal extension.[3]

REFERENCES

1. Grossman H, Kirks DR: Pediatric oncology, in Bragg DG, Rubin P, Youker JE (eds): *Oncologic Imaging*. New York, Pergamon Press, 1985, pp 549–571.
2. Moss AA: Computed tomography of the adrenal glands, in Moss AA, Gamsu G, Genant HK (eds): *Computed Tomography of the Body*. Philadelphia, WB Saunders Co, 1983, pp 837–876.
3. Anderson RE, Bragg DG, Youker JE: Brain and spinal cord neoplasms, in Bragg DG, Rubin P, Youker JE (eds): *Oncologic Imaging*. New York, Pergamon Press, 1985, pp 23–45.

CASE 73

HISTORY

A 57-year-old woman presenting with a history of night sweats and a left inguinal nodule. The inguinal nodule was biopsied, and a diagnosis of nodular, mixed-cell (non-Hodgkin's) lymphoma was made. A staging CT examination (Figure 73.1) was performed, during which the patient developed an allergic reaction to the contrast material. An MR examination was requested as a baseline for comparison with subsequent exams.

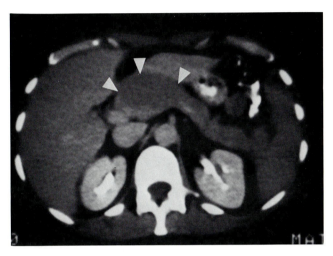

Figure 73.1. Enhanced axial CT scan through the pancreas.

QUESTIONS

1. What are your differential considerations?

_____

_____

2. What MR techniques would you use?

	1	2	3
a. Coil	___	___	___
b. Centering point	___	___	___
c. Imaging plane(s)	___	___	___
d. Contrast	___	___	___
e. Slice thickness	___	___	___

3. What do you expect to find?

_____

_____

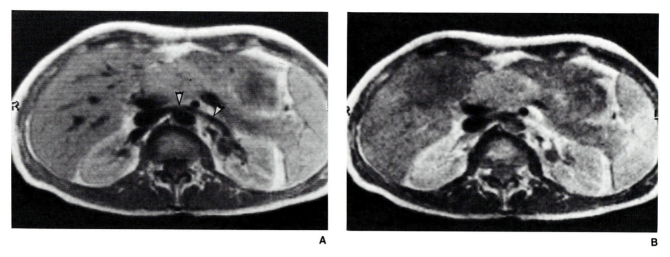

Figures 73.2A (SE 1000/28) and **73.2B** (SE 1000/56). Axial scans through the body of the pancreas.

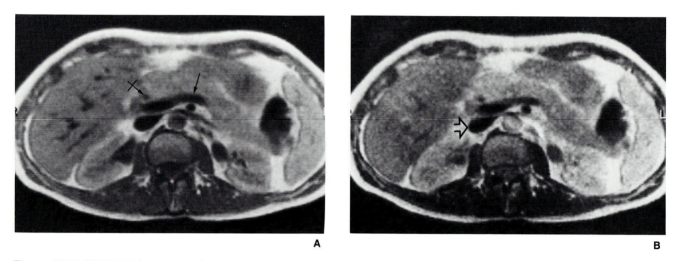

Figures 73.3A (SE 1000/28) and **73.3B** (SE 1000/56). Axial scans 1 cm inferior to Figure 73.2.

MR TECHNIQUES

a. Coil   Body
b. Centering point   Epigastrium
c. Imaging plane   Axial
d. Contrast   Mild T1W and mild T2W
e. Slice thickness   Routine

In light of the CT findings, a mildly T1-weighted sequence was chosen in an effort to accentuate the difference in intensities between the pancreas and the mesenteric fat. T1-weighted sequences are also the most effective way of evaluating abdominal and pelvic lymphadenopathy. Because shorter TR times limit the number of sections obtained, several sequences may be required to examine a large area.

MR FINDINGS

Figure 73.1. There is a relatively well defined and slightly lobulated mass involving the head and a portion of the body of the pancreas. The density of the mass is similar to that of the pancreatic parenchyma. Note the enhancement of the splenic vein outlining the posterior portion of the pancreas.

Figures 73.2 and 73.3. The mass seen in Figure 73.1 is well demonstrated on these mild T1WIs. This mass has an intensity slightly greater than that of the pancreatic parenchyma and is brighter on the second echo image, indicating a prolonged T2. The intensity pattern of the mass is relatively homogeneous. The common bile duct (crossed arrow) is not dilated and is seen as a signal void area just lateral to the mass. Note how well the splenic vein (solid arrow), left renal vein (arrowheads), and inferior vena cava (open arrowhead) are demonstrated. The unusual high signal intensity seen within the lumen of the aorta is probably due to a combination of diastolic pseudogating and even-echo rephasing.[1]

DIFFERENTIAL DIAGNOSIS

The differential diagnosis for a mass in the pancreatic region includes *focal pancreatitis, pancreatic tumor,* and *peripancreatic adenopathy*. Since most pathologic processes involving the pancreas increase both the T1 and the T2 relaxation times, differentiating between these entities on the basis of MR (or CT) findings alone is not possible.

Focal pancreatitis is unlikely in this patient because she did not have any abdominal symptoms and her serum amylase level was normal.

Pancreatic carcinoma or other pancreatic neoplasms are certainly strong considerations in this case. The lack of biliary ductal obstruction, however, would be unusual for a mass this size located in the head of the pancreas. In addition, in this patient with known non-Hodgkin's lymphoma, a simultaneous primary pancreatic tumor would be uncommon.

Although a metastasis to the pancreatic parenchyma may be considered, this would be an unusual site of involvement by non-Hodgkin's lymphoma.[3] In addition, lymphoma tends to infiltrate and would likely present as diffuse enlargement of the pancreas rather than as a focal lesion. Therefore, the most likely diagnosis in this case is *peripancreatic adenopathy* due to lymphoma. In our experience, peripancreatic adenopathy is less likely to cause biliary ductal dilatation than pancreatic tumor or focal pancreatitis. This is only a minor differential point, however.

The patient received chemotherapy for approximately 5 months. She returned for a follow-up MR scan (Figure 73.4). The mass has decreased significantly in size in the interim, and only minimal residual disease is seen. This is identifiable only by the subtle intensity difference between the tumor (arrowhead) and the remainder of the pancreas.

Comment

One distinct advantage of MRI compared with CT is illustrated in this case; that is, the tumor may be demonstrated without the use of intravenous contrast material. In patients with contrast allergy, this allows follow-up examinations without the need of premedication or the risk of a serious reaction.

One may consider percutaneous needle biopsy of this mass for cytologic examination. The inability to guide needle biopsy is one of the major disadvantages of MRI compared with CT. This disadvantage is less pertinent in this case, as lymphoma is difficult to diagnose by fine needle aspiration.

Final Diagnosis

Peripancreatic adenopathy secondary to non-Hodgkin's lymphoma.

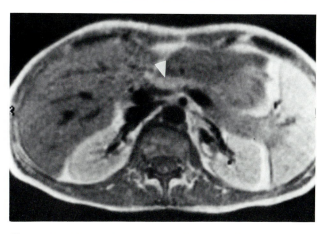

Figure 73.4 (SE 2000/28). Axial scan through the body of the pancreas performed 5 months after the initial scan.

SUMMARY OF MR FINDINGS FOR ABDOMINAL LYMPHOMA

1. Enlarged nodes in the retroperitoneal, retrocrural, mesenteric, and peripancreatic area, as well as in the splenic, renal, and hepatic hili.[3] Figure 73.5 is an MR scan from another patient with lymphoma, demonstrating retroperitoneal, retrocrural, and left renal hilar adenopathy.

2. The intensity of nodes is slightly higher than that of the skeletal muscle and liver parenchyma, especially on the second echo image, indicating a prolonged T2 relaxation time. Benign and malignant adenopathy cannot be differentiated on the basis of T1 and T2 values, and one must rely on size and morphologic criteria.[4]

3. Non-Hodgkin's lymphoma has a greater tendency than Hodgkin's lymphoma to cause mesenteric adenopathy.

4. One may see splenomegaly as a result of splenic involvement. A normal-size spleen does not exclude involvement, however.[2] Focal alteration in splenic signal intensity is a reliable indicator of splenic disease.

5. Hepatic infiltration may not be detectable by MR examination.[5] Hepatic involvement almost always occurs in the presence of splenic involvement.[2]

REFERENCES

1. Bradley WG, Waluch V: Blood flow: Magnetic resonance imaging. *Radiology* 1985;154:443–450.

2. Jones SE: The importance of staging in the management of the malignant lymphomas, in Carter SK, Glatstein E, Livingston RB (eds): *Principles of Cancer Treatment.* New York, McGraw-Hill Book Co, 1982, pp 790–799.

3. Jeffrey RB: Computed tomography of lymphovascular structures and retroperitoneal soft tissues, in Moss AA, Gamsu G, Genant HK (eds): *Computed Tomography of the Body.* Philadelphia, WB Saunders Co, 1983, pp 907–954.

4. Dooms GC, Hricak H, Moseley ME, et al: Characterization of lymphadenopathy by magnetic resonance relaxation times: Preliminary results. *Radiology* 1985;155:691–697.

5. Weinreb JC, Brateman L, Maravilla KR: Magnetic resonance imaging of hepatic lymphoma. *AJR* 1984;143:1211–1214.

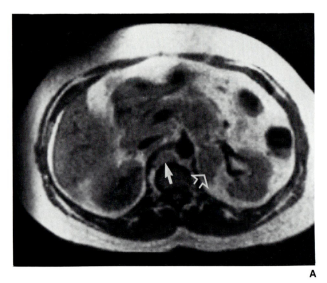
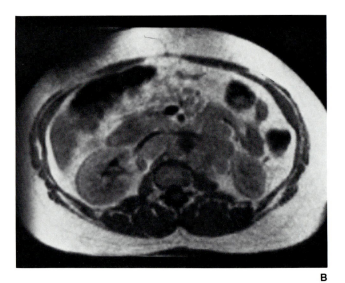

A   B

Figures 73.5A and **B** (SE 1000/28). MR scans from another patient with lymphoma. (A) Axial scan through the crura of the diaphragm demonstrating retrocrural (closed arrow) and left renal hilar adenopathy (open arrow). (B) Axial scan through the midabdomen demonstrating mesenteric, retroperitoneal, and left renal hilar adenopathy.

CASE 74

HISTORY

A 72-year-old man with bilateral ureteral obstruction requiring surgical release of the right ureter and stent placement within the left ureter. Medical history is notable for recurrent migraine headaches that required the prolonged use of methysergide. A CT of the abdomen was performed 5 months ago and is shown in Figure 74.1. The CT was complicated by the development of a contrast reaction. MRI was requested as a follow-up study and as a baseline for comparison with subsequent exams.

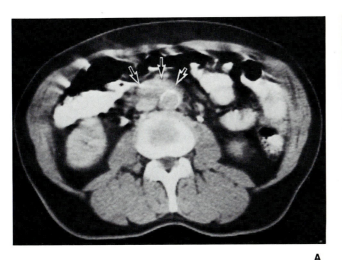
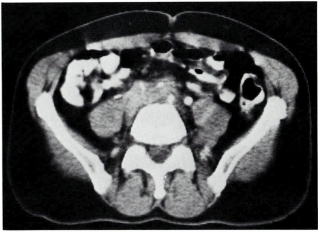

A   B

Figure 74.1(A). Enhanced CT scan through the lower pole of the right kidney. **(B)** Enhanced CT scan at the level of the umbilicus.

QUESTIONS

1. What are your differential considerations?

   _____

   _____

2. What MR techniques would you use?

	1	2	3
a. Coil			
b. Centering point			
c. Imaging plane(s)			
d. Contrast			
e. Slice thickness			

3. What do you expect to find?

   _____

   _____

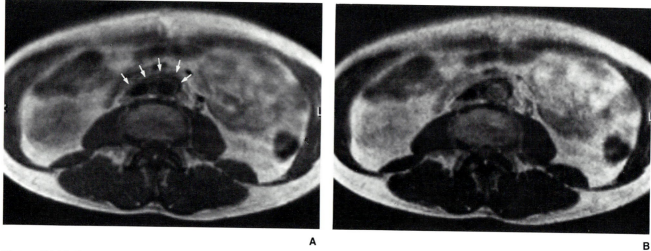

A

B

Figures 74.2A (SE 1000/28) and **74.2B** (SE 1000/56). Axial scans through the same level as Figure 74.1A.

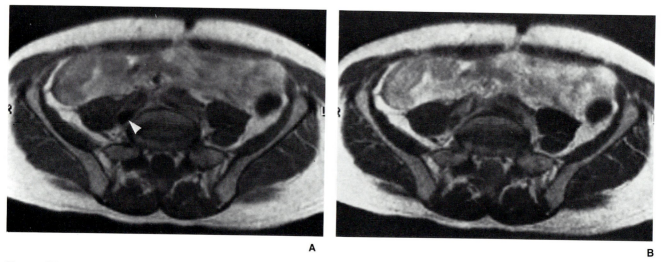

A

B

Figures 74.3A (SE 1000/28) and **74.3B** (SE 1000/56). Axial scans at the level of the umbilicus.

MR TECHNIQUES

a. Coil   Body
b. Centering point   Midabdomen
c. Imaging plane   Axial
d. Contrast   Mild T1W and mild T2W
e. Slice thickness   Routine

Since visualization of the retroperitoneum is the primary goal of this study, using mild T1 weighting is helpful in accentuating the contrast differences between soft tissue structures and the adjacent retroperitoneal fat. Axial images allow for direct comparison with the previous CT and provide important cross-sectional relationships.

MR FINDINGS

Figure 74.1. In A, there is a small, enhancing soft tissue mass (arrows) in the retroperitoneum obliterating the fascial planes around the aorta and the inferior vena cava (IVC). In B, a similar mass lesion is seen enveloping the vessels of the bifurcation.

Figure 74.2. There is an intermediate intensity mass (arrows) encircling the aorta and the IVC. On the first echo image, note the absence of signal within the lumen of the aorta and IVC due to flow void phenomena. On the second echo image, however, there is increased signal within the aorta. This finding is thought to represent a combination of diastolic pseudogating and even-echo rephasing.[1] In addition, note that the calcification within the wall of the aorta is well demonstrated in CT but poorly seen on the MR scan.

Figure 74.3. There is a band of intermediate intensity soft tissue similar in configuration to that seen on CT. The right common iliac vein (arrowhead) is readily identified.

DIFFERENTIAL DIAGNOSIS

The major considerations for this retroperitoneal lesion are *malignant lymphadenopathy*, *retroperitoneal sarcoma*, and *retroperitoneal fibrosis*. As with CT, differentiating between these three entities is often difficult. The symmetric involvement in this case makes retroperitoneal sarcoma less likely since this tumor generally arises from one side of the body; it tends to involve the retroperitoneum asymmetrically (see Case 75). In the past, several findings have been proposed as distinguishing features between lymphadenopathy and retroperitoneal fibrosis. These include margin definition, shape, area of involvement, medial displacement of the ureters, and contrast enhancement; however, all these criteria have been found to be unreliable.[2] A more consistent distinguishing feature, if present, is anterior displacement of the great vessels, which is not usually seen with retroperitoneal fibrosis.

We have noted that MRI may be more specific in distinguishing these two entities based on signal intensity differences. One may assume that fibrous tissue would possess lower proton density than lymphadenopathy and therefore may have lower signal intensity on spin echo images. We have observed this to be true in a limited number of cases. This is largely anecdotal, however, and further studies in this regard are needed. An example of malignant lymphadenopathy causing displacement of the aorta is seen in Figure 74.4. Note that the signal intensity of the nodes is greater than the signal intensity of retroperitoneal fibrosis as seen in Figures 74.2 and 3, even though similar pulsing sequences have been used on both cases.

The causes of retroperitoneal fibrosis are numerous and include drug therapy, radiation, aneurysm leakage, urinoma, and idiopathic causes. In this case, retroperitoneal fibrosis is

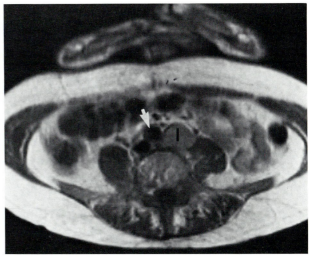

A

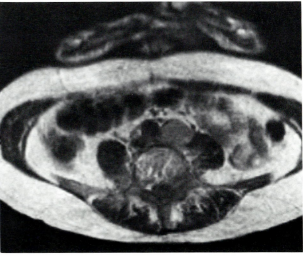

B

Figures 74.4A (SE 1000/28) and **74.4B** (SE 1000/56). Axial sections in a patient with malignant lymphoma (l). Note the rightward and anterior displacement of the aorta (arrow).

most certainly due to methysergide use. Pertinent negative findings are the absence of an aneurysm, urine extravasation, or radiation changes in the peritoneal fat and the vertebral bodies (see Case 51).

Final Diagnosis

Retroperitoneal fibrosis.

SUMMARY OF MR FINDINGS FOR RETROPERITONEAL FIBROSIS

1. Retroperitoneal soft tissue mass enveloping the great vessels.

2. Anterior displacement of the great vessels may serve to differentiate between lymphadenopathy and retroperitoneal fibrosis.
3. Medial ureteral displacement (not seen in this case) is usually present.
4. MR signal intensity differences may be a useful distinguishing feature.

REFERENCES

1. Bradley WG, Waluch V: Blood flow. Magnetic resonance imaging. *Radiology* 1985;154:443–450.
2. Degesys GE, Dunnick NR, Silverman PM, et al: Retroperitoneal fibrosis: Use of CT in distinguishing among possible causes. *AJR* 1986; 146:57–60.

CASE 75

HISTORY

A 57-year-old woman presenting with a 1-week history of left upper quadrant pain. CT examination showed a large mass in the left upper quadrant. Percutaneous needle biopsy was performed under CT guidance. Examination of the specimen revealed only fibrous tissue.

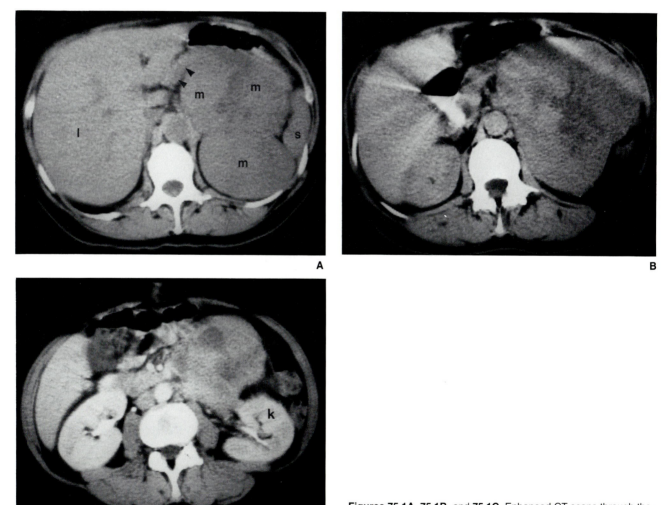

Figures 75.1A, 75.1B, and **75.1C.** Enhanced CT scans through the upper abdomen.

QUESTIONS

1. What are your differential considerations?

_____

_____

2. What MR techniques would you use?

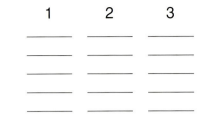

	1	2	3
a. Coil			
b. Centering point			
c. Imaging plane(s)			
d. Contrast			
e. Slice thickness			

3. What do you expect to find?

_____

_____

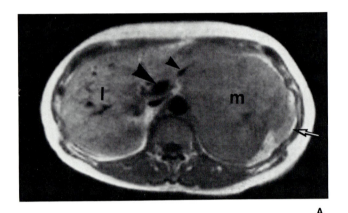

A

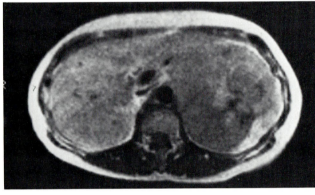

B

Figures 75.2A (SE 1000/28) and **75.2B** (SE 1000/56). Axial scans through the pancreatic bed.

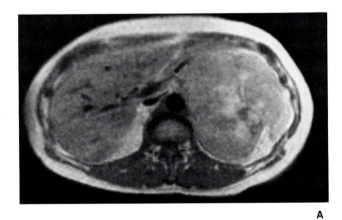

A

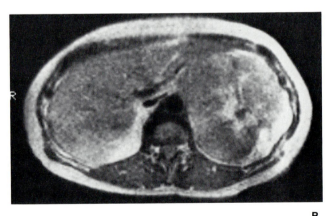

B

Figures 75.3A (SE 2000/28) and **75.3B** (SE 2000/56). T2-weighted axial scans through the same level.

MR TECHNIQUES

		1	2
a.	Coil	Body	Body
b.	Centering point	Xyphoid	Xyphoid
c.	Imaging planes	Axial	Axial
d.	Contrast	Mild T1W and mild T2W	Mild to moderate T2W
e.	Slice thickness	Routine	Routine

Our initial sequence was performed with T1 weighting. In this case, a TR of 1,000 mseconds was used and provided ten images with each image covering 1 cm. An alternative pulsing sequence with a shorter TR would provide greater T1 weighting and possibly improved contrast discrimination between the mass, liver, spleen, and adjacent retroperitoneal structures.

The second pulsing sequence was performed with T2 weighting to provide additional T2 information.

MR FINDINGS

Figure 75.1. There is a well-circumscribed mass (m) with slightly inhomogeneous density in the left upper quadrant of the abdomen. The contour of the mass is lobulated. The proximal third of the pancreas (arrowheads) is displaced anteromedially. The remainder of the pancreas is poorly seen and cannot be distinguished from the mass. The mass appears to enhance to the same degree as the liver (l) and spleen (s). The left kidney (k) does not appear to be involved by the mass.

Figure 75.2. On this moderate T1WI, the mass (m) is hypointense relative to the liver (l) and spleen (arrow). The pancreas is poorly seen on MRI compared with CT, being obscured by the adjacent liver and nonopacified stomach. The main portal vein (large arrowhead) and the splenic vein (small arrowhead), which form the posterior border of the pancreas, are better demonstrated on MRI than on contrast-enhanced CT. Also note the normal appearance of the aorta and inferior vena cava.

Figure 75.3. With more T2 weighting, the mass appears more heterogeneous and contains a central area of increased intensity, indicating possible central necrosis. This area of necrosis was also seen on CT as an area of low density. The remainder of the tumor is isointense compared with the liver parenchyma on both the first and second echo images.

DIFFERENTIAL DIAGNOSIS

The most difficult aspect in this case is determining the origin of this mass. The possible sites of origin include the pancreas, stomach, adrenal, kidney, and retroperitoneum.

Pancreas. Despite the size of the lesion and rapid onset of symptoms, the well-defined border of this tumor suggests that it may be slow growing. This finding excludes *pancreatic carcinoma*, which is usually a very aggressive infiltrating tumor. The predominately solid nature of this mass excludes *cystadenocarcinoma* of the pancreas. Most hormonally active islet cell tumors of the pancreas, including *insulinoma* and *gastrinoma*, tend to present early and are typically much smaller than the mass seen in this case. Hence, of all the pancreatic tumors, the only one that should be considered in this case is a nonsecreting islet cell tumor, which is rare.[1]

Stomach. *Leiomyosarcoma* of the stomach wall may present as a well-defined exophytic tumor in the left upper quadrant. It would be unusual, however, for a leiomyosarcoma to attain this size without undergoing significantly more necrosis or causing obstructive symptoms.[2]

Renal. The mass was shown in Figure 75.1C to be anterior to the left kidney and appeared to be separated from the kidney. This virtually excludes tumors of renal origin.

Adrenal. Most large adrenal tumors tend to displace the adjacent kidney inferiorly and laterally and have a propensity for invading the subcrural space. Neither of these features is observed in this case. Adrenal carcinoma cannot be completely excluded, however.

Retroperitoneal Tumors. Most retroperitoneal tumors are soft tissue sarcomas. These tumors usually grow slowly, are frequently encapsulated, and are recognized only when they reach significant size. The clinical symptoms may include pressure effect on the GI tract, urinary tract, or adjacent nerves. Of all the retroperitoneal sarcomas, *liposarcoma* is the most common type. *Fibrosarcoma* is the next most common; it tends to be well differentiated and has the best prognosis. Radiographically, the retroperitoneal tumors appear similar and generally cannot be differentiated. At times, however, a large *liposarcoma* may present with a large amount of fat and may be diagnosed on CT or MRI. The well-differentiated fibrous tissue seen in the specimen obtained by the needle biopsy is most in keeping with a *fibrosarcoma*.[3]

At surgery, a large, irregularly lobulated, and well-encapsulated mass weighing 1,235 g was removed. Pathologically, this was found to be a large retroperitoneal fibrosarcoma.

Final Diagnosis

Retroperitoneal fibrosarcoma.

SUMMARY OF MR FINDINGS FOR RETROPERITONEAL SOFT TISSUE SARCOMA

1. Large, well-encapsulated mass located in the retroperitoneum.
2. The T1 and T2 relaxation times of soft tissue malignancies were found to be much longer than those of surrounding normal tissues.[4] Hence, they have low

intensity on T1-weighted images and high signal intensity on T2-weighted images.

3. One may see central areas of necrosis.

4. Regional lymph node involvement is observed in 5% to 20% of cases.[3]

REFERENCES

1. Federle MP, Goldberg HI: Computed tomography of the pancreas, in Moss AA, Gamsu G, Genant HK (eds): *Computed Tomography of the Body*. Philadelphia, WB Saunders Co, 1983, pp 699–762.

2. Wong WS, Goldberg HI: Gastric, small bowel, and colorectal cancer, in Bragg DG, Rubin P, Youker JE (eds): *Oncologic Imaging*. New York, Pergamon Press, 1985, pp 243–285.

3. Koehler PR: Adrenal and retroperitoneal tumors, in Bragg DG, Rubin P, Youker JE (eds): *Oncologic Imaging*. New York, Pergamon Press, 1985, pp 343–361.

4. Reiser M, Rupp N, Heller HJ, et al: MR in the diagnosis of malignant soft tissue tumors. *Eur J Radiol* 1984;4:288–293.

CASE 76

HISTORY

A 70-year-old woman presenting with a 3-month history of right upper quadrant pain. Physical examination revealed a slightly tender 8-cm mass in the right upper quadrant. Her stool was positive for occult blood. An abdominal ultrasound was performed (Figure 76.1). MRI was requested for further evaluation.

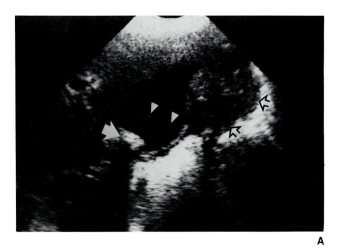
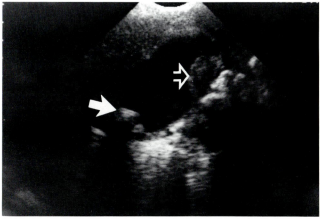

A   B

Figure 76.1. "Real-time" longitudinal sector scans through the right upper quadrant.

QUESTIONS

1. What are your differential considerations?

   _____

   _____

2. What MR techniques would you use?

	1	2	3
a. Coil			
b. Centering point			
c. Imaging plane(s)			
d. Contrast			
e. Slice thickness			

3. What do you expect to find?

   _____

   _____

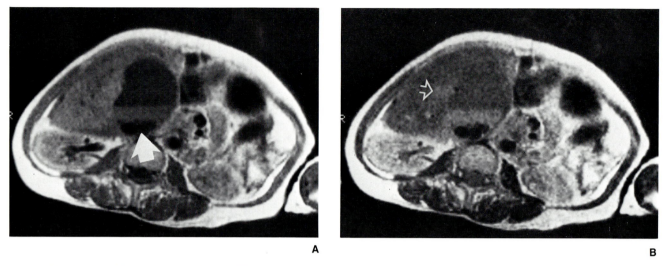

A

B

Figures 76.2A (SE 1000/28) and **76.2B** (SE 1000/56). Axial scans through the inferior portion of the right lobe of the liver.

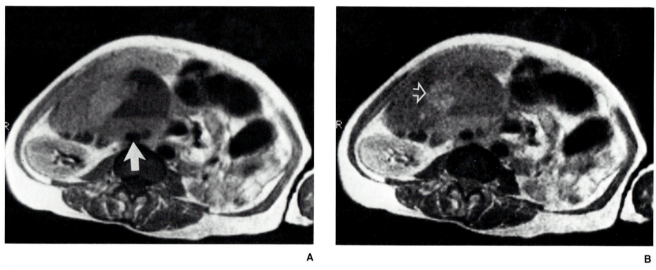

A

B

Figures 76.3A (SE 1000/28) and **76.3B** (SE 1000/56). Axial scans 1 cm inferior to Figure 76.2.

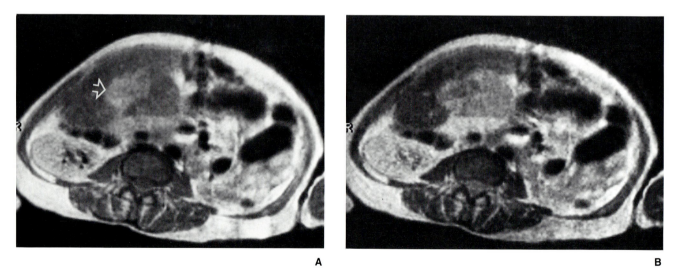

A

B

Figures 76.4A (SE 2000/28) and **76.4B** (SE 2000/56). Axial scans through the same level as Figure 76.3.

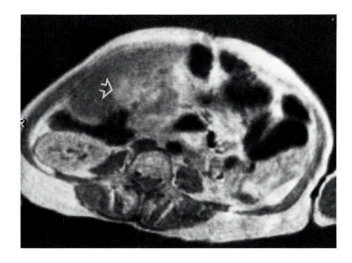

Figure 76.5 (SE 2000/28). Axial scan 1 cm inferior to Figures 76.3 and 76.4.

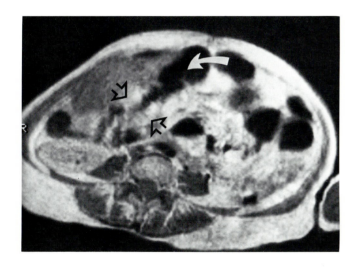

Figure 76.6 (SE 2000/28). Axial scan 1 cm inferior to Figure 76.5.

MR TECHNIQUES

	1	2
a. Coil	Body	Body
b. Centering point	6 cm inferior to the xyphoid process	
c. Imaging planes	Axial	Axial
d. Contrast	Mild T1W and mild T2W	Mild to moderate T2W
e. Slice thickness	Routine	Routine

A mildly T1-weighted image was performed to provide anatomic detail and contrast between fat and other soft tissues. The second pulsing sequence was performed to obtain T2 information and to cover a larger portion of the upper abdomen. In general, the axial plane is the best imaging plane for the abdomen.

MR FINDINGS

Figure 76.1. The gallbladder is slightly distended. There are hyperechoic areas (closed arrow) with acoustic shadowing in the dependent portion of the gallbladder consistent with cholelithiasis. The presence of sludge is indicated by the presence of a fluid–fluid level (arrowheads). In addition, there is an echogenic solid mass (open arrows) located in the fundal portion of the gallbladder. On real-time examinations, the mass appeared to extend laterally and was adherent to the gallbladder.

Figures 76.2 and 76.3. The gallstones are seen as several signal void foci (closed arrow) in the dependent portion of the gallbladder. The fluid–fluid (sludge and bile) level within the gallbladder is slightly better demonstrated by MRI than by ultrasound. Note that the signal intensity of the bile is low, indicating a poorly functioning gallbladder lacking the ability to concentrate bile. The mass seen on ultrasound is shown as an ill-defined lesion (open arrow) in the lateral aspect of the gallbladder. The mass is almost isointense with the liver parenchyma on the first echo image but becomes hyperintense to the liver on the second echo image, indicating prolongation of T2.

Figure 76.4. With more T2 weighting, the mass (open arrow) is hyperintense relative to the liver parenchyma on both the first and second echo images. The mass is better defined on this sequence because of the greater intensity difference between the mass and the liver.

Figures 76.5 and 76.6. The mass (open arrows) appears to extend to the lowermost aspect of the right lobe of the liver. Within the region of the mass, there is abrupt narrowing of the transverse colon, which is seen as a low intensity tubular structure (curved arrow).

DIFFERENTIAL DIAGNOSIS

The findings just described could represent either an inflammatory or neoplastic process. The presence of multiple gallstones and sludge within the gallbladder suggest the possibility of *acute cholecystitis* with a *pericholecystic inflammatory mass* (phlegmon). The patient's prolonged and relatively mild symptomatology would be unusual, however, for an inflammatory mass associated with acute cholecystitis.

Gallbladder carcinoma is another consideration. Carcinoma of the gallbladder, however, is usually associated with chronic cholecystitis,[1] which generally results in a small, shrunken gallbladder with a markedly thickened wall and numerous gallstones. In this case, the gallbladder is slightly distended, and its wall is only minimally thickened. Hence, gallbladder carcinoma is also not likely.

A *hepatoma* or a *hepatic metastasis* in the right lobe of the liver may cause these findings. As discussed in Case 70, most hepatomas present as multiple nodules, similar to hepatic metastases. The solitary nature of this mass shown on both MRI and ultrasound argues somewhat against either of these diagnoses. Neither diagnosis can be excluded solely on the basis of MR or ultrasound findings, however.

The fact that the mass can be traced from the gallbladder fossa inferiorly to an abruptly narrowed transverse colon suggests the possibility of a colon carcinoma with invasion of the gallbladder fossa. The presence of occult blood in the stool and the chronicity of the patient's symptom are compatible with this diagnosis.

At surgery, a large transverse colon carcinoma invading the gallbladder fossa was seen. The lesion was found to be unresectable. A colostomy was performed.

Comment

As discussed in the introductory section, ultrasound is the imaging modality of choice for examining the gallbladder. The nonspecificity of MR signal intensity is well illustrated in this case. Without the help of ultrasound, the solid or cystic nature of the mass cannot be determined by MRI. Both inflammatory and neoplastic disease processes can cause the described changes. None of the preceding diagnoses can be excluded on the basis of MR findings alone.

In general, carcinoma of the transverse or sigmoid colon is poorly demonstrated on MRI or CT because these segments of the colon are suspended on mesenteries, and the movements of these structures make imaging difficult.[2] In this case, the tumor had invaded the gallbladder fossa, fixing the colon to the liver and gallbladder and, thus, making MR imaging of the lesion possible.

One advantage of MRI is its ability to demonstrate the functional abnormality of the gallbladder. In a normally functioning gallbladder, the bile should have a higher signal intensity than the adjacent liver tissue (after eight hours of fasting).[3] In this case, the bile has a lower signal intensity than the adjacent liver tissue, suggesting a poorly functioning gallbladder. The presence of gallstones and sludge is also consistent with a poorly functioning gallbladder.

Final Diagnosis

Carcinoma of the transverse colon with invasion of the gallbladder fossa.

SUMMARY OF MR FINDINGS FOR CARCINOMA OF THE COLON

1. Most lesions are generally poorly seen with MRI, especially when they are in the transverse or sigmoid colon, unless they are of considerable size, as in this case.
2. The exam may demonstrate diffuse or focal thickening of the wall of the colon.
3. The intensity of the mass is higher on T2-weighted images, indicating prolongation of T2.

4. Mesenteric and/or retroperitoneal adenopathy may be demonstrated. (For examples of retroperitoneal and mesenteric adenopathy, see Case 73.)
5. The tumor may be locally invasive. (For radiographic staging, see Case 78.)

REFERENCES

1. Moss AA: Computed tomography of the hepatobiliary system, in Moss AA, Gamsu G, Genant HK (eds): *Computed Tomography of the Body*. Philadelphia, WB Saunders Co, 1983, pp 599–698.
2. Moss AA, Thoeni RF: Computed tomography of the gastrointestinal tract, in Moss AA, Gamsu G, Genant HK (eds): *Computed Tomography of the Body*. Philadelphia, WB Saunders Co, 1983, pp 535–598.
3. Loflin TG, Simeone JF, Mueller PR, et al: Gallbladder bile in cholecystitis: In vitro MR evaluation. *Radiology* 1985;157:457–459.

9

PELVIC IMAGING

In contrast to its utility in abdominal imaging, MRI has proven effective in pelvic imaging. Respiratory and cardiac motion artifact are not seen in the pelvis, and peristalsis is less marked. The combination of multiplanar imaging and superb contrast resolution is extremely helpful in defining the spread of tumors within the pelvis. In the pelvis as in the abdomen, flow phenomena are useful in differentiating vessels from lymphadenopathy. In patients who have multiple surgical clips following pelvic surgery (e.g., radical cystectomy or retroperitoneal node dissection), MRI has been shown to be less susceptible to metallic artifacts than CT. The disadvantages of using MRI within the pelvis, rather than CT or ultrasound, are similar to what has been described with regard to the abdomen. Specifically, these are the relatively higher cost and the lack of adequate small-bowel and large-bowel contrast.

The pelvic viscera usually have a slightly greater intensity than adjacent skeletal musculature, which has a moderately long T1 and a short T2. With increasing TR, a slight increase in muscle intensity is seen, but the intensity is consistently less than that of adjacent soft tissue. The perivisceral fat is of high intensity on all pulsing sequences and provides a natural contrast to the adjacent bowel or other pelvic organs.[1]

BLADDER TUMORS

The distinct advantage of MRI compared with other imaging modalities is its ability to define fascial planes, which is essential in determining tumor extension.

As in CT and ultrasound, in MRI the patient should be scanned with a distended bladder, so that the bladder wall can be adequately identified and characterized. Selection of a proper pulsing sequence allows the urine to be differentiated from the bladder wall. For instance, on a T1-weighted sequence (TR 500 mseconds and TE 30 mseconds), urine is hypointense compared with the bladder wall. With increasing T2 weighting (TR of 2,000 mseconds and TE of 60 mseconds), the intensity of urine approaches that of the bladder wall. With heavier T2 weighting, urine appears hyperintense because of its longer T2. The bladder wall remains relatively lower in intensity on heavily T2-weighted images because of its shorter T2.

Preliminary work has suggested that tumors may be differentiated from the bladder wall by using both T1- and T2-weighted images, so that the changing intensities of mass allow its differentiation from the bladder muscle. Sagittal and/or coronal images have been shown to be especially helpful. The most important task in the evaluation of bladder tumors is to define possible extravesicular extension. Extension into the perivesicular fat is best demonstrated using T1-weighted sequences, because of the optimal contrast differences between tumor and perivesicular fat, which has a short T1.

RECTAL CARCINOMA

Rectal carcinoma is still best detected by conventional means, such as barium enema, clinical examination, and sigmoidoscopy. The major role of MRI or CT is to define tumor extension, nodal disease, and distant metastases. Imaging in all three orthogonal planes is helpful in determining tumor invasion into the perirectal soft tissue. By using T1-weighted sequences, the lower intensity tumor may be differentiated from high intensity fat. Determining the integrity of the levator sling is important in the evaluation of tumor resectability and can be accurately accomplished with coronal or sagittal sequences. MRI may also help in the detection of tumor recurrence, and its accuracy may approach that of CT.

PROSTATIC TUMORS

Early experience suggested that an heterogeneous signal pattern of the prostate gland on MR examination was indicative of prostate tumor. Since tumors have prolonged T1 and T2 values, they produce focal decreased intensity on T1-weighted images and increased intensity on T2-weighted images. Benign prostatic hypertrophy was thought to produce a homogeneous appearance. More recent work, however, has proven these distinctions invalid. There have been several examples of benign nodular hyperplasia producing a heterogeneous appearance indistinguishable from that of prostatic carcinoma. Signal heterogeneity within a gland may be due to several causes, including tumor, nodular hyperplasia, prostatitis, abscess, or prior biopsy.[1,2]

With prostatic tumors, as with other pelvic malignancies, the main role of MRI is in tumor staging via depiction of extraprostatic invasion and pelvic adenopathy. Multiplanar imaging aids in defining tumor extent. Preliminary work has suggested that MRI is at least as accurate as CT in staging this tumor.[2]

FEMALE PELVIS[3]

Uterus[4]

The normal uterus has three distinct layers of varied intensity. The high intensity central zone is thought to represent the endometrium. This is separated from the intermediate intensity myometrium by a band of low intensity thought to be the stratum basale. The cervix also has three distinct zones. The central high intensity zone is thought to represent cervical mucus. The next layer is a low intensity band assumed to be stromal tissue of the endocervix. The third layer is the muscularis of the cervix, which has an intermediate intensity.

A recent study has demonstrated that differences in uterine size, shape, and signal intensity may reflect degrees of hormonal stimulation. For example, patients taking oral contraceptives tend to have a higher signal within the myometrium and a reduced endometrial width compared with nontreated women. Also, the intensity pattern and size of the myometrium and endometrium may vary between the proliferative and secretory phases of the reproductive cycle.[4]

On T1-weighted images, uterine myomas generally have a decreased signal intensity and a heterogeneous signal pattern when compared with the adjacent normal uterus. Fibroids may have variable intensity patterns, however, ranging from isointense to rarely hyperintense compared with normal uterine tissue. The increased signal intensity in some lesions may be secondary to degeneration, hemorrhage, or other unknown factors. Carcinomas of the endometrium produce irregular, increased signal intensity on T2-weighted images but may be difficult to separate from degenerated fibroids. Periuterine tumor extension and/or adenopathy may be demonstrated in cases of endometrial carcinoma.

Ovaries[3,5,6]

Normal ovaries have intermediate intensity on T1-weighted sequences and show a slight increase in intensity (approaching that of fat) with increasing repetition times. It is often difficult to separate normal adnexa from adjacent bowel loops. On T1-weighted images, *functional cysts* may have a low signal intensity compared with adjacent normal ovarian tissue because of the relatively longer T1 of the lesions. *Dermoids* have a generally increased intensity on both T1- and T2-weighted sequences due to their fat content. A heterogeneous pattern may be seen because of the presence of other elements, such as hair and teeth. Associated calcification, which can be readily seen on other imaging modalities, may be difficult to detect with MRI.

Endometriomas have, in general, no pathognomonic findings. The intensity of these lesions may vary from hyperintense to hypointense compared with that of the normal uterus. This variability is likely related to varying chronicity of hemorrhage within the cysts. *Cystadenomas* and *cystadenocarcinomas* also have varying intensities depending on their content. Cystadenocarcinomas have been reported to have mixed signal characteristics, reflecting both the fluid and solid components of the tumor. In general, it is not possible to determine if a tumor of the ovary is benign or malignant on the basis of MR findings alone. Inflammatory masses, such as tubo-ovarian abscesses, are usually indistinguishable from other masses of the adnexa and may have variable signal intensity. As in CT and ultrasound, in MRI the morphology and clinical history are important considerations in making these diagnoses.

Pregnancy[7,8]

The U.S. Food and Drug Administration has given its preliminary approval for MR imaging of the pregnant patient. Our institutional criteria are as follows:

1. The prenatal MR examination is strongly indicated (e.g., imaging maternal CNS tumor).
2. CT is definitely contraindicated (e.g., contrast allergy or radiation dose to the fetus).
3. Ultrasound is not diagnostic.
4. The patient has been fully informed of the possible effects of MRI on the fetus.

Obviously, more flexibility can be applied when the pregnancy is going to be terminated. MR imaging has been reported useful in the detection of fetal anomalies, such as hydronencephaly, hydrocephalus, and genitourinary tract pathology. Placental pathology and trophoblastic disease have also been imaged effectively.

It has been suggested that MRI may be useful in the detection of intrauterine growth retardation (IUGR). In this condition, there is a generalized deficiency of fetal fat. If subcutaneous fat can be detected on an MR scan, IUGR is essentially excluded.[9] Much work is still needed in this area, however.

Others have shown that MRI is as accurate as CT pelvimetry in determining pelvic dimensions.[10] MRI has the advantage of not using ionizing radiation, which may be harmful to the fetus.

REFERENCES

1. LiPuma JP, Bryan PJ: Magnetic resonance imaging of the genitourinary tract, in Kressel HY (ed): *Magnetic Resonance Annual 1985*. New York, Raven Press, 1985, pp 149–196.

2. Bryan PJ, Butler HE, Nelson AD, et al: Magnetic resonance imaging of the prostate. *AJR* 1986;146:543–548.

3. Hricak H, Williams RD, Moon KL, et al: Magnetic resonance imaging of the female pelvis: Initial experience. *AJR* 1983;141:1119–1128.

4. Demas BE, Hricak H, Jaffe RB: Uterine MR imaging: Effects of hormonal stimulation. *Radiology* 1986;159:123–126.

5. Butler H, Bryan PJ, LiPuma JP, et al: Magnetic resonance imaging of the abnormal female pelvis. *AJR* 1984;143:1259.

6. Dooms GC, Hricak H, Tscholakoff D: Adnexal structures: MR imaging. *Radiology* 1986;158:639–646.

7. McCarthy SM, Stark DD, Filly RA, et al: Obstetrical magnetic resonance imaging: Maternal anatomy. *Radiology* 1985;154:421–425.

8. McCarthy SM, Filly RA, Stark DD, et al: Obstetrical magnetic resonance imaging: Fetal anatomy. *Radiology* 1985;154:427–432.

9. Stark DD, McCarthy SM, Filly RA, et al: Intrauterine growth retardation: Evaluation by magnetic resonance: Work in progress. *Radiology* 1985;155:425–427.

10. Stark DD, McCarthy SM, Filly RA, et al: Pelvimetry by magnetic resonance imaging. *AJR* 1985;144:947–950.

CASE 77

HISTORY

A 61-year-old man presenting with a 3-week history of gross hematuria. An excretory urogram revealed left-sided hydronephrosis and a filling defect within the bladder. Cystoscopy showed a large bladder tumor overlying the entire trigone, extending into the left lateral wall. MRI was requested to help define the extent of the lesion.

QUESTIONS

1. What MR techniques would you use?

	1	2	3
a. Coil	___	___	___
b. Centering point	___	___	___
c. Imaging plane(s)	___	___	___
d. Contrast	___	___	___
e. Slice thickness	___	___	___

2. What is the pattern of spread of bladder carcinoma?

_____

_____

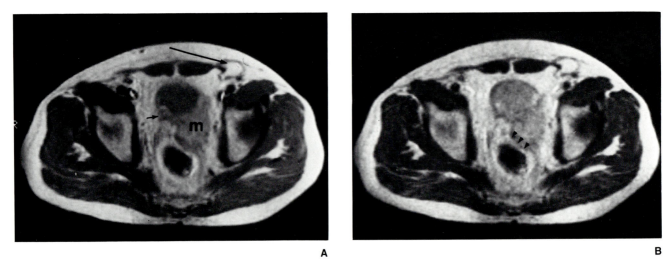

Figures 77.1A (SE 2000/28) and **71.1B** (SE 2000/56). Axial scans through the level of the seminal vesicles. (Reprinted with permission from *Radiology* (1985;154:443–450), Copyright © 1985, Radiological Society of North America Inc.)

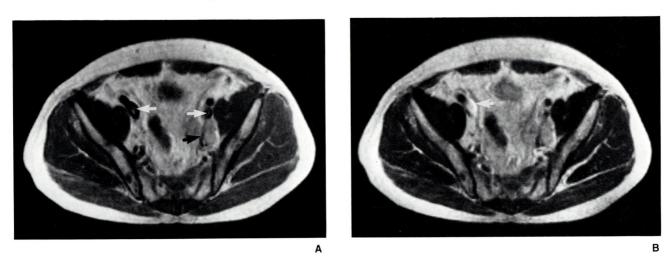

Figures 77.2A (SE 2000/28) and **77.2B** (SE 2000/56). Axial scans through the iliac fossa.

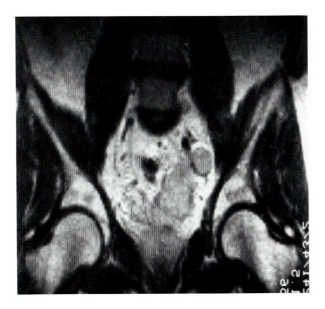

Figure 77.3 (SE 1500/56). Coronal scan through the midportion of the pelvis.

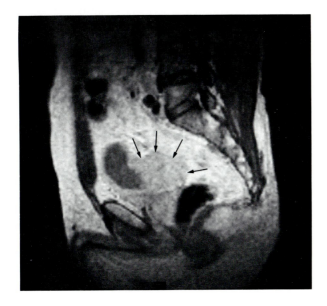

Figure 77.4 (SE 2000/28). Midsagittal scan of the pelvis.

MR TECHNIQUES

	1	2	3
a. Coil	Body	Body	Body
b. Centering point	ASIS*	Midcoronal	Midsagittal
c. Imaging planes	Axial	Coronal	Sagittal
d. Contrast		Mild to moderate T2W	
e. Slice thickness	Routine	Routine	Routine

*ASIS = anterior superior iliac spine

As discussed in the introductory section, urine is best separated from the bladder wall on T1WIs. Both T1- and T2-weighted images are needed, however, to differentiate tumor from bladder wall. Extension into the perivesicular fat is best demonstrated using T1-weighted sequences because of the optimal contrast differences between tumor and perivesicle fat, which has a short T1. Similarly, lymph nodes are most easily detected on T1-weighted axial sections.

All three imaging planes are needed to optimally define the extent of the tumor. The axial plane is important in demonstrating the adjacent organs (e.g., seminal vesicles or ovaries) and for detecting lymphadenopathy. The coronal view best demonstrates the integrity of the pelvic side walls. The sagittal view provides better demonstration of the midline structures, such as the uterus and the rectum. In addition, both the axial and coronal views allow evaluation of left-to-right symmetry within the pelvis. The sagittal and coronal views provide better appreciation of the longitudinal extent of the tumor.

MR FINDINGS

Figure 77.1. The posterior and left lateral wall of the bladder are diffusely thickened with a large exophytic mass (m) that projects posteriorly and encases the left seminal vesicle. The short arrow is pointing to the normal right seminal vesicle for comparison. The mass extends to (and possibly through) the serosa of the rectum (arrowheads). Note that the urine is hypointense compared with the tumor and surrounding fat on the first echo image but becomes nearly isointense with the tumor on the second echo image. The tumor margin is less well defined on the second echo image. The pelvic side walls do not appear to be involved. Also note the small, high intensity mass (long arrow) in the right inguinal canal, representing herniated mesenteric fat.

Figure 77.2. There is an enlarged node belonging to the medial or middle group of the left external iliac chain (black arrow). The node has an intermediate intensity and is better defined on the first echo image. Note the flow-related en-hancement within the external iliac veins (white arrows) on the first echo image, which becomes much more intense on the right side of the second echo image due to even-echo rephasing.

Figure 77.3. The enlarged, left external iliac node and the diseased left seminal vesicle are again demonstrated on this coronal image. The perivesicle fat along the pelvic side wall is preserved and is best demonstrated on the coronal view.

Figure 77.4. The superior (arrows) extent of the tumor is better appreciated on this midline sagittal scan.

DISCUSSION

As in the case of other pelvic tumors, MRI (or CT) does not contribute significantly to the detection of bladder carcinoma. The major role of MRI (or CT) is to provide more precise preoperative staging and to allow serial postoperative follow-up examinations for early detection of recurrence. The single most important prognostic factor for patients with invasive transitional cell carcinoma is the degree of bladder wall invasion. The 5-year survival rate for patients with superficial tumor is 50% to 80%, while in those with deep invasion, it is only 6% to 23%.[1] Unfortunately, at the present time, neither MRI nor CT is able to differentiate the different layers of the bladder wall; and thus, neither modality is capable of determining the degree of invasion of the bladder wall. Therefore, in terms of staging, the role of MRI and CT is relegated to the detection of local spread to adjacent organs and nodal metastasis.

Local Extension. Initially, the tumor tends to spread radially through the wall of the bladder and then circumferentially through the muscular layer. The perivesicle fat, seminal vesicles, prostate, and obturator internus muscles are frequently involved. In women, the tumor occasionally invades the uterus or cervix. The ureters and urethra may also be involved if the tumor arises close to these structures.

Lymphatic Spread. There is a tendency for tumors to spread to the external iliac nodes, especially to the medial or middle group, as in this case. Bladder carcinomas may rarely spread to the hypogastric (internal) iliac nodes.

Hematogenous Spread. Bladder carcinomas tend to metastasize to the liver, lung, and skeleton.

In this case, the tumor has spread radially around the posterior wall of the bladder, the trigone, left ureter, left seminal vesicle, the left external iliac node, and possibly the anterior portion of the rectum. By clinical staging criteria (see following), this tumor is considered to be stage D_1.

Final Diagnosis

Invasive transitional cell carcinoma of the bladder.

SUMMARY OF MR FINDINGS FOR BLADDER CARCINOMA[1-3]

1. Polypoid or asymmetric thickening of the wall of the bladder.
2. The tumor may be differentiated from the bladder wall by using both T1- and T2-weighted images.
3. Local extension to the adjacent organs.
4. Spread to the external iliac nodes.
5. Clinical staging system:
   Stage O: Carcinoma in situ
   Stage A: Invasion of the lamina propria
   Stage B_1: Invasion of superficial muscular layer
   Stage B_2: Invasion of deep muscular layer
   Stage C: Invasion of perivesical fat
   Stage D_1: Extension to pelvic viscera and/or regional nodes
   Stage D_2: Widespread lymphadenopathy and/or distant metastases

Note: Stages 0 to B_2 cannot be differentiated by MRI or CT.

REFERENCES

1. Balfe DM, Heiker JP, McClennan BL: Bladder cancer, in Bragg DG, Rubin P, Youker JE (eds): *Oncologic Imaging*. New York, Pergamon Press, 1985, pp 389–404.

2. Li Puma JP, Bryan PJ: Magnetic resonance imaging of the genitourinary tract, in Kressel HY (ed): *Magnetic Resonance Annual 1985*. New York, Raven Press, 1985, pp 149–196.

3. Fisher MR, Hricak H, Crooks LE: Urinary bladder MR imaging: Part I. Normal and benign conditions. *Radiology* 1985;157:467–470.

CASE 78

HISTORY

A 56-year-old man presenting with hematochezia. Sigmoidoscopy revealed a large mass encircling the lower rectum. Histologic examination of the biopsied specimen revealed adenocarcinoma of the rectum. MRI was requested to help define the extent of the lesion.

QUESTIONS

1. What MR techniques would you use?

	1	2	3
a. Coil	_____	_____	_____
b. Centering point	_____	_____	_____
c. Imaging plane(s)	_____	_____	_____
d. Contrast	_____	_____	_____
e. Slice thickness	_____	_____	_____

2. What do you expect to find?

_____

_____

Source: Courtesy of Valley MRI, Phoenix, AZ.

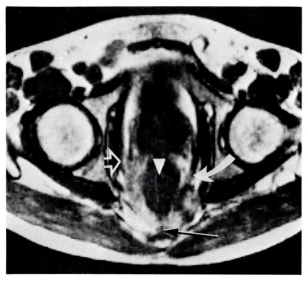

Figure 78.1 (SE 500/28). Axial scan 5 cm above the anal verge.

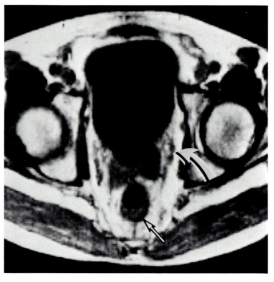

Figure 78.2 (SE 500/28). Axial scan 3 cm above Figure 78.1.

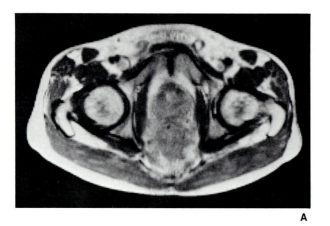

A

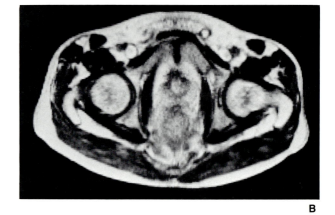

B

Figures 78.3A (SE 1500/28) and 78.3B (SE 1500/56). T2-weighted axial scans through the same level as Figure 78.1.

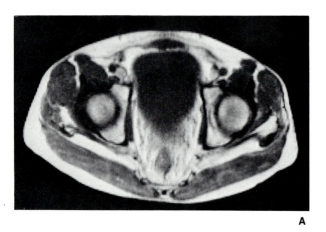

A

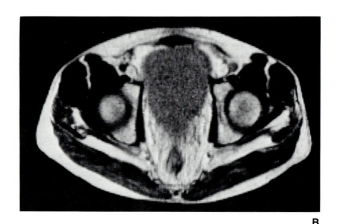

B

Figures 78.4A (SE 1500/28) and 78.4B (SE 1500/56). T2-weighted axial scans through the same level as Figure 78.2.

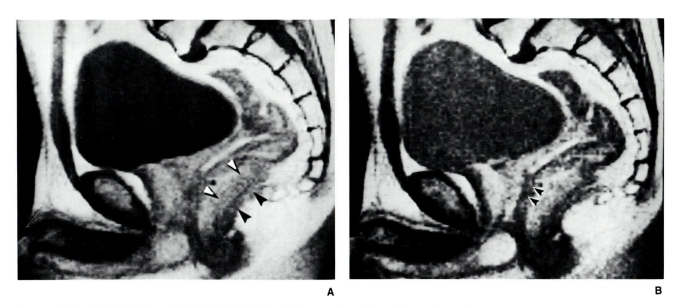

Figures 78.5A (SE 1000/28) and **78.5B** (SE 1000/56). Sagittal scans through the midline of the pelvis.

MR TECHNIQUES

	1	2	3	4
a. Coil	Body	Body	Body	Body
b. Centering point	Pubic symphysis	ASIS*	Midline	Midcoronal
c. Imaging planes	Axial	Axial	Sagittal	Coronal
d. Contrast	Moderate T1W	Mild T2W	Mild T1W and mild T2W	Mild T1W and mild T2W
e. Slice thickness	Routine	Routine	Routine	Routine

*ASIS = anterior superior iliac spine

As discussed in the introductory section, imaging in all three orthogonal planes is useful in determining the extent of tumor invasion into the perirectal soft tissues. The axial images are useful in assessing tumor spread to the pelvic sidewalls, perirectal fat, and lymph nodes. The coronal images (not shown) are useful in assessing the integrity of the levator sling, which is important in determining tumor resectability. The sagittal images are useful in the evaluation of midline structures, such as the prostate, uterus, bladder, rectum, and the presacral space.

The T1-weighted sequences were performed to provide better anatomic definition and to accentuate the differences in intensities between skeletal muscle, lymph nodes, abnormal and normal perirectal fat, and tumor. A mildly T2-weighted sequence was also performed to obtain additional T2 information and to possibly differentiate tumor from rectal wall.

MR FINDINGS

Figure 78.1. On this T1WI, the rectal wall is thickened circumferentially. The normal thickness of the distended rectal wall should be less than 5 mm.[1] The lumen of the rectum (white arrowhead) is barely visible and is seen as a linear area of absent signal outlined by a thin layer of slightly higher intensity material, probably representing mucus. The perirectal fat, which is normally homogeneous and high in intensity, has a heterogeneous, intermediate intensity pattern due to tumor infiltration. The left levator ani muscle is poorly seen and involved by tumor. The right levator is indistinct posteriorly (curved arrow) due to tumor infiltration. The tumor has spread to the presacral area (straight arrow). In addition, the tumor has extended to and possibly involves the right obturator internus muscle (open arrow).

Figure 78.2. More superiorly, only the posterior wall of the rectum (short white arrow) is thickened. The seminal vesicles are normal in size and do not appear to be involved.

The perirectal fat has a more normal, high intensity pattern at this level; however, there are numerous, ill-defined, low intensity linear structures (curved arrow) scattered throughout the perirectal and periprostatic fat. These structures probably represent dilated lymphatic channels.

Figure 78.3. On this mild T2WI, the tumor has a higher signal intensity, especially on the second echo image, indicating prolongation of T2. The tumor margin is less well defined than on the T1WI (Figure 78.1) because its higher signal intensity decreases the contrast with surrounding fat.

Figure 78.4. The seminal vesicles are less well visualized on this T2WI. The low intensity tubular structures seen in Figure 78.2, however, are slightly better demonstrated on this scan.

Figure 78.5. Both the rectum and the prostate gland are well demonstrated on this midline sagittal scan. The intensity pattern of the prostate is normal, and the organ does not appear to be involved by tumor. Diffuse thickening of the rectal wall is again demonstrated (short white arrows). Denonvilliers' fascia (white arrowheads), which separates the rectum from the prostate gland, is better seen on the second echo image and is intact. Note the spondylolisthesis and disc degeneration at L-5–S-1.

DISCUSSION

The major role of MRI in the evaluation of rectal carcinoma, as with prostate carcinoma, is to define the extent of the tumor. Although the primary rectal tumor may occasionally be demonstrated by MRI, the detection of the tumor is best accomplished with physical examination, sigmoidoscopy, and/or barium enema. Like CT, MRI cannot determine whether a tumor is localized to the mucosa or has extended to the muscularis. Hence, the frequently applied Duke's staging system cannot be used with MRI or CT.[2] A modified CT staging system based on the thickness of the rectal wall and spread to adjacent and distant organs has been proposed;[1] this system is also applicable to MRI (see following).

In rectosigmoid carcinoma, determining the lower margin of tumor is very important in planning the surgical approach. For those tumors located more than 12 cm above the anal verge, a simple intra-abdominal approach is used. For those tumors located less than 7 cm from the anal verge, an abdominal-perineal approach is needed. For those tumors located between 7 and 12 cm above the anal verge, the surgical approach is variable.[2]

Tumor recurrence is a difficult problem in the management of patients with rectosigmoid carcinoma. Thirty percent of patients have a pelvic recurrence. The site is usually in the posterior pelvic and presacral area for men and in the posterior vaginal wall/rectal-vaginal pouch for women. Both MRI and CT are useful in evaluating these areas. CT has the advantage, however, in being able to direct needle biopsy, which may be needed to differentiate scar tissue from tumor recurrence.

There has not been a large series examining the accuracy of MRI in staging primary or recurrent rectal tumor. Because of the higher soft tissue contrast resolution and the multiplanar capability of MRI, its accuracy is expected to approach or possibly surpass that of CT.

In this case, the lower margin of the tumor is less than 7 cm from the anal verge by both MR and clinical examination. This finding mandates an abdominal-perineal surgical approach. The tumor has also extended beyond the perirectal fat to involve the levator ani muscles as well as the right pelvic side wall. By CT staging criteria, this would be a stage IIIB lesion.

Final Diagnosis

Rectal carcinoma (stage IIIB by cross-sectional imaging staging system).

SUMMARY OF MR FINDINGS FOR RECTAL CARCINOMA

1. Diffuse or focal thickening of the rectal wall.

2. As for most pathologic processes, the T1 and T2 relaxation times of the tumor and involved tissues are increased. Hence, they are of low intensity on T1WIs and of high intensity on T2WIs.

3. If infiltrated by tumor, the perirectal fat becomes inhomogeneous and lower than normal in intensity.

4. One may detect adenopathy and/or dilated lymphatic channels.

5. Cross-sectional imaging staging system:[1]
   Stage I: Intraluminal polypoid mass
   Stage II: Wall thickening (more than 0.5 cm)
   Stage IIIA: Invasion of surrounding tissue with or without lymph node involvement (without extension to pelvic side walls)
   Stage IIIB: Extension to the pelvic side walls
   Stage IV: Presence of distant metastases

REFERENCES

1. Moss AA, Thoeni RF: Computed tomography of the gastrointestinal tract, in Moss AA, Gamsu G, Genant HK (eds): *Computed Tomography of the Body*. Philadelphia, WB Saunders Co, 1983, pp 535–598.
2. Wong WS, Goldberg HI: Gastric, small bowel, and colorectal cancer, in Bragg DG, Rubin P, Youker JE (eds): *Oncologic Imaging*. New York, Pergamon Press, 1985, pp 243–285.

CASE 79

HISTORY

A 58-year-old man was found to have a nodule on the right side of the prostate on rectal examination. A transrectal biopsy of the lesion revealed prostate carcinoma. MRI was requested to define the extent of the lesion.

QUESTIONS

1. What are your differential considerations?

_____

_____

2. What MR techniques would you use?

	1	2	3
a. Coil	___	___	___
b. Centering point	___	___	___
c. Imaging plane(s)	___	___	___
d. Contrast	___	___	___
e. Slice thickness	___	___	___

3. What do you expect to find?

_____

_____

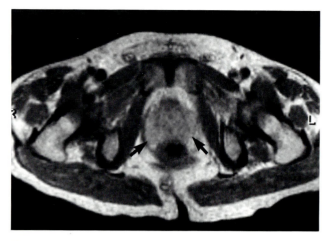

Figure 79.1 (SE 2000/28). Axial scan through the midportion of the prostate gland.

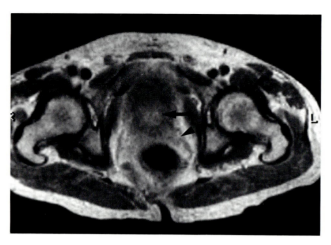

Figure 79.2 (SE 2000/28). Axial scan through the superior aspect of the prostate gland.

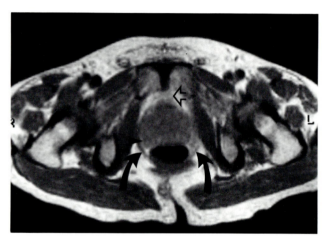

Figure 79.3 (SE 1000/28). Axial scan through the same level as Figure 79.1.

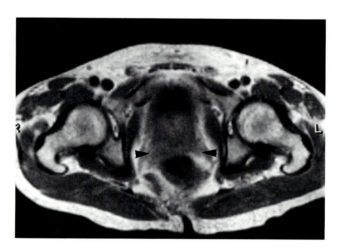

Figure 79.4 (SE 1000/28). Axial scan through the same level as Figure 79.2.

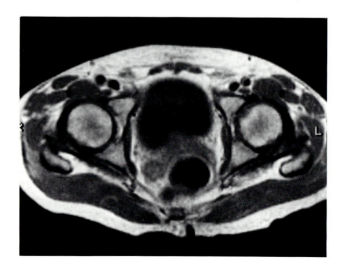

Figure 79.5 (SE 1000/28). Axial scan through the seminal vesicles.

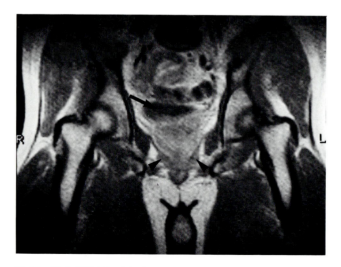

Figure 79.6 (SE 1500/28). Coronal scan through the prostate.

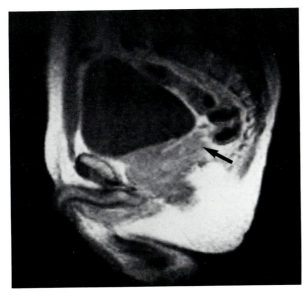 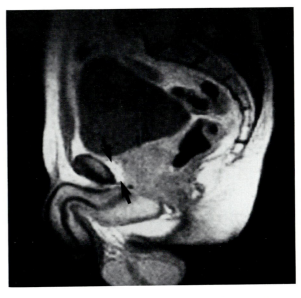

Figure 79.7 (SE 1000/28). Sagittal scan 1 cm to the right of the midline.

Figure 79.8 (SE 1000/28). Sagittal scan through the midline.

MR TECHNIQUES

	1	2	3	4
a. Coil	Body	Body	Body	Body
b. Centering point	ASIS*	ASIS*	ASIS*	ASIS*
c. Imaging planes	Axial	Axial	Coronal	Sagittal
d. Contrast	Mild and moderate T2W	Mild T1W and mild T2W		
e. Slice thickness	Routine	Routine	Routine	Routine

*ASIS = anterior superior iliac spine

For optimal staging of prostatic carcinoma, the prostate gland should be visualized in all three orthogonal planes. The axial plane shows the lateral and posterior periprostatic fat best. The anterior fat in the space of Retzius is best demonstrated on the sagittal scan. The coronal scan is best for visualizing the levator ani muscles that separate the perineum from the true pelvis.[1]

The first pulsing sequence with T2 weighting provides T2 information about the prostate gland and has an additional benefit of covering a large area with a single pulsing sequence. The latter three pulsing sequences were chosen with mild T1 weighting to provide better anatomic definition, which is important in defining tumor extent.

MR FINDINGS

Figure 79.1. On this moderate T2WI, the prostate gland has a heterogeneous intensity pattern with a slightly lower intensity centrally and a higher intensity peripherally. A discrete nodule is not identified; however, there is slight asymmetry (arrows) in the posterolateral aspect of the gland. Note the prostate gland has a significantly higher signal intensity than the skeletal muscles on this sequence.

Figure 79.2. There is an ill-defined, 2.5-cm, high intensity nodule (arrow) located centrally in the superior aspect of the prostate gland. The lower portion of the left seminal vesicle (arrowhead) is seen on this section and is slightly prominent. The right seminal vesicle is not well demonstrated on this image because its intensity is similar to that of the surrounding fatty tissue.

Figure 79.3. With more T1 weighting, the prostate gland has a lower signal intensity, and the inhomogeneity of the signal pattern seen on Figure 79.1 is less well appreciated. The anatomic details of the prostate gland and the bulge (arrowhead) in the right posterolateral aspect of the gland, however, are better demonstrated on this image. Note the anterior fat (open arrow) in the space of Retzius and the levator ani muscles (curved arrows).

Figure 79.4. With more T1 weighting, the central high intensity nodule seen in Figure 79.2 is slightly better defined. The lower portions of both seminal vesicles (arrowheads) are seen on this image and are noted to be prominent.

Figure 79.5. One centimeter superior to Figure 79.4, both seminal vesicles are shown to be enlarged, suggesting tumor infiltration.

Figure 79.6. The levator ani muscles (arrowheads) are well demonstrated on this coronal image and do not appear to be involved by tumor. Note the urine-filled bladder (arrow) has a low signal intensity on this T1-weighted image.

Figure 79.7. The posterior and superior extension of the tumor into the right seminal vesicle (arrow) is well demonstrated on this parasagittal scan.

Figure 79.8. On this midsagittal scan, the fascial plane separating the posterior aspect of the prostate from the anterior aspect of the rectum is not seen, suggesting tumor involvement. Note the anterior fat in the space of Retzius (arrows) is best demonstrated on this scan.

DISCUSSION

As discussed in the introductory section, the main role of MRI in the management of patients with prostate carcinoma is to help define the extent of tumor involvement (rather than to detect intracapsular disease). A good understanding of the natural history and pattern of spread of this common tumor may help to optimize this staging process.

The majority of prostate carcinomas are adenocarcinomas, and they frequently arise in the periphery of the posterior lobe of the gland, which is easily accessible by rectal digital examination. Because of this peripheral location, however, the periurethral area is usually not involved and the patients are not symptomatic until very late in the course of the disease. In addition, the tumor frequently arises in multiple peripheral sites simultaneously. Hence, most patients who come to medical attention present with very advanced disease.[2]

The tumor may spread to other organs by direct extension, lymphatic spread, or hematogenous dissemination.[2] Direct extension into the seminal vesicles and the bladder is quite common. In contradistinction, direct extension into the rectum is relatively rare because Denonvilliers' fascia, which separates the prostate from the rectum, is quite strong.

The lymphatics of the prostate drain into the internal and external iliac nodes as well as the nodes in the presacral area. The group of nodes that are most commonly involved by tumor are the medial chain of the external iliac group, the "obturator" nodes, which are adjacent to the obturator nerve. The next most common group is the presacral nodes. Involvement of the para-aortic nodes is always associated with pelvic nodal disease. Several investigators have examined the use of CT in detecting lymph node involvement. The major shortcoming of CT is its lack of sensitivity to nodes that are involved by tumor but remain normal in size.[3] The great hope for MRI is that it may eventually be able to make this distinction because of greater contrast. Unfortunately, recent studies have shown that MRI is also insensitive in the detection of normal size but diseased nodes.[1]

Hematogenous dissemination is believed to occur independent of lymphatic spread. The most frequent site of metastases is bone, with a propensity for the lumbar spine. A possible explanation for this is the free communication between the periprostatic venous plexus and the lumbar epidural veins. Metastases to the spine may be detectable on MRI (see Case 50).

In this case, MRI has shown extension of tumor to both seminal vesicles that was confirmed at surgery. The lack of a definable fascial plane separating the tumor from the rectum (Figure 79.8) suggests possible rectal involvement; at surgery, however, the rectum was found to be free of tumor (emphasizing the point that failure to see a fascial plane on MRI or CT does not necessarily indicate involvement). In addition, microscopic involvement of one of the internal iliac nodes was found that had not been detected on MRI.

Final Diagnosis

Prostate carcinoma with direct extension to both seminal vesicles.

SUMMARY OF MR FINDINGS FOR PROSTATE CARCINOMA[1]

1. Heterogeneous signal intensity. This is a nonspecific finding, however. Some patients with benign prostatic hypertrophy or prostatitis may have heterogeneous signal pattern within the prostate, and some prostate carcinomas may have a homogeneous signal pattern.[1]
2. Nodules

   a. Some may be well defined

   b. Some may be poorly defined
   c. Decreased signal intensity relative to the rest of the prostate on T1WIs
   d. Mixed relative intensity, though predominantly increased, on T2WIs.

3. Extension into periprostatic fat is seen as areas of decreased signal intensity in contrast with the high signal of fat.
4. Enlarged nodes have a signal intensity greater than that of skeletal muscle on both T1WIs and T2WIs. Adenopathy is better demonstrated on T1-weighted images, however.
5. American Urologic Staging System:[2]

   A_1: No clinical disease; less than three fragments contains tumor.

   A_2: No clinical disease; greater than three fragments contains tumor.

   B_1: Palpable nodule confined to one lobe.

   B_2: Tumor involving both lobes; invasion of, but not through, the capsule.

   C_1: Penetration of capsule; minimal extension.

   C_2: Extensive local disease; ureteral/bladder obstruction.

   D_1: Nodal metastases not clinically appreciated. Widespread metastases not clinically appreciated.

   D_2: Nodal metastases clinically manifest. Widespread metastases clinically manifest.

REFERENCES

1. Bryan PJ, Butler HE, Nelson AD, et al: Magnetic resonance imaging of the prostate. *AJR* 1986;146:543–548.
2. Balfe DM, Heiken JP, McClennan BL: Prostatic cancer, in Bragg DG, Rubin P, Youker JE (eds): *Oncologic Imaging.* New York, Pergamon Press, 1985, pp 405–424.
3. Golimbu M, Morales P, Al-askari P, et al: CAT scanning in staging of prostate cancer. *Urology* 1981;18:305.

CASE 80

HISTORY

A postmenopausal woman presents with pain in her midpelvis. The uterus was noted to be enlarged on physical examination. A CT scan is shown in Figure 80.1.

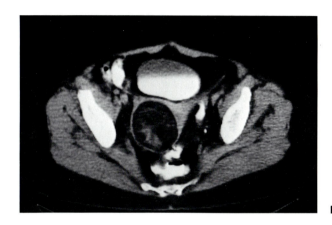

Figure 80.1. Enhanced CT scan through the midpelvis.

QUESTIONS

1. What are your differential considerations?

_____

_____

2. What MR techniques would you use?

	1	2	3
a. Coil	____	____	____
b. Centering point	____	____	____
c. Imaging plane(s)	____	____	____
d. Contrast	____	____	____
e. Slice thickness	____	____	____

3. What do you expect to find?

_____

_____

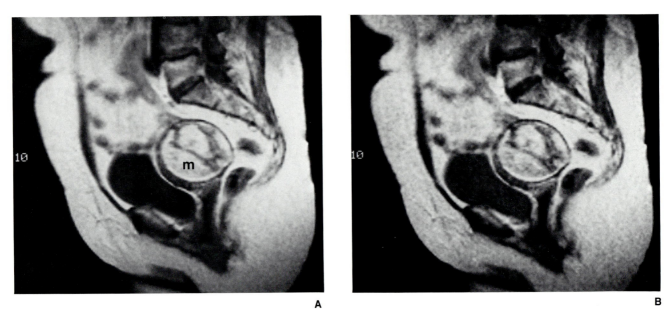

A
B

Figures 80.2A (SE 1000/30) and **80.2B** (SE 1000/60). Midsagittal sections.

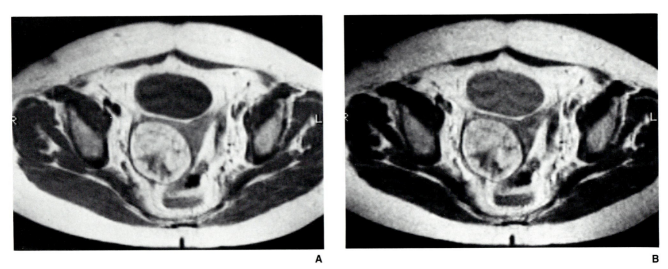

A
B

Figures 80.3A (SE 1500/28) and **80.3B** (SE 1500/56). Axial MR scans through the midpelvis.

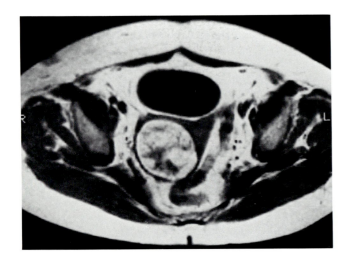

Figure 80.4 (SE 500/30). Axial section through the same level.

MR TECHNIQUES

		1	2	3
a.	Coil	Body	Body	Body
b.	Centering point	ASIS	ASIS	ASIS
c.	Imaging planes	Sagittal	Axial	Axial
d.	Contrast	Mild T1W	Mild T2W	Moderate T1W
e.	Slice thickness	Routine	Routine	Routine

The sagittal plane was first used since it is helpful in evaluating midline structures (e.g., prostate, uterus, rectum, sacrum), in determining the longitudinal extent of lesions, and in centering for any additional scans in either the axial or coronal planes. The contrast was selected to provide sufficient T1 weighting on the first echo. When combined with a second echo, some T2 weighting is possible for screening for prolonged T2 lesions. Also, with mild T1 weighting, the TR is sufficiently long so that the coverage—in this example, 10 cm—is adequate.

The second plane is the standard imaging plane for the pelvis because its axial anatomy is familiar to most radiologists and allows symmetric comparison of the two sides of the pelvis. Such comparison is important in both the detection and diagnosis of pathology. For further tissue characterization, both T1 weighting and T2 weighting were performed.

A coronal scan may occasionally be helpful for additional anatomic detail (e.g., pelvic side wall invasion). In any case, we recommend scanning the pelvis in at least two orthogonal planes.

MR FINDINGS

Figure 80.1. There is a well-defined, heterogeneous mass in the right/midpelvis that appears to be compressing and displacing the uterus. This mass originates in the region of the broad ligament and has low attenuation consistent with fat. No calcifications were visualized.

Figure 80.2. On the MR scan, the mass (m) is shown to have components of relatively high intensity similar to the surrounding pelvic fat, indicating it has a relatively short T1 and a long T2. Heterogeneity is again noted. The uterus appears atrophic consistent with the patient's age.

Figures 80.3 and 80.4. Similar findings compared with those of the CT study are noted. On all pulsing sequences, the main component of the mass is similar to fat in signal intensity. No other masses were identified, and there was no evidence of adenopathy.

DIFFERENTIAL DIAGNOSIS

The preceding findings are characteristic of a dermoid tumor (see typical findings later). However, other differential considerations should include:

1. **Endometriomas.** These lesions have been reported to have prolonged T2, probably related to their cystic component, and have high signal intensity on T2-weighted images. Different endometriomas, however, may show different signal intensities on a T1-weighted image because of differing T1 values. This is thought to be related to differences in iron content.[1,2] Endometriomas can be quite difficult to separate from dermoids on MRI (see Case 81). In some cases, the presence of calcifications within the tumor may help in this distinction.

2. **Cystadenoma.** Although most types of cystadenomas are predominately cystic and appear similar on sonogram, they may have quite different MR appearances. Depending on their protein content, they have been reported to have variable T1 and T2 values, which at times may simulate those of a dermoid tumor.[1,2] Calcification would be unusual for this tumor, however (see Case 83).

3. **Ovarian Cyst.** The short T1 of the preceding mass would be atypical for an uncomplicated ovarian cyst. A cyst with hemorrhage, however, may appear quite similar to a dermoid or an endometrioma.

4. **Tubo-ovarian Abscess.** Since these may have a significant cystic component, they also may have a prolonged T2 and high intensity on T2-weighted images. Because of their proteinaceous component, they also may have a shortened T1. The relative lack of symptoms is against this diagnosis, however.

It should be noted that the use of MRI in diagnosing gynecologic pathology should be considered secondary at this time. Ultrasound, being less expensive and nonionizing, should still be the primary imaging modality. In addition, the preceding entities may be more easily distinguished on the basis of sonographic findings since ultrasound is more sensitive than MRI in the detection and differentiation of the various components of cystic masses.

Final Diagnosis

Dermoid.

SUMMARY OF MR FINDINGS FOR DERMOID[1-3]

1. May have quite a heterogeneous intensity pattern because of their variable components of hair, fat, calcification, and fluid.

2. Generally, they are of high intensity on most pulsing sequences, indicating a shortened T1 and a prolonged T2, probably due to their significant fat content.
3. Calcifications may be seen as a signal void focus but generally are difficult to detect on MRI alone because of the modality's relative insensitivity to calcification (see Figure 80.5).

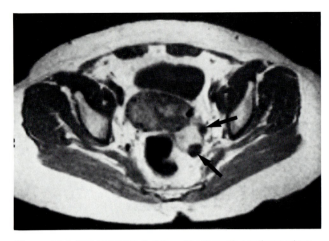

Figure 80.5 (SE 1500/28). Axial section through another patient with a dermoid tumor. Note the foci of low signal intensity (arrows) along the left lateral and inferior wall of the mass representing calcification.

REFERENCES

1. Butler H, Bryan PJ, LiPuma JP, et al: Magnetic resonance imaging of the abnormal female pelvis. *AJR* 1984;143:1259–1266.
2. Bryan PJ, Butler HE, LiPuma JP, et al: NMR scanning of the pelvis: Initial experience with a 0.3 T system. *AJR* 1983;141:1111–1118.
3. Hricak H, Alpers C, Crooks LE, et al: Magnetic resonance imaging of the female pelvis: Initial experience. *AJR* 1983;141:1119–1128.

CASE 81

HISTORY

A 30-year-old woman with a history of infertility and irregular menses presenting with bilateral adnexal masses.

QUESTIONS

1. What are your differential considerations?

   _____

   _____

2. What MR techniques would you use?

	1	2	3
a. Coil	____	____	____
b. Centering point	____	____	____
c. Imaging plane(s)	____	____	____
d. Contrast	____	____	____
e. Slice thickness	____	____	____

3. What do you expect to find?

   _____

   _____

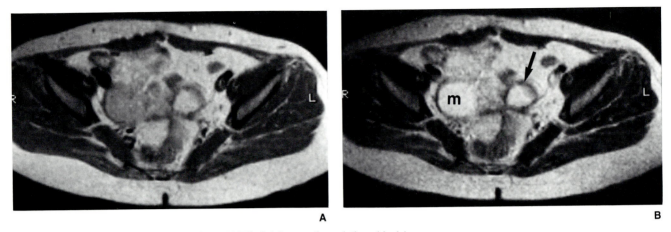

A   **B**

Figures 81.1A (SE 2000/28) and **81.1B** (SE 2000/56). Axial scans through the midpelvis.

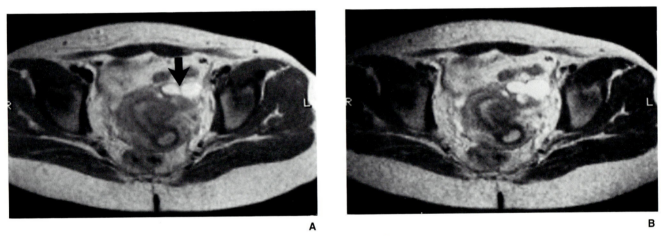

A   **B**

Figures 81.2A (SE 2000/28) and **81.2B** (SE 2000/56). Axial scans 2 cm inferior to Figure 81.1.

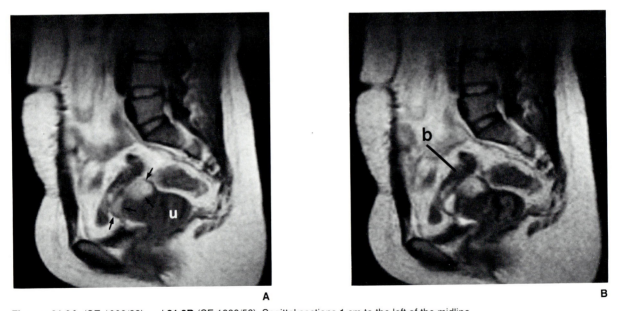

A   **B**

Figures 81.3A (SE 1000/28) and **81.3B** (SE 1000/56). Sagittal sections 1 cm to the left of the midline.

410/PRACTICAL MAGNETIC RESONANCE IMAGING

MR TECHNIQUES

		1	2
a.	Coil	Body	Body
b.	Centering point	ASIS*	Midline
c.	Imaging planes	Axial	Sagittal
d.	Contrast	Mild and moderate T2W	Mild T1W and mild T2W
e.	Slice thickness	Routine	Routine

*Anterior superior iliac spine.

See introductory section and Case 80 on imaging technique of the pelvis.

MR FINDINGS

Figure 81.1. There is a 3.5-cm, well-defined mass (m) in the right adnexal area. The mass has an intermediate intensity on the first echo image but becomes more intense on the second echo image, indicating a prolonged T2 compared with that of surrounding soft tissues. There is an additional 2.5-cm, well-circumscribed mass (arrow) in the left adnexal area. Compared with the right-sided lesion, this mass is slightly more intense on the first echo image but becomes similar in intensity on the second echo image.

Figure 81.2. There are two well-defined smaller masses (arrow) located anterior and to the left of the uterus. Compared with the lesions seen in Figure 81.1, the signal intensity of these smaller masses is greater on both the first and second echo images.

Note the typical appearance of the uterus, with the three distinct layers, as described in the introductory section.

Figure 81.3. On this moderate T1W1, the left adnexal masses (arrows) seen in Figures 81.1 and 81.2 are shown to be in close proximity to the uterus (u). The tubular low intensity structure (b) immediately anterior to the masses represents a nonopacified loop of bowel.

DIFFERENTIAL DIAGNOSIS

The diagnostic consideration for multiple pelvic masses with varying signal intensities in a young female is largely limited to endometriosis. It is conceivable that these masses could represent multiple abscesses secondary to pelvic inflammatory disease. However, the anterior and superior distribution of these lesions, preservation of the surrounding fascial planes, and relative lack of clinical symptoms would be atypical for this diagnosis. Although the signal intensities of cystadenomas may vary depending on the protein content (described in Case 82), the separate locations of these tumors makes cystadenoma very unlikely. Similar arguments hold true for multiple follicular cysts and dermoid tumors.

There are two distinct forms of endometriosis.[1] The more common type is the infiltrating form, which presents as multiple small implants on the peritoneal lining. Clinically, this type usually presents with diffuse pelvic pain that worsens with menses. The second type presents as multiple focal masses, and clinically, affected patients are usually less symptomatic. The first type is difficult to visualize on ultrasound, CT, or MRI and is best diagnosed by laparoscopy. The second type is more readily identifiable on any of these three imaging modalities.

The MR intensity characteristics of endometriomas can vary depending on the cyst protein content and the presence of hemorrhage.[2] (See introductory section.)

Final Diagnosis

Multiple endometriomas.

SUMMARY OF MR FINDINGS FOR ENDOMETRIOSIS

As discussed in the differential diagnosis section, only one of the two forms of endometriosis is demonstrable on MRI.

1. Well-defined masses of varying sizes.
2. Variable signal intensity patterns with homogeneous texture.
3. The size and intensity of the lesions may change on serial examinations depending on the clinical course and the menstrual cycle.

REFERENCES

1. Athey PA: Adnexa: Nonneoplastic cysts, in Athey PA, Hadlock FP (eds): *Ultrasound in Obstetrics and Gynecology.* St. Louis, CV Mosby Co, 1985, pp 206–221.
2. Butler H, Bryan PJ, LiPuma JP, et al: Magnetic resonance imaging of the abnormal female pelvis. *AJR* 1984;143:1259.

CASE 82

HISTORY

A 34-year-old woman presenting with a large abdominal/pelvic mass. She noted a mass in her pelvis 1 year previously. She also complained of shortness of breath and bipedal edema. An ultrasound examination is shown in Figure 82.1.

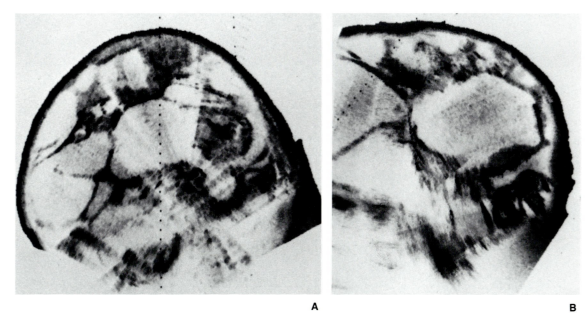

A   B

Figures 82.1A (transverse) and **82.1B** (longitudinal). Sonograms of the lower abdomen and pelvis.

QUESTIONS

1. What are your differential considerations?

   _____

   _____

2. What MR techniques would you use?

	1	2	3
a. Coil	___	___	___
b. Centering point	___	___	___
c. Imaging plane(s)	___	___	___
d. Contrast	___	___	___
e. Slice thickness	___	___	___

3. What do you expect to find?

   _____

   _____

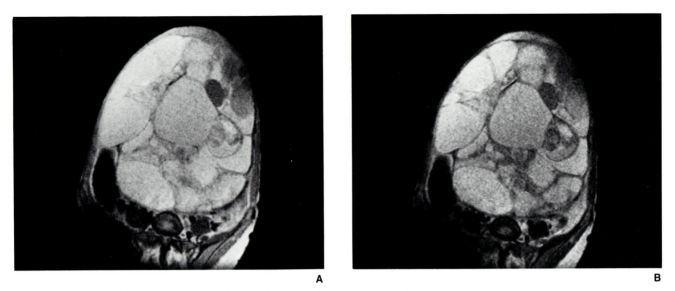

Figures 82.2A (SE 2000/28) and **82.2B** (SE 2000/56). Axial scans through the lower abdomen.

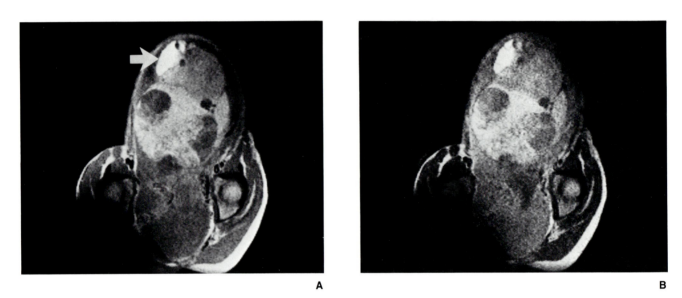

Figures 82.3A (SE 1000/28) and **82.3B** (SE 1000/56). Axial scans through the pelvis.

MR TECHNIQUES

		1	2
a.	Coil	Body	Body
b.	Centering point	Umbilicus	ASIS*
c.	Imaging planes	Axial	Axial
d.	Contrast	Mild and moderate T2W	Mild T1W and mild T2W
e.	Slice thickness	Routine	Routine

*ASIS = anterior superior iliac spine

Because the patient experienced significant respiratory distress when supine, she was placed in the left lateral decubitus position within the body coil. A T2WI was chosen to cover a large area (20 cm) of the abdomen without the need for repositioning the patient between acquisitions. In the pelvis, the area to be examined is smaller; hence, a shorter TR was chosen. In addition, more T1 weighting allowed further tissue characterization and increased sensitivity to the presence of hemorrhage. With these two sequences, we were able to examine the bulk of the mass within a reasonable period of time.

Ideally, sagittal scans would have been performed to better define midline structures as well as the superior and inferior extent of the tumor. However, the patient was not able to tolerate additional examination.

MR FINDINGS

Figure 82.1. There is a large complex mass with both cystic and solid components, extending from the deep pelvis to the upper abdomen. The cystic components of the mass have multiple septations and a heterogeneous echo pattern.

Figures 82.2 and 82.3. Similar findings are shown with the MR images. The septations are well demonstrated, and the cystic components are noted to have varying signal intensities, reflecting different concentrations of protein. Note the focal area of high signal intensity (arrow) in Figure 82.3A, indicating significant T1 shortening possibly because of the presence of methemoglobin. The tumor margins are well defined by MRI.

Compared with MRI, ultrasound is more accurate in determining the cystic nature of a mass, particularly if there is elevated protein concentration. The advantage of MRI in this case is its ability to demonstrate the retroperitoneal structures and tumor margins.

DIFFERENTIAL DIAGNOSIS

In view of the preceding findings, the differential is largely limited to ovarian neoplasms, such as cystadenomas or cystadenocarcinomas. The presence of fine echogenic material and high protein content indicate that the tumor may be mucus producing, such as a pseudomucinous cystadenoma. *Pseudomucinous cystadenoma* is the most common type of ovarian cystic mass and is composed of epithelial cells that secrete mucin. These cysts may vary in size, ranging to 30 cm. In fact, the more massive ovarian tumors tend to be of this type.

On gross examination, the capsule of the tumor appears to be smooth, lobulated, and glistening. Internally, there are multiple cystic compartments of varying sizes separated by thick septa. The fluid may be mucoid, viscid, transparent, and/or cloudy. Hemorrhage and necrosis are frequently seen.[1]

Following the MR examination, the patient underwent surgery. A 10-kg tumor with the gross pathologic characteristics just described was removed. Histologic examination confirmed the diagnosis of pseudomucinous cystadenoma.

A rare complication of this entity is *pseudomyxoma peritonei*, presumably due to rupture of the tumor with implantation of the epithelial cells within the abdominal cavity. This was not present during surgery.

Final Diagnosis

Pseudomucinous cystadenoma.

SUMMARY OF MR FINDINGS FOR PSEUDOMUCINOUS CYSTADENOMA[1,2]

1. A well-encapsulated, multiseptated complex tumor.
2. Variable intensity pattern depending on the protein content.
3. Hemorrhage may be demonstrated.
4. Compared with MRI, ultrasound is more accurate in distinguishing between the cystic and solid nature of the mass.
5. Rarely, ascites may also be seen.

REFERENCES

1. Netter FH: Pseudomucinous cystadenoma, in *The CIBA Collection of Medical Illustrations: Reproductive System.* CIBA, Summit, NJ, 1970, vol 2, p 200.
2. Dooms GC, Hricak H, Tscholakoff D: Adnexal structures: MR imaging. *Radiology* 1986;158:639–646.

CASE 83

HISTORY

A 43-year-old woman presents with urinary frequency and urgency. A large, complex pelvic mass with predominate cystic components was seen on pelvic sonogram.

QUESTIONS

1. What are your differential considerations?

   _____

   _____

2. What MR techniques would you use?

	1	2	3
a. Coil	____	____	____
b. Centering point	____	____	____
c. Imaging plane(s)	____	____	____
d. Contrast	____	____	____
e. Slice thickness	____	____	____

3. What do you expect to find?

   _____

   _____

Source: Courtesy of Arthur Radow, MD, Glendale, AZ.

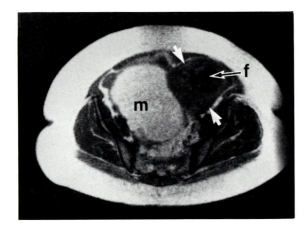

Figure 83.1 (SE 1000/28). Axial scan through the midsacrum.

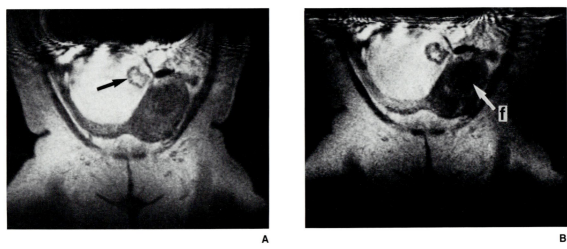

A   B

Figures 83.2A (SE 1500/28) and **83.2B** (SE 1500/56). Coronal scans through the anterior third of the pelvis.

MR TECHNIQUES

	1	2
a. Coil	Body	Body
b. Centering point	ASIS*	ASIS*
c. Imaging planes	Axial	Axial
d. Contrast	Mild T1W and mild T2W	Mild to moderate T2W
e. Slice thickness	Routine	Routine

*Anterior superior iliac spine

Axial images were acquired with moderate T1 weighting (TR = 1,000 mseconds) to provide tissue characterization of the lesion previously identified on pelvic sonogram. With this relatively short TR, the entire pelvis cannot be examined with one pulsing sequence; hence, a second sequence was performed in the coronal projection with a TR of 1,500 mseconds.

MR FINDINGS

Figure 83.1. There is a well-defined, homogeneous mass (m) measuring 12 cm by 12 cm by 9 cm in the right false pelvis. The signal intensity is high, indicating T1 shortening. In addition, there is a mass (arrows) with a signal intensity similar to that of skeletal muscle in the left side of the pelvis. There is also a well-circumscribed, low intensity area (f) within this mass.

Figure 83.2. On this coronal image with a slightly longer TR, the masses just mentioned are again demonstrated. Within the larger mass in the right false pelvis, there is a 4 cm by 2 cm mural nodule (arrow) with mixed signal intensity. The mass within the left side of the pelvis appears to be an enlarged uterus with a large myoma (f) represented by the central area of low signal intensity.

DIFFERENTIAL DIAGNOSIS

The differential diagnosis for this large pelvic mass would include a functional ovarian cyst, a cystadenoma, a cystadenocarcinoma, or a dermoid tumor. Although endometrioma or pelvic abscess could be considered, they usually do not attain this large a size without causing significant clinical symptoms. The presence of a mural nodule excludes a functional ovarian cyst and also would make a cystadenoma less likely.

The high signal intensity on the moderately T1-weighted axial images is suggestive of either fat or subacute hemorrhage. Therefore, a hemorrhagic cystadenocarcinoma or dermoid would be the most likely diagnosis. On surgery, a large cystadenocarcinoma containing brownish fluid, consistent with subacute hemorrhage, along with a smaller solid mass was found.

Final Diagnosis

Cystadenocarcinoma of the ovary.

SUMMARY OF MR FINDINGS FOR CYSTADENOCARCINOMA OF THE OVARY[1,2]

1. A complex pelvic mass with both solid and cystic components.
2. The signal intensity of the cystic components reflects its fluid content, which may have varying amounts of protein and/or hemorrhage.
3. When septation is demonstrated, cystadenomas may be distinguished from dermoid tumors.

REFERENCES

1. Butler H, Bryan PJ, LiPuma JP, et al: Magnetic resonance imaging of the abnormal female pelvis. *AJR* 1984;143:1259.
2. Dooms GC, Hricak H, Tscholakoff D: Adnexal structures: MR imaging. *Radiology* 1986;158:639–646.

CASE 84

HISTORY

A 32-year-old gravida 2, para 1 woman whose uterus was found to be larger than anticipated for her menstrual age. The patient's beta-HCG level was markedly elevated.

QUESTIONS

1. What are your differential considerations?

   _____

   _____

2. What MR techniques would you use?

	1	2	3
a. Coil	___	___	___
b. Centering point	___	___	___
c. Imaging plane(s)	___	___	___
d. Contrast	___	___	___
e. Slice thickness	___	___	___

3. What do you expect to find?

   _____

   _____

Source: Courtesy of Arthur Radow, MD, Glendale, AZ.

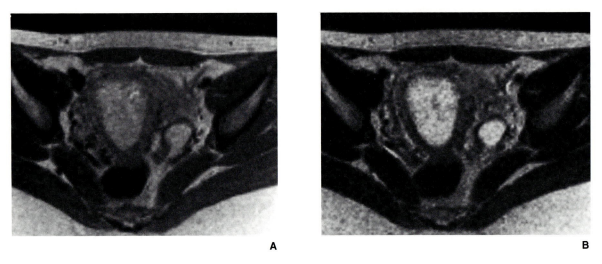

A　　　　　　　　　　　　　　　　　**B**

Figures 84.1A (SE 2000/28) and **84.1B** (SE 2000/56). Axial scans through the uterus.

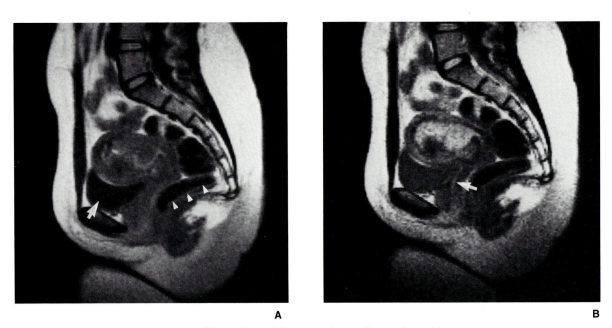

A　　　　　　　　　　　　　　　　　**B**

Figures 84.2A (SE 1000/28) and **84.2B** (SE 1000/56). Midline sagittal scans through the pelvis.

MR TECHNIQUES

	1	2
a. Coil	Body	Body
b. Centering point	ASIS*	Midline pelvis
c. Imaging planes	Axial	Sagittal
d. Contrast	Mild and moderate T2W	Mild T1W and mild T2W
e. Slice thickness	Routine	Routine

*Anterior superior iliac spine

The first pulsing sequence provides T2 information about the uterine content and has the additional benefit of multiple slices, which cover a larger area with a single pulsing sequence. The second pulsing sequence was chosen with mild T1 weighting to provide better anatomic definition. The axial plane is the standard imaging plane of the abdomen and pelvis and allows comparison of right–left symmetry. The sagittal images are useful in evaluating the midline structures of the pelvis.

MR FINDINGS

Figure 84.1. The uterine cavity is filled with a mass with a heterogeneous signal intensity. The intensity of the mass is greater on the second echo image, indicating a prolonged T2 compared with the surrounding soft tissue. No discernible normal fetal structures are identified.[1] A 3-cm high intensity, well-circumscribed mass is also seen in the left adnexa.

Figure 84.2. On this mild T1WI, a moderately enlarged uterus is shown to be posterior and superior to the bladder (arrow) and anterior to the colon (arrowheads). The cervix is not well seen, but the vagina is readily identified (small arrow, Figure 84.2B). Heterogeneous soft tissue is again demonstrated within the uterine cavity, which has increased signal intensity compared with urine, indicating T1 shortening.

DIFFERENTIAL DIAGNOSIS

The abnormal signal intensit pattern of the uterine contents and the markedly elevated HCG leve suggest that this most likely represents a *molar pregnancy*. This is not a *normal pregnancy* since amniotic fluid should have the same signal characteristic as urine in the bladder. An *incomplete abortion* should also be considered and could conceivably have this appearance; however, in that case, the HCG level should be low.

The left adnexal mass most likely represents a theca-lutein cyst. In general, these cysts are bilateral and septated. This adnexal mass may also represent a corpus-lutein cyst, however. MRI is not able to differentiate between these two entities.

Occasionally, vaginal bleeding can be associated with a molar pregnancy, and subacute hemorrhage may be identified within the mass.[2]

Final Diagnosis

Molar pregnancy.

SUMMARY OF MR FINDINGS FOR MOLAR PREGNANCY

1. Uterus larger than expected for gestational age.
2. Signal intensity of uterine contents not typical for normal amniotic fluid.

   a. Heterogeneous intensity.
   b. T2 may be prolonged compared with that for the surrounding soft tissue, and the T1 is shorter than that of urine.

3. Adnexal masses representing theca-lutein cysts.
4. Hemorrhage may be demonstrated around the mass.
5. Normal fetal structures not identifiable.

REFERENCES

1. Weinreb JC, Lowe T, Cohen JM, et al: Human fetal anatomy: MR imaging. *Radiology* 1985;157:715–720.
2. Weinreb JC, Lowe TW, Santos-Ramos R, et al: Magnetic resonance imaging in obstetric diagnosis. *Radiology* 1985;154:157–161.

Appendix A

LISTING OF CASES

IMAGE CONTRAST VS. TR AND TE AT 0.35 AND 1.5T

CONTRAST	0.35T		1.5T	
	TR*	TE*	TR*	TE*
Heavy T1	TR ≤ 300	min	TR ≤ 400	min
Moderate T1	300 < TR ≤ 800	min	400 < TR ≤ 1200	min
Mild T1	800 < TR ≤ 1000	min	1200 < TR ≤ 1800	min
Proton density	TR > 2000	min	TR > 3000	min
Mild T2	1000 < TR ≤ 2000	30 < TE < 50	1500 < TR ≤ 3000	30 < TE < 50
Moderate T2	TR ≤ 2000	50 < TE < 70	TR ≤ 3000	50 < TE < 70
Heavy T2	TR ≥ 2000	TE ≥ 70	TR ≥ 3000	≥ 70

*All times in mseconds
min = minimum TE available

427

Appendix B-2
SLICE THICKNESS

Description	Thickness (mm)
Thick	> 10
Routine	7–10
Thin	4–6
Very thin	3 or less

Appendix B-3
SPATIAL RESOLUTION

Type	Resolution (mm)
Routine	> 1.0
High	.75–.95
Very high	< .75

Appendix C

SUMMARY OF MR PROTOCOLS FOR ADULTS

Region	Indication/Structure	Coil	Plane	Thickness
Brain				
	General screening	Head	Axial	Routine
	AVM/Aneurysm	Head	Axial	Thin
			Coronal	Thin
	Facial pain	Head	Axial	Thin
	Headaches	Head	Axial	Routine
	Hearing loss/Vertigo	Head	Axial	Thin
			Axial	Thin-very thin
	Hydrocephalus	Head	Axial	Routine
			Sagittal	Thin
	Memory loss	Head	Axial	Routine
	Multiple sclerosis	Head	Axial	Thin
	Psychiatric disorder	Head	Axial	Routine
	Seizures	Head	Axial or Coronal	Routine
	Stroke	Head	Axial	Routine-thin
	Subdural hematoma	Head	Axial	Routine
			Coronal	Routine
	Hemispheric lesion	Head	Axial	Routine-thin
			Coronal	Routine-thin
	Brainstem lesion	Head	Axial	Routine-thin
			Sagittal	Thin
	Skull base lesion	Head	Axial	Routine-thin
			Coronal	Thin
	Vertex lesion	Head	Coronal	Routine-thin
			Axial	Thin
	Foramen magnum lesion	Head	Axial	Thin
			Sagittal	Thin
	Pineal mass	Head	Axial	Thin
			Sagittal	Thin
	Sellar mass	Head	Axial	Thin
			Sagittal	Thin-very thin
			Coronal	Thin-very thin

Center	Coverage (cm)	Contrast	Comments
			All head studies include a "survey" sequence of the entire brain.
CML	15	Mild to moderate T2W	
CML	15	Mild to moderate T2W	
Lesion	5-10	Mild to moderate T1W	
EAC	20	Mild to moderate T2W	Include parotid glands
CML	15	Mild to moderate T2W	
CML	15	Mild to moderate T2W	
EAC	4-5	Moderate T1W	
CML	15	Mild to moderate T2W	
Mid-sagittal	4-5	Moderate T1W	
CML	15	Mild to moderate T2W	
CML	20	Mild to moderate T2W	Include upper cervical cord
CML	15	Mild to moderate T2W	
CML or Mid-Coronal	15	Mild to moderate T2W	
CML	15	Mild to moderate T2W	May need heavy T2 or T1 weighting to confirm acute or subacute hemorrhage
CML	15	Mild to moderate T2W	
Lesion	5-10	Moderate T1W	
CML	15	Mild to moderate T2W	
Lesion	5-10	Moderate T1W	
EAC	15	Mild to moderate T2W	
Mid-sagittal	4-5	Moderate T1W	
EAC	15-20	Mild to moderate T2W	
Lesion	5-10	Mild to moderate T1W	
Mid-coronal	15	Mild to moderate T2W	
Lesion	5-10	Moderate T1W	
EAC	15	Mild to moderate T2W	
Foramen magnum	4-5	Moderate T1W	
CML	15	Mild to moderate T2W	
Mid-sagittal	4-5	Moderate T1W	
CML	15	Mild to moderate T2W	
Mid-sagittal	4-5	Moderate T1W	
Sella	4-5	Moderate T1W	

Region	Indication/Structure	Coil	Plane	Thickness
Brain (cont)				
	Cavernous sinus	Head	Axial	Thin
			Coronal	Thin
	Optic Chiasm/Tracts	Head	Axial	Thin
			Coronal	Thin
			Sagittal	Thin
Orbits	Intra-orbital mass	Head or Surface	Axial	Thin-very thin
			Coronal	Thin-very thin
	Intrabulbar lesion	Head or Surface	Axial	Thin-very thin
			Axial or Coronal	Thin-very thin
Spine Cord	Screening	As indicated	Sagittal	Thin-very thin
	Arachnoiditis	As indicated	Sagittal	Thin-very thin
			Axial	Thin
	Dysraphism	As indicated	Sagittal	Thin-very thin
			Axial	Routine-thin
	Herniated disc	Surface	Sagittal	Thin-very thin
			Axial	Thin-very thin
	Intraspinal mass	As indicated	Sagittal	Thin-very thin
			Axial or Coronal	Routine-thin
	Metastases	As indicated	Sagittal	Thin-very thin
			Axial or Coronal	Thin-very thin
	Multiple sclerosis	As indicated	Sagittal	Thin-very thin
			Axial or Coronal	Thin-very thin

Center	Coverage (cm)	Contrast	Comments
CML	15	Mild to moderate T2W	
Sella	4-5	Moderate T1W	
CML	15	Mild to moderate T2W	
Sella	4-5	Moderate T1W	
Mid-sagittal	4-5	Moderate T1W	
CML	4-5	Mild to moderate T1W	
Mid-orbit	4-5	Mild to moderate T1W	
Globe	4-5	Mild to moderate T1W	
Globe		Mild to moderate T2W	
			The choice of a volume vs. a surface spine coil should depend on desired signal-to-noise, field of view, and depth of focus. Sagittal sequence coverage should be adequate to include the entire width of the spine (4-5 cm in the cervical and upper thoracic region and 6-8 cm in the lower thoracic and lumbosacral region). Sagittal sequence centering should allow evaluation of the level(s) of interest and reference to a segmental landmark, ie, the C2 or S1 vertebral bodies. Axial and coronal sequence coverage and centering should be adequate to include the level(s) of interest and to define the superior and inferior extent of any lesion.
As indicated	4-8	Mild T1W to mild T2W	
As indicated	4-8	Mild T1W to mild T2W	
As indicated	As indicated	Mild T1W to mild T2W	
As indicated	4-8	Mild T1W to mild T2W	
As indicated	As indicated	Moderate T2W	
As indicated	4-8	Mild T1W to mild T2W	
As indicated	As indicated	Mild T1W to mild T2W	
As indicated	4-8	Mild T1W to mild T2W	
As indicated	As indicated	Mild to moderate T2W	
As indicated	4-8	Mild to moderate T1W	
As indicated	As indicated	Mild to Moderate T2W	
As indicated	4-8	Mild to moderate T2W	Include T2-weighted brain examination
As indicated	/.s indicated	Mild to moderate T2W	

Region	Indication/Structure	Coil	Plane	Thickness
Spine/ Cord (cont)				
	Myelomeningocele	As indicated	Sagittal Axial	Thin-very thin Thin-very thin
	Osteomyelitis/Discitis	As indicated	Sagittal Sagittal	Thin-very thin Thin-very thin
	Scar vs. disc	Surface	Sagittal Axial	Thin-very thin Thin-very thin
	Spinal stenosis	As indicated	Sagittal Axial	Thin-very thin Thin-very thin
	Syringomyelia (non-neoplastic)	As indicated	Sagittal Axial	Thin-very thin Routine-thin
	Tethered cord	As indicated	Sagittal Axial	Thin-very thin Thin-very thin
	Transverse myelitis	As indicated	Sagittal Axial or Coronal	Thin-very thin Thin
	Trauma	As indicated	Sagittal Axial	Thin-very thin Thin
	Vascular malformation	Surface	Sagittal Axial	Thin-very thin Thin-very thin
Head/ Neck				
	Skull base	Head	Axial Coronal	Thin Thin
	Nasopharynx/Infra- temporal fossa	Head	Axial Coronal	Thin Thin
	Nasal cavity	Head	Axial Coronal or Sagittal	Thin Thin
	Oropharynx/Tongue	Head	Axial Coronal	Thin Thin
	Larynx/Hypopharynx	Surface	Axial Coronal Sagittal	Thin Thin Thin
	Paranasal Sinuses	Head	Axial Coronal	Thin Thin
	Salivary Glands	Head or Surface	Axial	Thin

Center	Coverage (cm)	Contrast	Comments
As indicated	4-8	Mild T1W to mild T2W	
As indicated	As indicated	Moderate T1W	
As indicated	4-8	Moderate T1W	
As indicated	4-8	Moderate T2W	
As indicated	4-8	Mild T1W to mild T2W	
As indicated	As indicated	Mild to moderate T2W	
As indicated	4-8	Mild T1W to mild T2W	
As indicated	As indicated	Mild T1W to mild T2W	
As indicated	4-8	Mild T1W to mild T2W	Include foramen
As indicated	As indicated	Moderate T1W	magnum to exclude Chiari malformation
As indicated	4-8	Mild T1W to mild T2W	
As indicated	As indicated	Moderate T1W	
As indicacted	4-8	Mild to moderate T2W	
As indicated	As indicated	Mild to moderate T2W	
As indicated	4-8	Mild T1W-mild T2W	
As indicated	As indicated	Mild T1W-mild T2W	
As indicated	4-8	Mild T1W-mild T2W	May need gating to eliminate CSF flow artifacts
As indicated	As indicated	Mild T1W-mild T2W	
EAC	15	Mild to moderate T2W	If evaluation of cervical adenopathy is indicated in any head/neck case, obtain additional, appropriately centered, T1-weighted axial sections
Lesion	5-10	Moderate T1W	
Angle of jaw	15	Mild to moderate T2W	
Lesion	5-10	Moderate T1W	
EAC	15	Mild to moderate T2W	
Lesion	5-10	Mild to moderate T1W	
Angle of jaw	15	Mild to moderate T2W	
Mid-tongue	10-15	Mild to moderate T2W	
Thyroid cartilage	10-15	Mild to moderate T1W	
Mid-larynx	7-10	Mild to moderate T1W	
Mid-sagittal	4-5	Mild to moderate T1W	
Inf. orbital rim	10-15	Mild to moderate T2W	
Mid-sinus	7-10	Mild to moderate T1W	
Angle of jaw	10-15	Mild to moderate T2W	

Region	Indication/Structure	Coil	Plane	Thickness
Head/ Neck (cont)				
	Thyroid/Parathyroid	Surface	Axial	Thin
			Sagittal or Coronal	Thin
	Temporomandibular joint	Surface	Sagittal	Thin-very thin
Thorax				
	Brachial plexus	Body	Axial	Routine
			Coronal	Routine
	Superior mediastinum	Body	Axial	Routine
			Coronal	Routine
	Inferior mediastinum	Body	Axial	Routine
			Coronal	Routine
	Hilar mass	Body	Axial	Routine
			Coronal	Routine
Cardiac				
	Congenital anomaly	Body	Axial	Routine-thin
			Coronal or Sagittal	Routine-thin
	Coronary artery/Bypass graft patency	Body	Axial	Thin
	Myocardial infarct/ Myocarditis	Body	Axial	Routine
			Axial	Routine
	Wall motion	Body	Axial	Routine
	Pericardial disease	Body	Axial	Routine
			Coronal	Routine
	Thoracic aorta	Body	Axial	Routine
			Sagittal/ oblique	Thin
Abdomen				
	Liver/Spleen	Body	Axial	Routine
			Axial	Routine

Center	Coverage (cm)	Contrast	Comments
Thyroid cartilage	10-15	Mild to moderate T2W	
Mid-thyroid	7-10	Mild to moderate T1W	
EAC	3-4	Mild to moderate T1W	Two sequences (mouth open and closed) required for each side of interest
Clavicular heads	10	Mild to moderate T1W	
Lesion	10	Mild to moderate T1W	
Sternal notch	10-15	Mild to moderate T1W	
Anterior chest	5-10	Moderate T1W	
Mid-sternum	10-15	Gated every beat	
Mid-chest	5-10	Gated every beat	
Mid-sternum	10-15	Gated every beat	
Mid-chest	5-10	Gated every beat	
Mid-sternum	10-15	Gated every beat	
Mid-chest	10	Gated every beat	
Aortic root	5-10	Gated every beat	May need localizing scan for appropriate centering
Mid-ventricle	5-10	Gated every beat	
Mid-ventricle	5-10	Gated every other beat	
Mid-ventricle	5-10	Gated every beat	Obtain midventricular sections in systole and diastole. If constrictive pericarditis is suspected, obtain mid-atrial sections in systole and diastole.
Mid-sternum	10	Gated every beat	
Mid-chest	5-10	Gated every beat	
Mid-sternum	10-15	Gated every beat	
Aortic arch	5-10	Gated every beat	
Xyphoid	15-20	Moderate to heavy T1W	Use oral contrast (250 cc of 5% ferrous solution)
Xyphoid	15-20	Mild to Moderate T2W	

Region	Indication/Structure	Coil	Plane	Thickness
Abdomen (cont)				
	Pancreas	Body	Axial Axial	Routine Routine
	Renal/Adrenal	Body	Coronal Axial	Routine Routine
	Retroperitoneum	Body	Axial	Routine
Pelvis				
	Adnexa	Body	Axial Axial or Coronal	Routine Routine
	Bladder	Body	Axial Axial or Coronal Sagittal	Routine Routine Routine
	Prostate	Body	Axial Axial or Coronal Sagittal	Routine Routine Routine
	Rectum	Body	Axial Sagittal	Routine Routine
	Renal transplant	Body	Coronal Axial	Routine Routine
	Sacral plexus	Body	Axial	Routine
	Uterus	Body	Axial Sagittal	Routine Routine
Muscu-loskeletal				
	Hips/Shoulders-avascular necrosis	Body	Coronal Axial	Routine-thin Routine-thin
	Knees-internal derangement	Surface or Head	Sagittal Coronal	Thin-very thin Thin-very thin
	Bone tumor	As indicated	Axial Coronal or Sagittal	Routine-thin Routine-thin
	Soft tissue tumor	As indicated	Axial Coronal or Sagittal	Routine-thin Routine-thin

Center	Coverage (cm)	Contrast	Comments
Sub-xyphoid	10-15	Mild to moderate T1W	
Sub-xyphoid	10-15	Mild to moderate T2W	
Mid-kidney	10-15	Mild to moderate T1W	
Mid-kidney	10-15	Mild to moderate T2W	
As indicated	As indicated	Mild to moderate T1W	
Mid-pelvis	10-15	Mild to moderate T1W	
Adrexa	10-15	Mild to moderate T2W	
Lower pelvis	10-15	Mild to moderate T2W	
Bladder	10	Moderate T1W	
Mid-sagittal	5-10	Moderate T1W	
Lower pelvis	10-15	Mild to moderate T2W	
Prostate	10	Moderate T1W	
Mid-sagittal	5-10	Moderate T1W	
Lower pelvis	10-15	Mild to moderate T1W	Rectal contrast optional
Mid-sagittal	5-10	Moderate T1W	
Transplant	10-15	Moderate T1W	
Transplant	10-15	Mild to moderate T2W	
Lower pelvis	10-15	Mild to moderate T1W	
Lower pelvis	10-15	Mild to moderate T2W	
Mid-sagittal	5-10	Moderate T1W	
As indicated	10	Mild to moderate T1W	
As indicated	10	Mild to moderate T1W	
As indicated	10	Mild to moderate T1W	
As indicated	10	Mild to moderate T1W	Two or three sagittal sequences may be needed to include both menisci and cruciates.
As indicated	10-20	Mild to moderate T1W	
As indicated	5-10	Mild T1W–T2W	
As indicated	10-20	Mild to moderate T2W	
As indicated	5-10	Mild T1W–T2W	

GLOSSARY

Bandwidth	Range of frequencies in spin echo. Noise increases with square root of bandwidth.
CML	Canthomeatal line.
Coherence	Precessing in phase. Coherent precession generates the transverse component of magnetization, which is detectable by the RF coil.
Cryomagnet	Superconducting magnet that requires no electrical power once field is established. Superconductivity is a property of some substances whereby there is no electrical resistance at temperatures approaching absolute zero. Requires liquid helium to maintain low temperatures.
Deoxyhemoglobin	A paramagnetic form of hemoglobin in magnetically susceptible acute hemorrhage with short T2.
Diastolic Pseudogating	Cause of high intraluminal signal due to chance synchronization of cardiac and MR cycles.
Echo Delay Time	(TE) Time between 90-degree RF pulse and midpoint of spin echo.

Even-Echo Rephasing	Cause of high intraluminal signal during slow flow due to rephasing phenomenon on even-numbered spin echos when there is slow laminar flow through gradient.
FID	Free induction decay. Signal emitted by precessing transverse magnetization following 90-degree RF pulse. The decay envelope is determined by an exponential time constant T_2 in an ideal, perfectly uniform, external magnetic field. (In reality, the decay envelope is determined by a constant T_2 that includes nonuniformities in the external field.)
Flow-Related Enhancement	High signal produced by slowly flowing blood as fully magnetized (unsaturated) protons enter first slice of multislice imaging volume.
Fourier Transform	Representation of any shape by a sum of sines and cosines.
Gauss	A unit of magnetic field strength. The earth's magnetic field is approximately 0.5 Gauss at the surface (1 kilogauss = 10^3 Gauss; tesla = 10^4 Gauss).

Gradient Coils	Room temperature (resistive) electromagnetic coils generating magnetic fields that are superimposed on the main magnetic field to cause spatial variation in the field strength.
Gyromagnetic Ratio	Ratio of magnetic moment to angular momentum (indicated by γ). Constant for a given nucleus. 42.58 MHz per tesla for hydrogen nucleus (single proton).
Inversion Recovery	180°–90° pulse sequence producing T1-weighted images.
Magnetic Moment	The torque exerted on magnets or spinning, charged particles causing north–south alignment when placed in an external magnetic field.
Magnetization	Net effect of magnetic moments of an ensemble (large group) of protons precessing in a magnetic field. Presence of magnetization indicates degree of alignment of individual magnetic moments with external field. It is this group phenomenon that is observed following RF pulse sequence.
Methemoglobin	A paramagnetic form of hemoglobin that results from oxidative denaturation of deoxyhemoglobin. Causes T1 shortening by dipole–dipole interaction in 3 to 4 days.
Paramagnetism	Unpaired electrons cause substance to be attracted to stronger part of magnetic field (as opposed to diamagnetic substances). Dipole–dipole interaction causes T1 shortening followed by T2 shortening. Magnetic susceptibility effects lead to T2 shortening only.
Partial Saturation	Short TR spin echo acquisition.
Precession	Wobbling of top in earth's gravitational field or proton in external magnetic field. Precessional frequency given by Larmor equation:

$$\Omega = \gamma \, \mathbf{B}$$

The precessional frequency Ω (which is also frequency of RF pulse that causes resonance and is frequency of emitted MR signal) is determined by strength of local magnetic field $\mathbf{B}$ (sum of imposed static field, gradient field, and any significant internal fields that may be present in substance) and gyromagnetic ratio Υ.

Proton Density Weighted Image	Long-TR, short-TE image emphasizing proton density differences.
Quench	Loss of superconductivity in a cryomagnet. Usually results from failure to maintain environment at near absolute zero temperatures with liquid helium. Results in release of heat as magnet becomes resistive.
Relaxation	Process by which molecules in excited state (e.g., following 90 degree RF pulse) return to lower energy state. Mechanisms for relaxation depend on physical state of substance and are anisotropic (i.e., different in transverse and longitudinal directions).
spin lattice	(Thermal, longitudinal) relaxation; characterized by exponential time constant T_1:

$$M_z = M_o\,(1 - e^{-t/T_1})$$

Exchange of energy of excited hydrogen nucleus with any other molecules in lattice. Thermal effects (i.e., kinetic energy) prominent. Determines time to become initially magnetized after sample placed in magnetic field. Determines time for recovery of longitudinal magnetization M_z to equilibrium value M following RF pulse. T_1 of tissues dependent on water content.

spin-spin	(Transverse) relaxation: characterized by exponential time constant T_2:

$$M_{xy} = M_o e^{-t/T_2}$$

Exchange of energy of excited hydrogen nucleus with other precessing protons. Determines amplitude of spin echo.

Repetition Time TR	Time between 90-degree pulses that initiate spin echo sequences for a given slice.
Resistive Magnet	Air or iron core, room temperature electromagnet drawing electrical power and generating heat.

Resonance	Rapid, stimulated flipping between upper and lower (parallel and anti-parallel, north and south) energy states; exchange of energy with environment at discrete levels (quantum mechanical model). Process by which nuclei absorb RF energy when transmitted radio frequency matches precessional frequency (classical mechanical model).
RF Coil	Antenna for transmitting radiofrequency (RF) pulses and receiving MR signal (FID or spin echo). Saddle coil design used when main field is along body's axis (i.e., most superconducting magnets). Solenoidal coils used when main field is perpendicular to body's axis (e.g., permanent or vertical field, four-coil magnet).
RF Pulse	Short burst of radiofrequency energy generated by RF oscillator and transmitted by RF coil. Frequency to cause resonance determined by strength of local magnetic field. Duration and amplitude of RF pulse causes rotation of magnetization M about axis of RF coil. Typical rotations are quarter and half cycle (i.e., 90 degrees and 180 degrees), although lower flip angles are used in certain fast scanning techniques.
Saturation Recovery	Also called "repeated FID." 90-degree to 90-degree pulse sequences with less T1 discrimination than inversion recovery.
Shim Coils	Room temperature (resistive) electromagnetic coils used to reduce nonuniformities in main field.
Signal-to-Noise Ratio	The intensity of the NMR signal above random thermal noise is improved by sampling a larger volume or by performing multiple signal averages.
Spin	Property of nuclei with odd number of neutrons, protons, or both. Nuclei with spin have a magnetic moment and can display the NMR phenomenon.
Spin Echo	A signal produced following a 90-degree to 180-degree pulse sequence. The spin echo is actually two mirror image FIDs back to back. Its amplitude is determined by the T_2 of the substance.
Tesla	The standard unit of magnetic field strength; equivalent to 10,000 Gauss.
T1W	T1-weighting.
T1-weighted image (T1WI)	Short-TR, short-TE image emphasizing T1 differences.
T2W	T2-weighting.
T2-weighted image (T2WI)	Long-TR, long-TE image emphasizing T2 differences.

Note: Page numbers in italics indicate illustrations or tabular material.

413. See also Ultrasound
Sonography. *See* Ultrasound
Spatial resolution, 1, 11–12, 20–22, 23, *429*
  MRI compared to CT, 335
Speech, slurred, 87
Spinal canal, extension of tumor into, 327
Spinal cord, 45. *See also* Head and neck
  abnormalities (T1- and T2-weighted images for), 255
  adhesions, 255
  astrocytoma of, 251
  cervical, *111*, 238
  cervicothoracic, *250*
  cystic tumor of, 239
  enlargement and alteration of signal intensity of, 251
  focal areas of low signal intensity within proximal cervical, 239
  fusiform enlargement of upper thoracic, 251
  glioma of, 253
  head coil for, 251
  imaging technique for, 225–26
  inflammatory disease of, 226
  lesions of, 45
  MRI for evaluation of, 226
  MR protocols for, *434–37*
  myelomalacia of, 255
  paresthesia referable to disease of, 44
  proximal thoracic, *238*
  radiculopathy, 226–27
  sagittal plane for, 225
  screening of, 239
  swelling of, 251
  syrinx of, 239
  tethering of, 231
  trauma to, 226
  tumors of, 226
  upper thoracic, *250*
Spine. *See also* Head and neck
  atropic and displaced distal, 255
  disease of the bony, 227
  injury to bony, 226
  lower lumbar, *234*
  lumbar, *242, 254, 362, 363*
  lymphoma of, *248*
  metastatic disease of, 247
  midlumbar, *230*
  midthoracic, 246
  MR protocols for, *434–37*
  osteoporosis and, 255
  screening examination of, 45, 255
  T1 shortening in, 255
  thoracic, *254*
  thoracolumbar, *230*
  vascular abnormality in, 226
Spin echo, 1, 6, 8–11
  signal intensities and, 181
Spin echo sequence
  minimizing motion artifacts with heavily T1-weighted, 335
  multiple, *3*
Spin echo signal, 10, *20*
  generation of, 3
Spleen
  scan of liver and, *353*
  T1 weighting with shortened TR for, 375

Spondylolisthesis
  L-4 on L-5, 241
  L-5–S1, 396
Sternotomy sutures, 30
Stomach, leiomyosarcoma of wall of, 375
Streak artifacts, 42, 111
Stroke, 89, 90
Subarachnoid space, 255
Subcortical arteriosclerotic encephalopathy (SAE), 93
Subdural effusion, 82
Subdural hematoma, 81, 82
Subendocardial infarction (SEMI), 298
Sugioka's procedure, 273
Sulcus, compressed and displaced cerebral, 81
Superventricular level axial scans, *36, 92, 96*
Supralaryngeal level, *222*
Swallowing, difficulty in, 187
Swelling, right arm, 323, 325
Symmetry, assessment of right-left, 37, *423*
Syndrome
  Horner, 329
  infantile hypercalcemia, 311, 314
  Klippel-Feil, 45
  multiple midline tumor, 155
  Parinaud's, 153
  William's, 314
Synovial fluid, 257
Synovitis, atlantoaxial, 260
Syringomyelia, 45
  nonneoplastic, 226
Syrinx, 239

T

T1 contrast, effect of variable TR on, *8*
T1 relaxation time, 2, 377
  measurement of, 6
  physical basis for, 3–6
T1 shortening, 65, 73, 78, 81, 82, 134
T1-weighted images, 335, 337, 338
  contrast on mild, 201, 206
  decreased signal on, 227
  degrees of, 19–20, 82
  motion artifacts and, 335
  with short TR for contrast between mass, liver, spleen, and retroperitoneal structures, 375
  with short TR, short TE to differentiate fat from tumor, 182
T2*, 19
T2 contrast, effect on variable echo delay time on, *8*
T2 decay, *7*
T2 prolongation, 124, 193
T2 relaxation time
  measurement of, 6
  physical basis for, 3–6
  prolonged, 220, 332
T2 shortening, pathological, 140
T2 weighting
  for detecting demyelinating diseases, 107
  for detecting pulmonary nodules, 325
  to differentiate CSF from brain parenchyma, 116

  to differentiate normal from abnormal muscle, 278
  to differentiate tumor from normal tissue, 182, 219
  to distinguish urine from bladder wall, 383, 390
  every-other-heartbeat gating and, 305
TE. *See* Echo delay time (TE)
Temperomandibular joint (TMJ), 184
Tendons, 258
Teratoma, 333
Thigh, *282, 290*
  pain in, 281
Thin slices
  anatomic detail and, 65, 294
  linear abnormality detection and, 53
  for major intracranial vessels, 58
  to minimize partial volume averaging of small lesions, 107
  for small lesions, 107, 111
Thoracic inlet, 183
Thorax, MR protocols for, *438–39*
Thromboembolism, infarcts secondary to, 151
Thrombosis
  high intraluminal signal from, 183
  sinus, 211
Thrombus, 14
  mural (heart), 305
Thymoma, 333
Thyroid bed, *219*
Tinnitus, pulsatile, 207
tissue characterization, 32. *See also*
  Normal tissue; Pathological tissue; *names of specific tissues*
  MR sequence for, 42, 85
  T2-weighted pulsing sequence for normal vs. tumor, 219
Tongue, 183
  carcinoma of, 206
  mass on, 203
  neoplasm of, 206, 216
  paresis of, 195
  scan through, *204, 205*
TR
  advantages of long, 359
  for gated acquisitions, 294
  heart rate and, 305
Transplants, heart, 301
Transverse magnetization, loss of, 3
Transverse magnetization decay, 3
Trauma, 259
  extremity, 283
  pericardial effusion and, 305
  spinal, 226
Trigeminal neuralgia, 111
Trigeminal nuclei, MS plaques within, *110, 112*
Trophoblastic disease, 385
Tube, dysfunction of Eustachian, 191
Tuber cinerium, hamartoma of, *135*
Tuberculosis, pericardial effusion and, 305
Tumors. *See also* Malignancy
  bladder, 383, 387, 390
  brain, 9, *10*
  brainstem, 111
  cardiac, 299, 305
  contrast by mild T1 weighting, 201, 206
  CT for examining, 31, 325
  dermoid, *9*, 407–408, 411, 419

  detection of, 159, 258, 325
  differentiating from fat, 182, 223
  differentiating from muscle, 182
  differentiating from normal tissue, 219, 359
  flowing blood simulating, *210*
  giant cell, *286*
  glomus, 183, *209*
  glomus jugulare, 211
  hemorrhage with, 65
  infiltration of femur by, 287
  infiltrating (with transglottic extension), 219
  invasion of pericardial soft tissue, 396
  intracranial, 31
  jugulotympanic glomus, 211
  laryngeal, 220
  loss of fascial planes between adjacent organs and, 359–60
  mediastinal, 301, 325
  metastasizing of, 390
  MRI to examine, 325
  MRI to stage, 338, 359
  lymph node involvement in head and neck, *233*
  neurogenic, 193
  ovarian, 415
  pancoast, 329–30
  paralaryngeal, 220
  pineal region, 155
  prostate, 384
  pyriform sinus, 219
  rectum, 384, 393, 396–97
  recurrence of, 396
  retroperitoneal, 375–76
  salivary gland, 193
  soft-tissue component of, 287
  spinal, 235
  spinal cord, 226
  spread of, 390
  staging of, 338, 359, 390, 391, 397, 402
  superior sulcus, 329
  suspected, 29
  thyroid, 219
  T2-weighted pulsing sequence to distinguish normal tissue from, 219
  T2-weighted to distinguish renal parenchyma from, 359
  vascular, 61
  Wilm's, 364

U

Ultrasound
  for abdomen and pelvis, *413*
  for determining cystic nature of a mass, 415
  for evaluating gallbladder diseases, 337, 380
  for evaluating gynecologic pathology, 407
Umbilicus, CT scan at level of, *369*
Upper convexity of brain, CT and MR scans of, *80*
Uremia, 305
Urinary frequency and urgency, 417
Urine, T2 weighting to distinguish from bladder wall, 383
Urogram, excretory, 361

Uterus, 384, *422*
  abnormal signal intensity pattern
    for contents of, 423

V

Variables
  to describe image quality, 18
  improvement and worsening of, 17
Vascular abnormalities, evaluating, 30
Vascular clips, 30
Vascular malformation with
    hematoma, MR findings for, 65
Vasculitis, infarcts secondary to, 151
Vaso-occlusive disease, 29–30
Veins, 13
  AVM calcifications and abnormal,
    61
  hepatic, *9, 312*
  pulmonary, 297
  systemic, 297
Vena cava, inferior, 355
Venous angioma, 53
Ventricles (brain)
  coronal section at level of third, *48*
  deformity of, 81
  enlargement of, *119,* 120

fourth, 45, 159
lateral, *36, 41, 72, 80, 88, 92,* 96,
    106, 114, 119, 145, *150, 158*
  superior lateral, *106*
  third, *48,* 49, *114, 133, 137,* 140
Ventricles (heart), *304, 308*
  left, *295, 296,* 298, 299, 300
  right, *295,* 298
Ventricular areas,
  lateral, 41, *123*
  third, *48*
Ventricular bodies, 37
Ventricular morphology, sequence to
    define abnormal, 49
Ventricular septal defect (VSD), 309
Ventricular shunt, 120, *139*
Vermian lesion, superior, 73
Vermis, cerebellar (hemorrhagic foci
    in), 70
Vertebra, 247, *248, 254,* 329
Vertebral column. *See* Spine
Vertebrobasilar infarct, 93
Vertex, cranial, 30
Vision loss, left temporal, 131
Visual problems, 95, 153, 195
Vocal cords, *218*
Volume element (voxel), 1

Vomiting, 141. *See also* Nausea
Voxel volume, 22, *23*

W

Water
  T1 of hydration-layer vs. bulk
    phase, 5
  T1 relaxation time of, 3–4
  T2 prolongation and increase
    content of, 124
Watershed infarct, MR findings for,
    97
Weakness
  extremity, 105, 145
  right side, 67
White matter
  adjacent to frontal horns, 37
  age-related infarction of deep, 37

  demyelinating process and, 124
  high intensity periventricular
    lesions of, *124*
  intensity of, 8, *124,* 125
  low attenuation with periventricular,
    123

metastases and midline, 148
multiple high-intensity foci
    symmetrically distributed in
    periventricular, 93
periatrial, 147–48
periventricular, 93
radiation-related changes in, *124,*
    125
vasogenic edema in, 151
Wrist, *273*

X

X-ray computed tomography (CT)
  bladder carcinoma and, 390
  bony changes demonstrated by, 329
  brightness of lesion on, 69
  compared with MR, 1, 2, 29–30, 42,
    181, 182, 183, 216, 321, 325, 333,
    335, 351
  contrast resolution of, 351
  needle biopsy guiding and, 367
  preferred over MR imaging, 30–31,
    129, 181, 182, 329, 337, 367
  rectal tumor recurrence and, 396